.

Obstetrics and Gynecology: A Case-Based Approach

Obstetrics and Gynecology: A Case-Based Approach

Editor: Annabelle Coleman

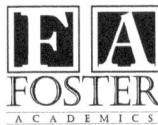

FOSTER
ACADEMICS

www.fosteracademics.com

www.fosteracademics.com

FA FOSTER
ACADEMICS

Cataloging-in-Publication Data

Obstetrics and gynecology : a case-based approach / edited by Annabelle Coleman.
          p. cm.
Includes bibliographical references and index.
ISBN 978-1-63242-665-9
1. Obstetrics. 2. Gynecology. 3. Obstetrics--Case studies.
4. Gynecology--Case studies. I. Coleman, Annabelle.
RG524 .O27 2019
618.2--dc23

Foster Academics,
118-35 Queens Blvd., Suite 400,
Forest Hills, NY 11375, USA

ISBN 978-1-63242-665-9 (Hardback)

Contents

Preface

Obstetrics and gynecology is a medical field encompassing the subspecialties of gynecology and obstetrics. Gynecology is concerned with the overall health of the female reproductive system, including the uterus, vagina and the ovaries, while obstetrics is concerned with pregnancy, childbirth and the postpartum period. Practitioners of this field are adept at the care and management of pregnancy as well as the female reproductive organs. Some of the specialties of this discipline are reproductive endocrinology and infertility, maternal-fetal medicine, female pelvic medicine and reconstructive surgery, pediatric and adolescent gynecology, etc. This book unravels the recent studies in the field of obstetrics and gynecology. It will also provide interesting topics for research, which interested readers can take up. It is appropriate for students seeking detailed information in this area as well as for experts.

This book has been the outcome of endless efforts put in by authors and researchers on various issues and topics within the field. The book is a comprehensive collection of significant researches that are addressed in a variety of chapters. It will surely enhance the knowledge of the field among readers across the globe.

It gives us an immense pleasure to thank our researchers and authors for their efforts to submit their piece of writing before the deadlines. Finally in the end, I would like to thank my family and colleagues who have been a great source of inspiration and support.

Editor

Spontaneous Ruptured Pyomyoma in a Nulligravid Female: A Case Report and Review of the Literature

S. Read [iD][1] and J. Mullins[2]

[1]UConn Health, Department of OB/GYN, Farmington, CT, USA
[2]Hartford Hospital, Department of OB/GYN, Hartford, CT, USA

Correspondence should be addressed to S. Read; susan.h.read@gmail.com

Academic Editor: Mehmet A. Osmanağaoğlu

Introduction. Pyomyoma, or suppurative leiomyoma, is a rare complication of uterine fibroids. It occurs most commonly in the setting of pregnancy, the immediate postpartum period, or postmenopausal status. It may also arise after recent uterine instrumentation, after uterine artery embolization, or in immunocompromised patients. The most likely cause of pyomyoma is vascular compromise followed by bacterial seeding from direct, hematogenous, or lymphatic spread. Diagnosis is difficult, as the condition is rare, presents with vague symptoms, and is difficult to identify on imaging. Definitive diagnosis is only possible with surgery. Pathology shows a degenerating fibroid with hemorrhage, necrosis, cystic degeneration, and/or inflammatory change. Cultures of the pus contained within often show polymicrobial infection. *Case Presentation.* Our patient is a 24-year-old nulligravid female who presented with a surgical abdomen, fever, hypotension, and leukocytosis. She had no significant prior medical or surgical history, no history of uterine instrumentation, and no history of pelvic infection; she was not currently sexually active at the time of presentation. She was taken to the operating room, where she underwent diagnostic laparoscopy. This showed a ruptured pyomyoma originating in the left broad ligament. She then underwent laparoscopic myomectomy. She was transferred to the ICU intubated; she slowly recovered on IV antibiotics and was discharged home on postoperative day 10. *Discussion.* Pyomyoma is a rare condition and is even rarer in premenopausal patients without recent history of pregnancy or uterine instrumentation. This demonstrates an unusual case of spontaneous pyomyoma in the absence of risk factors, other than a history of known fibroids. Pyomyoma should be considered as a diagnosis in patients with sepsis, history of fibroids, and no other identifiable source of infection.

1. Introduction

Leiomyomata are a common benign smooth muscle neoplasm in women, occurring in 20-30% of premenopausal women [1]. The cumulative incidence is approximately 70% in Caucasian women and may be as high as 80% in Afro-Caribbean women [2]. Pyomyoma, or suppurative leiomyoma, is a rare condition that occurs with infection of a leiomyoma. The infected leiomyoma generally shows suppurative inflammation, containing pus with neutrophils and necrotic exudate [3]. Most cases in premenopausal women occur during pregnancy or the immediate postpartum period, after uterine instrumentation [3], or as a result of cervical stenosis [4]. Only four cases have been reported as being diagnosed during pregnancy [5]. Cases in postmenopausal women are likely the result of immune or vascular compromise, such as in the setting of diabetes, hypertension, or atherosclerotic disease [3]. Infections are generally polymicrobial and are thought to arise from the lower genital tract, by direct spread—for example, by contact with the endometrial cavity in a C-section [6]—or by hematogenous/lymphatic spread [1, 3, 7]. Cases in the immediate postpartum period or after uterine instrumentation, e.g., after a D&C, are thought to be most likely the result of ascending infection [1]. Use of instrumentation in the case of postpartum hemorrhage, including intrauterine balloons, also increases risk of infection, while hemorrhage increases risk of infarction of fibroids [8]. Recently, uterine artery embolization (UAE) has become more popular as a treatment for fibroids, as it offers an alternative to traditional surgical and medical therapies [3, 9]. After its introduction in 1996, there have been multiple case reports of pyomyoma forming after UAE [9–12]. This is thought to be a result of uterine and leiomyomatous ischemia [9]. The mechanism of pyomyoma formation is most likely infarction followed by necrosis, with subsequent infection and pus formation [9].

Diagnosis of pyomyoma is difficult, as it is a relatively rare condition and may develop over an extended period of time [4]. Patients typically present with abdominal pain and fever; the triad that should raise suspicion is sepsis, history of fibroids, and absence of another source of infection [1, 9]. However, the presentation in postmenopausal women may be similar to malignancy, with symptoms of abdominal distension/bloating, anorexia, and change in stools [13]. CA-125 may also be elevated [14]. Imaging is often nonspecific; diagnosis cannot truly be made until the time of surgery [14]. Ultrasound shows heterogeneous uterine masses, sometimes with cystic components or air [1, 3]. Abulafia et al. (2010) proposed that an anechoic halo of normal myometrium surrounding the mass may be highly suggestive or even pathognomonic for pyomyoma on ultrasound. CT shows a similar picture but may better demonstrate calcifications, free peritoneal air, and fluid with the density of purulent material [15]. MRI has not been shown to be helpful in diagnosis. The differential diagnosis includes pyometra, tuboovarian abscess, an infected ectopic pregnancy, malignancy, perforated viscus, or degenerating fibroids [2, 8]. The most feared complication of a pyomyoma is rupture, followed by sepsis and death [9]. Rupture is suggested on imaging by disruption of the wall of the pyomyoma, along with free intraperitoneal fluid and air [1]. Mortality rate estimates range from 6% to 21% in the era of antibiotics [5, 8, 14, 16]. Prior to the development of antibiotics in 1945, the mortality rate was 29% according to case series [17]. During pregnancy, occurrence of a pyomyoma may result in spontaneous abortion, preterm labor, preterm premature rupture of membranes (PPROM), or postpartum hemorrhage [17].

Due to the nonspecific presentation of pyomyoma, initiation of appropriate treatment is frequently delayed [16]. Treatment of pyomyoma is almost always surgical. It may be managed with hysterectomy or myomectomy, depending on the location of the pyomyoma and the severity of the patient's condition [1]. Perioperative antibiotics are also necessary; conservative treatment with antibiotics alone is generally ineffective [15]. On occasion, conservative management is possible with drainage and antibiotics. Laubach et al. (2011) presented a case series in which management was successfully performed with drainage by interventional radiology and IV antibiotic therapy in two of three cases. Chen et al. (2014) performed a literature review and found that in 48 cases, 32 underwent hysterectomy, 10 underwent myomectomy, and 6 underwent drainage. The patient's menopausal status and desire for future fertility should be taken into consideration when deciding which approach to take for management [15]. When possible, myomectomy alone is an important treatment option for women desiring maintenance of their fertility [16].

Pathology shows a degenerating fibroid containing hemorrhage, necrosis, or calcification [3]. The pyomyoma may demonstrate a "capsule" on imaging, which on pathology appears as a flattened layer of smooth muscle cells [3]. Cystic degeneration, hyaline change, and acute inflammatory change may also be present [18]. Cultures of the pus from the pyomyoma generally demonstrate polymicrobial infection; the most commonly isolated organisms are *Staphylococcus* species, but *Streptococcus* sp., *E. coli*, *Pasteurella multocida*, and other organisms may also be identified [1, 3, 13, 19]. A case of *Candida*-related pyomyoma has also been described [20].

2. Case Presentation

Our patient is a 24-year-old nulligravid female with uncertain last menstrual period who presented to the emergency department (ED) with 12 hours of diffuse abdominal pain, worse in the left lower quadrant. She had intermittent nausea with one episode of emesis. She denied fevers or chills. She noted intermittent vaginal spotting, but no abnormal vaginal discharge. She had been seen two months previously for menorrhagia and was told at that time she had a possible fibroid; she was started on Depo-Provera for her menorrhagia. She denied any significant medical or surgical history. She denied any history of diabetes, HIV, or other immunocompromise. She denied any history of IUD placement or other uterine instrumentation. She had not been sexually active in several months and had no history of sexually transmitted infections.

She was initially febrile to 100.9F in the ED; within a few hours her temperature increased to 103.6F, she became tachycardic to the 140s, and was hypotensive to the 80s/50s. Her WBC count was 17.8. Urine pregnancy and HIV tests were negative. Blood glucose was 164 on admission. She was started on IV fluids and pressors and was given doses of cefepime, ceftriaxone, doxycycline, and metronidazole. CT abdomen/pelvis with contrast showed an 8.1 x 5.5 x 5.6 cm heterogeneous mass in the deep left pelvis that was inseparable from the uterus and broad ligament; it had an incomplete solid ventral surface and was thought to represent a hemorrhagic or infarcted fibroid (Figure 1). No internal calcifications or fat was seen. Fat stranding and fluid were visible surrounding the mass. There was no pneumoperitoneum. Given the severity of the patient's condition and her hemodynamic instability, she was taken to the operating room for an exploratory laparoscopy.

Intraoperatively, pus was noted throughout the abdomen and the patient's bowel was edematous and filled with gas. Multiple pus pockets were seen in the patient's pelvis. A large left broad ligament leiomyoma was noted and appeared to be leaking pus (Figures 2 and 3). A myomectomy was performed laparoscopically, and the patient's abdomen was washed out.

She was then taken to the ICU intubated on pressors. She was kept on tobramycin and clindamycin for a presumed tuboovarian abscess. She was extubated on postoperative day 2 but continued to require supplemental oxygen and pressors. She also continued to spike fevers to 101.3F and was persistently tachycardic to the 140s. Infectious disease recommended switching to ceftriaxone and

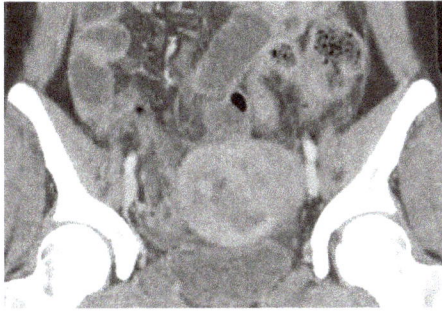

FIGURE 1: Heterogeneous pelvic mass on CT.

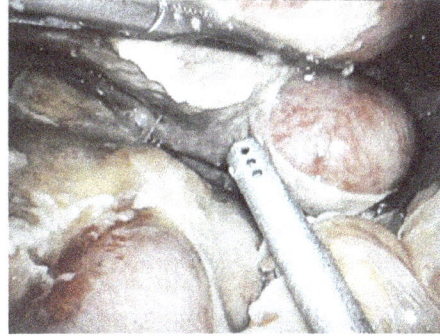

FIGURE 3: The uterine fundus is seen on the right hand side of the image. The pyomyoma is at the top of the image.

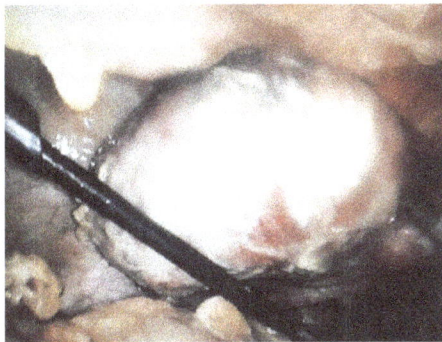

FIGURE 2: The left broad ligament pyomyoma. Purulent material is visible along the abdominal wall and bowel.

metronidazole at that time. She was afebrile by postoperative day 4 and remained afebrile with the exception of one isolated elevated temperature on postoperative day 8. Her tachycardia resolved. Blood glucose remained within normal limits. She was transitioned to oral antibiotics and discharged home in good condition on postoperative day 10.

Pathology showed a 128-gram leiomyoma with partial ischemic changes and nonspecific inflammation. A gram stain of the pus showed many neutrophils and gram-negative rods; a culture of the purulent fluid showed no growth, indicating an anaerobic infection.

3. Discussion

Pyomyoma is a rare complication of leiomyomata and is generally seen in the context of pregnancy, postmenopausal status, or uterine instrumentation. This case is a rare exception, as the patient had no recent uterine instrumentation, was nulligravid, and had no reason to exhibit vascular compromise. No records were available from the time when her diagnosis of fibroids was made, so the size of her fibroid at the time of diagnosis is unknown. It is possible that she had rapid growth of the fibroid leading to ischemic changes, degeneration, and subsequent seeding with normal vaginal flora.

Pyomyoma should be suspected in cases of sepsis, history of fibroids, and no other clear source of infection, as was the case in this patient. For many patients found to have pyomyoma, symptoms may develop insidiously, and they may present with only a fever [21]. Imaging showed a heterogeneous pelvic mass, and culture of the pus from the pyomyoma showed no growth, indicating likely polymicrobial anaerobic infection. Surgical management was successfully performed laparoscopically; however, it would have also been reasonable to perform a laparotomy, which could have obtained a better washout. Luckily for this young, nulliparous patient, the pyomyoma was in her left broad ligament, and a fertility-sparing myomectomy was possible as a result. Fertility-sparing surgery should always be attempted if feasible, if the patient is premenopausal and desires future fertility, or if her childbearing wishes are unknown [15]. This patient did have a ruptured pyomyoma diagnosed at the time of surgery; luckily, she presented to the ED before she became hemodynamically unstable, and we were able to manage her appropriately.

In a review of 41 cases of pyomyoma diagnosed since 1986 (Table 1), 14 cases were treated with myomectomy (34%), 20 were treated with hysterectomy (49%), and the remainder were treated with IV antibiotics or minor procedures.

All patients received IV antibiotics during the course of their treatment. Of the 41 patients, only one patient died; she had been treated with IV antibiotics alone. The outcome of one of the patients was not reported. Since 2010, 10 of 25 cases were treated with hysterectomy (40%) [1–3, 5, 6, 8–19, 21–26], and only 2 of 11 patients under age 40 (18%) were treated with hysterectomy, so there may be a trend toward managing cases with conservative surgical treatments for fertility preservation purposes. The majority of cases were in premenopausal women or were associated with pregnancy, uterine artery embolization, or uterine instrumentation (e.g., IUD in place, D&E). Our patient is unique because of her young age, nulliparity, and lack of any prior uterine procedures or recent known infection. To our knowledge, this is the only known case to occur in a premenopausal woman without any history of uterine instrumentation or immunocompromise or in the peripartum period.

TABLE 1: List of reviewed cases.

Citation Number	Author	Age	Relevant History	Treatment	Outcome
[3]	Ono	69	Postmenopausal	Hysterectomy	Unknown
[1]	Bagga	26	Post SAB	Myomectomy	Alive
[15]	Chen ZHY	46	Prior C-section (remote)	Hysterectomy	Alive
[9]	Obele	37	UAE	Hysterectomy	Alive
[18]	Goyal	42	Diabetic	Hysterectomy	Alive
[2]	Demaio	Unknown	Postpartum	Myomectomy	Alive
[14]	Iwahashi	53	IUD	Hysterectomy	Alive
[13]	Chen JR	69	Postmenopausal	Myomectomy	Alive
[16]	Pinton	28	Post SAB	Myomectomy	Alive
[8]	Kaler	28	Postpartum w/ PPH, intrauterine balloon	Myomectomy	Alive
[21]	Del Borgo	37	Postpartum	Myomectomy	Alive
[17]	Sirha	37	Postpartum	Hysterectomy	Alive
[6]	Shiota	36	C-section	Myomectomy	Alive
[10]	Rosen	47	UAE, untreated *Trichomonas* infection	Hysterectomy	Alive
[11]	Pinto	36	UAE	Drainage	Alive
[5]	Kobayashi	28	Pregnant	Myomectomy	Alive
[22]	Shaaban	30	Post C-section	Myomectomy	Alive
[23]	Liu	42	Myomectomy (remote)	Marsupialization	Alive
[24]	Stroumsa	41	D&E	IV antibiotics	Alive
[19]	Zangeneh	47	Perimenopausal; chronic endometritis on pathology	Hysterectomy	Alive
[25]	Laubach	31	D&E	Drainage	Alive
		35	C-section	Drainage	Alive
		31	C-section, surgical site infection	Drainage followed by hysterectomy	Alive
[12]	Abulafia	48	UAE	Hysterectomy	Alive
[26]	Lee	46	Unknown	Hysterectomy	Alive
[27]	Fletcher	44	Diabetic, PID	Hysterectomy	Alive
[28]	Nguyen	40	C-section, chorioamnionitis	Hysterectomy	Alive
[29]	Patwardhan	38	Torsion of pedunculated fibroid	Myomectomy	Alive
[30]	Manchana	42	Perimenopausal; IUD	Hysterectomy	Alive
[31]	Calleja-Agius	30	C-section	Myomectomy	Alive
[32]	Sah	64	Postmenopausal	Hysterectomy	Alive
[33]	Mason	29	Postpartum	Myomectomy	Alive
[4]	Karcaaltincaba	36	Post SAB	Myomectomy	Alive
[20]	Lin	33	C-section, surgical site infection	Hysterectomy	Alive
[34]	Grune	44	Pregnant	Myomectomy	Alive
[35]	Genta	60	Postmenopausal, diabetes	Hysterectomy	Alive
[36]	Gupta	75	Postmenopausal	Hysterectomy	Alive
[37]	Yang	46	Bacteremia	Hysterectomy	Alive
[38]	Prahlow	31	Pregnancy, IV drug use	Hysterectomy	Alive
[7]	Greenspoon	49	Bacteremia	IV antibiotics	Deceased
[39]	Pritchard	37	Post SAB, laparotomy	Hysterectomy	Alive

SAB: spontaneous abortion; UAE: uterine artery embolization; PID: pelvic inflammatory disease; D&E: dilation and evacuation; IUD: intrauterine device; PPH: postpartum hemorrhage.

References

[1] R. Bagga, R. Rai, J. Kalra, P. K. Saha, and T. Singh, "An unusual cause of postabortal fever requiring prompt surgical intervention: A pyomyoma and its imaging features," *Oman Medical Journal*, vol. 32, no. 1, pp. 73–76, 2017.

[2] A. DeMaio and M. Doyle, "Pyomyoma as a Rare Source of Postpartum Sepsis," *Case Reports in Obstetrics and Gynecology*, vol. 2015, Article ID 263518, 2 pages, 2015.

[3] H. Ono, M. Kanematsu, H. Kato et al., "MR imaging findings of uterine pyomyoma: radiologic-pathologic correlation," *Abdominal Imaging*, vol. 39, no. 4, pp. 797–801, 2014.

[4] M. Karcaaltincaba and G. S. Sudakoff, "CT of a ruptured pyomyoma," *American Journal of Roentgenology*, vol. 181, no. 5, pp. 1375–1377, 2003.

[5] F. Kobayashi et al., "Pyomyoma during pregnancy: A case report and review of the literature," *Journal of Obstetrics and Gynaecology*, vol. 39, no. 1, pp. 383–389, 2013.

[6] M. Shiota, Y. Kotani, K. Ami, Y. Mizuno, Y. Ekawa, and M. Umemoto, "Uterus-sparing myomectomy for uterine pyomyoma following cesarean section," *Taiwanese Journal of Obstetrics and Gynecology*, vol. 52, no. 1, pp. 140-141, 2013.

[7] J. S. Greenspoon, M. Ault, B. A. James, and L. Kaplan, "Pyomyoma associated with polymicrobial bacteremia and fatal septic shock: Case report and review of the literature," *Obstetrical & Gynecological Survey* , vol. 45, no. 9, pp. 563–569, 1990.

[8] M. Kaler, R. Gailer, J. Iskaros, and A. L. David, "Postpartum Pyomyoma, a Rare Complication of Sepsis Associated with Chorioamnionitis and Massive Postpartum Haemorrhage Treated with an Intrauterine Balloon," *Case Reports in Obstetrics and Gynecology*, vol. 2015, Article ID 609205, 6 pages, 2015.

[9] C. C. Obele, S. Dunham, G. Bennett, J. Pagan, L. Y. Sung, and H. W. Charles, "A Case of Pyomyoma following Uterine Fibroid Embolization and a Review of the Literature," *Case Reports in Obstetrics and Gynecology*, vol. 2016, Article ID 9835412, 5 pages, 2016.

[10] M. L. Rosen, M. L. Anderson, and S. M. Hawkins, "Pyomyoma after uterine artery embolization," *Obstetrics & Gynecology*, vol. 121, no. 2, pp. 431–433, 2013.

[11] E. Pinto, A. Trovão, S. Leitão, C. Pina, F. K. Mak, and A. Lanhoso, "Conservative laparoscopic approach to a perforated pyomyoma after uterine artery embolization," *Journal of Minimally Invasive Gynecology*, vol. 19, no. 6, pp. 775–779, 2012.

[12] O. Abulafia, T. Shah, G. Salame et al., "Sonographic features associated with post-uterine artery embolization pyomyoma," *Journal of Ultrasound in Medicine*, vol. 29, no. 5, pp. 839–842, 2010.

[13] J.-R. Chen, T.-L. Yang, F.-H. Lan, and T.-W. Lin, "Pyomyoma mimicking advanced ovarian cancer: A rare manifestation in a postmenopausal virgin," *Taiwanese Journal of Obstetrics and Gynecology*, vol. 53, no. 1, pp. 101–103, 2014.

[14] N. Iwahashi, Y. Mabuchi, M. Shiro, S. Yagi, S. Minami, and K. Ino, "Large uterine pyomyoma in a perimenopausal female: A case report and review of 50 reported cases in the literature," *Molecular and Clinical Oncology*, vol. 5, no. 5, pp. 527–531, 2016.

[15] Z. H.-Y. Chen, H.-D. Tsai, and M.-J. Sun, "Pyomyoma: a rare and life-threatening complication of uterine leiomyoma," *Taiwanese Journal of Obstetrics and Gynecology*, vol. 49, no. 3, pp. 351–356, 2010.

[16] A. Pinton, G. Aubry, V. Thoma, I. Nisand, and C. Y. Akladios, "Pyomyoma after abortion: Uterus conserving surgery is possible to maintain fertility. Case report," *International Journal of Surgery Case Reports*, vol. 24, pp. 179–181, 2016.

[17] R. Sirha, A. Miskin, and A. Abdelmagied, "Postnatal pyomyoma: a diagnostic dilemma.," *BMJ Case Reports*, vol. 2013, 2013.

[18] S. Goyal, H. Mohan, R. S. Punia, and R. Tandon, "Subserosal pyomyoma and tubo-ovarian abscess in a diabetic patient," *Journal of Obstetrics & Gynaecology*, vol. 35, no. 1, pp. 101-102, 2015.

[19] M. Zangeneh, A. Alsadat Mahdavi, E. Amini, S. Davar Siadat, and L. Karimian, "Pyomyoma in a premenopausal woman with fever of unknown origin," *Obstetrics & Gynecology*, vol. 116, no. 2, pp. 526–528, 2010.

[20] Y.-H. Lin, J.-L. Hwang, L.-W. Huang, and H.-J. Chen, "Pyomyoma after a cesarean section," *Acta Obstetricia et Gynecologica Scandinavica*, vol. 81, no. 6, pp. 571-572, 2002.

[21] C. Del Borgo, F. Maneschi, V. Belvisi et al., "Postpartum fever in the presence of a fibroid: *Sphingomonas paucimobilis* sepsis associated with pyomyoma," *BMC Infectious Diseases*, vol. 13, no. 1, article 574, 2013.

[22] H. S. Shaaban, H. F. Choo, and J. W. Sensakovic, "A case of Staphylococcus lugdunensis related pyomyoma occurring after cesarean section," *Journal of Global Infectious Diseases*, vol. 3, no. 1, pp. 101-102, 2011.

[23] H.-S. Liu and C.-H. Chen, "Subserosal pyomyoma in a virgin female: Sonographic and computed tomographic imaging features," *Ultrasound in Obstetrics & Gynecology*, vol. 37, no. 2, pp. 247-248, 2011.

[24] D. Stroumsa, E. Ben-David, N. Hiller, and D. Hochner-Celnikier, "Severe clostridial pyomyoma following an abortion does not always require surgical intervention," *Case Reports in Obstetrics and Gynecology*, vol. 2011, Article ID 364641, 3 pages, 2011.

[25] M. Laubach, M. Breugelmans, M. Leyder, J. Demey, and W. Foulon, "Nonsurgical treatment of pyomyoma in the postpartum period," *Surgical Infections*, vol. 12, no. 1, pp. 65–68, 2011.

[26] S. R. Lee, B. S. Kim, and H.-S. Moon, "Magnetic resonance imaging and positron emission tomography of a giant multiseptated pyomyoma simulating an ovarian cancer," *Fertility and Sterility*, vol. 94, no. 5, pp. 1900–1902, 2010.

[27] H. Fletcher, R. Gibson, N. Williams, G. Wharfe, A. Nicholson, and D. Soares, "A woman with diabetes presenting with pyomyoma and treated with subtotal hysterectomy: a case report," *Journal of Medical Case Reports*, vol. 3, article 7439, 2009.

[28] Q. H. Nguyen and S. M. Gruenewald, "Sonographic appearance of a postpartum pyomyoma with gas production," *Journal of Clinical Ultrasound*, vol. 36, no. 3, pp. 186–188, 2008.

[29] A. Patwardhan and P. Bulmer, "Pyomyoma as a complication of uterine fibroids," *Journal of Obstetrics & Gynaecology*, vol. 27, no. 4, pp. 445-446, 2007.

[30] T. Manchana, N. Sirisabya, S. Triratanachat, S. Niruthisard, and Y. Tannirandorn, "Pyomyoma in a perimenopausal woman with intrauterine device," *Gynecologic and Obstetric Investigation*, vol. 63, no. 3, pp. 170–172, 2007.

[31] J. Calleja-Agius, P. O'Brien, J. Iskaros, and N. Calleja, "Pyomyoma," *Journal of Obstetrics & Gynaecology*, vol. 26, no. 7, pp. 709-710, 2006.

[32] S. P. Sah, A. K. Rayamajhi, and P. P. Bhadani, "Pyomyoma in a postmenopausal woman: A case report," *Southeast Asian Journal of Tropical Medicine and Public Health*, vol. 36, no. 4, pp. 979–981, 2005.

[33] T. C. Mason, J. Adair, and Y. C. Lee, "Postpartum pyomyoma," *Journal of the National Medical Association*, vol. 97, no. 6, pp. 826–828, 2005.

[34] B. Grüne, E. Zikulnig, and U. Gembruch, "Sepsis in second trimester of pregnancy due to an infected myoma. A case report and a review of the literature," *Fetal Diagnosis and Therapy*, vol. 16, no. 4, pp. 245–247, 2001.

[35] P. R. Genta, M. L. N. Dias, T. A. Janiszewski, J. P. Carvalho, M. H. Arai, and L. P. Meireles, "*Streptococcus agalactiae* endocarditis and giant pyomyoma simulating ovarian cancer," *Southern Medical Journal*, vol. 94, no. 5, pp. 508–511, 2001.

[36] B. Gupta, A. Sehgal, R. Kaur, and S. Malhotra, "Pyomyoma: A case report," *Australian and New Zealand Journal of Obstetrics and Gynaecology*, vol. 39, no. 4, pp. 520-521, 1999.

[37] C.-H. Yang and C.-K. Wang, "Edwardsiella tarda bacteraemia - Complicated by acute pancreatitis and pyomyoma," *Infection*, vol. 38, no. 2, pp. 124–126, 1999.

[38] J. A. Prahlow, J. O. Cappellari, and S. A. Washburn, "Uterine pyomyoma as a complication of pregnancy in an intravenous drug user," *Southern Medical Journal*, vol. 89, no. 9, pp. 892–895, 1996.

[39] J. G. Pritchard et al., "Streptococcus milleri pyomyoma simulating infective endocarditis," *Obstetrics & Gynecology*, vol. 68, no. 3, pp. 46S–49S, 1986.

2

Changes in Intra-Amniotic, Fetal Intrathoracic, and Intraperitoneal Pressures with Uterine Contraction: A Report of Three Cases

Daisuke Katsura ⓘ, Yuichiro Takahashi, Shigenori Iwagaki, Rika Chiaki, Kazuhiko Asai, Masako Koike, Shunsuke Yasumi, and Madoka Furuhashi ⓘ

Department of Fetal-Maternal Medicine, Nagara Medical Centre, 1300-7, Nagara, Gifu 502-8558, Japan

Correspondence should be addressed to Daisuke Katsura; katsuo14@belle.shiga-med.ac.jp

Academic Editor: Seung-Yup Ku

Intra-amniotic, fetal intrathoracic, and intraperitoneal pressures during pregnancy have been previously investigated. However, to our knowledge, changes in these pressures during uterine contractions have not been reported. Herein, we present three cases of polyhydramnios, fetal pleural effusion, and fetal ascites, in which intra-amniotic, fetal intrathoracic, intraperitoneal pressures increased with uterine contractions. These pressure increases may affect the fetal circulation. We suggest that managing potential premature delivery (e.g., with tocolysis) is important in cases with polyhydramnios and excess fluid in fetal body areas, such as the thorax, abdomen, and heart. The results of this preliminary study on intrafetal pressure measurements will be useful in performing fetal and neonatal surgeries in the future.

1. Introduction

Caldeyro-Barcia and Poseiro (1960) reported that uterine contractions (UCs) increases human intrauterine pressure [1, 2]. Intra-amniotic pressure during pregnancy has been reportedly measured via a transabdominal approach [3, 4]. However, to our knowledge, direct measurement of pathologic fetal intrathoracic and intraperitoneal pressures during pregnancy has not been systematically reported [5, 6]. In addition, association between fetal pressure and UCs has not been reported.

UCs cause a significant reduction in placental perfusion [7], and the association between impaired placental perfusion and fetal growth restriction is known [8]. Several physiological studies using fetal pulse Doppler have been reported [9, 10]. Furthermore, in fetal growth restriction, the umbilical artery (UA) pulsatility index (PI) was significantly high during UCs in cases with positive oxytocin challenge test [9]. Moreover, the inferior vena cava preload index (PLI) increased with UCs in normal pregnancy [10]. Therefore, UCs may indirectly affect fetal circulation, including preload and afterload. However, the direct effect of pressures on

the fetus remains unclear. This study reports three cases in which UCs increased intra-amniotic, fetal intrathoracic, and intraperitoneal pressures and discusses the potential effect of these pressures on the fetus.

2. Case Presentations

2.1. Ethical Approval. The study was accepted and approved by the Institutional Review Board and Ethical Committee of Nagara Medical Centre (IRB number: 28-19). All patients provided informed consent.

2.2. Case 1. Case 1 was a 30-year-old, gravida 2, para 1 woman. At week 22 of pregnancy, she was admitted to our hospital because of a monochorionic twin pregnancy with cervical dilatation, frequent UCs on cardiotocogram, and polyhydramnios. As intervention, tocolysis was performed. Although UCs were reduced, ultrasonography revealed a maximum vertical pocket (MVP) of 12 cm (although the MVP of the co-twin was 4 cm) and the patient had dyspnea; therefore, emergency amnioreduction was performed, and 2,000 mL of amniotic fluid was drained during tocolysis.

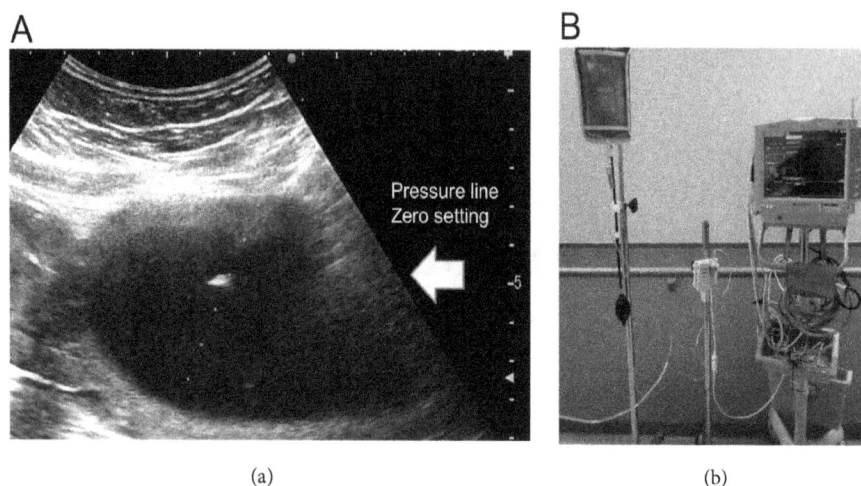

FIGURE 1: (A) Ultrasound and zero pressure level line setting during amnioreduction for polyhydramnios. (B) Circuit that includes a silicone stain-gauge transducer (DX-300, Nihon Koden) for measuring pressure.

Intra-amniotic pressure was measured during the procedure. A saline-filled line was attached at one end to the hub of the needle and at the other end to a silicone stain-gauge transducer (DX-300; Nihon Kohden Corporation, Tokyo, Japan). Readings were recorded at the needle tip and were recorded if they were stable for 10 s. A zero pressure level line setting was performed at the estimated vertical line using the ultrasound-guided needle tip level (Figure 1). Prior to this case, we did not perform this procedure for pressure measurement alone.

The intra-amniotic pressure was 16 mmHg before reduction, increased to 29 mmHg with UCs during reduction, and then declined to 9 mmHg after reduction. At this point, the Doppler of the recipient and donor showed the following results: UA PI, 1.42 and 1.54; middle cerebral artery (MCA) PI, 1.56 and 2.79; umbilical venous flow volume (UVFV), 149 and 110 mL/kg/min; ductus venosus (DV) PI, 0.74 and 0.65; cardiothoracic area ratio (CTAR), 24 and 30%; inferior vena cava PLI, 0.26 and 0.34. These data were within the normal limit, but the recipient had moderate tricuspid regurgitation. After amnioreduction, the Doppler of the recipient and donor showed the following results: UA PI, 1.18 and 1.79; MCA PI, 1.59 and 2.79; UVFV, 225 and 114 mL/kg/min; DV PI, 0.81 and 0.70. These data were within the normal limit, but the recipient's UA PI decreased mildly and UVFV increased. At week 25 of pregnancy, the MVPs of the donor and recipient were 1 and 15 cm, respectively. Therefore, the patient was diagnosed with stage II twin-to-twin transfusion syndrome, and fetoscopic laser photocoagulation was performed. Thereafter, caesarean section was performed due to labor onset at week 28 of pregnancy. Male neonates were born weighing 1573 and 1709 g, with Apgar scores of 5 and 4 at 1 min and 6 and 4 at 5 min, and umbilical arterial cord blood pH of 7.312 and 7.264, respectively. They were admitted to the neonatal intensive care unit because of prematurity and low birth weight and respiratory distress syndrome. The neonates responded well to the treatment.

2.3. Case 2. Case 2 was a 29-year-old, gravida 1, para 0 woman. Fetal ascites was observed at week 33 of pregnancy, and the patient was admitted to our hospital. Test results for maternal serum cytomegalovirus and parvovirus B19 IgM were negative. Abdominocentesis was performed for diagnosis, and 99 mL of ascitic fluid was drained, containing 92% lymphocytes; hence, diagnosis of chylous ascites was made. The subsequent pregnancy course was uneventful until term. However, abdominocentesis was performed again to reduce the risk of dystocia [11] at week 37 of pregnancy, with drainage of 510 mL of ascitic fluid during labor preparation. Tocolysis was performed for preventing UC only during the procedure. The fetal intraperitoneal pressure was 18 mmHg before drainage, 14 mmHg after drainage, and 32 mmHg when confirming UC on palpation. At this point, the fetal Doppler showed the following results: UA PI, 0.98; MCA PI, 1.08; and DV PI, 0.87. These values were within the normal limit. After abdominocentesis, the fetal Doppler showed the following results: UA PI, 0.65; MCA PI, 1.04; and DV PI, 0.59. These data were within the normal limit, but UA PI decreased. Thereafter, ascites recurred, and the mother had spontaneous premature rupture of membranes at week 38 of pregnancy. Caesarean section was performed due to cephalopelvic disproportion. A male neonate was born weighing 3117 g, with Apgar scores of 8 at 1 min and 9 at 5 min and umbilical arterial cord blood pH of 7.221. He was admitted to the neonatal intensive care unit for chylous ascites. Ascitic fluids were drained twice. However, although there was ascitic fluid retention, the amount did not increase. He was transferred to another hospital.

2.4. Case 3. Case 3 was a 30-year-old, gravida 1, para 1 woman. Fetal pleural effusion was observed at week 22 of pregnancy during a routine prenatal visit, and she was admitted to our hospital. Skin edema and ascites were not observed. Thoracentesis was performed, and 24 mL of the pleural fluid was drained, containing 95% lymphocytes;

hence, a diagnosis of chylothorax was made. Although the amniotic fluid index was normal, the intra-amniotic pressure remained as high as 20–22 mmHg because of frequent UCs on palpation even if tocolysis was performed for preventing UC during the procedure. The fetal intrathoracic pressure was 30 mmHg before and 19 mmHg after drainage. At this point, the fetal Doppler showed the following results: UA PI, 1.39; MCA PI, 1.57; UVFV, 72 mL/kg/min; DV PI, 0.58; CTAR, 17.1%; inferior vena cava PLI, 0.4; and TEI index (left/right ventricle), 0.474/0.581.These values indicate that CTAR was low and the right ventricle TEI index was mildly high. After thoracentesis, the fetal Doppler showed the following results: UA PI, 1.26; MCA PI, 1.42; UVFV, 73 mL/kg/min; DV PI, 0.63. These data were within the normal limit and did not change. Because pleural effusion recurred within 7 days after the first procedure, a thoracoamniotic shunt was inserted into the left pleural space 4 days after the first procedure according to the Japanese protocol for thoracoamniotic shunt [12]. Thereafter, the pleural effusion reduced and did not recur. Consequently, she was transferred to another hospital at week 26 of pregnancy.

3. Discussion

Few reports have assessed intra-amniotic, fetal intrathoracic, and intraperitoneal pressures. Table 1 presents a review of the previously reported pressures, as well as those presented in our cases [4–6]. Normal intra-amniotic pressure during pregnancy is believed to exponentially decrease with gestation, from 9 mmHg at 10 weeks to 5 mmHg at 30 weeks [3]. Additionally, normal intra-amniotic pressure was not significantly elevated in twin pregnancies [4]. Reports on fetal intrathoracic pressure in cases of congenital chylothorax revealed a correlation between increased intrathoracic pressure and ultrasonographic signs of mediastinal shift and diaphragm inversion [5]. Fetal intraperitoneal pressure during intrauterine transfusion in patients with Rhesus alloimmunization showed a basal pressure of 2.5 mmHg (95% confidence interval, 1.4–3.6), and the pressure in complicated intraperitoneal transfusion significantly increased compared to that in uncomplicated pregnancies [6]. To our knowledge, the association between fetal pressure and UCs has not been previously reported.

Pressures were previously measured near the uterine fundus [3, 4, 6]; however, in the present study, these pressures were measured at the tip of the needle, based on the methods used to measure adult central venous pressure [13, 14]. Considering these factors, our measured pressures were higher (approximately 3–5 mmHg) than those previously reported. Moreover, there was no difference in the normal control of intra-amniotic pressure between our methods (16 and 18 weeks; mean, 10.75 mmHg; range, 10–3 mmHg; four cases were measured during amniocentesis for amniotic diagnosis) and those of previous reports (16 and 18 weeks; lower limits, 2.2 and 2.2 mmHg, respectively; upper limits, 9.3 and 9.5 mmHg, respectively) [4], which suggests that our methodology is reliable (Table 1).

In our cases, intra-amniotic pressures increased with UCs and were higher than the normal range in cases with polyhydramnios [4]. Intra-amniotic pressure may increase because the intrauterine pressure caused by UCs exceeds the uterine tolerance and the amniotic fluid cannot escape. Intra-amniotic pressure >15 mmHg may be perceived as painful and uncomfortable if polyhydramnios is present [1, 2]. For example, in Case 1, the pressure was 16 mmHg and the mother had dyspnea. After amnioreduction, the pressure returned to the normal range, and the dyspnea resolved. According to Nicolini et al. [6], the increase in pressure due to excess fluid should return to the normal range once the excess fluid is removed. However, in Case 2, although the fluid was removed, the pressure remained higher than the normal range, possibly because the intra-amniotic pressure was increased due to polyhydramnios. Further, to our knowledge, normal fetal intrathoracic pressures have not previously been reported. In Case 3, after the pleural effusion was drained, intrathoracic pressure decreased and was equal to the intra-amniotic pressure. This may have occurred because the intra-amniotic pressure increased as a result of frequent UCs, which ultimately affected intrathoracic pressure.

Even with the amniotic fluid as cushioning, UC pressure on the fetus increased, as did the intrathoracic and intraperitoneal pressures. According to Pascal's principle, a change in pressure at any point in an enclosed fluid compartment at rest is transmitted undiminished to all points in the fluid. Thus, the increased intrathoracic and intraperitoneal pressures equally affect the intra-amniotic pressure, which is influenced by UCs and/or polyhydramnios. These pressures on the fetus squeeze the surrounding organs and blood vessels, possibly affecting fetal circulation. In these cases, although fetal flow velocity was within the normal limit, the pressures during uterine contractions might be changing. In Case 1, decreased intra-amniotic pressure decreased UA PI and increased UVFV, and, in Case 2, decreased fetal intraperitoneal pressure decreased UA PI. These suggested to improve fetal circulation.

We believe that management of potential premature delivery with tocolysis is important in cases with polyhydramnios and excess fluid in fetal body areas, such as the thorax, abdomen, and heart. The results of this preliminary study on intrafetal pressure measurements will be useful for performing fetal and neonatal surgeries in the future, such as judgment of adaptation of fetal thoracoamniotic shunt and neonatal thoracic drainage depending on fetal intrathoracic pressure, and for removal of fluid for improving fetal circulation and facilitating neonatal resuscitation depending on intra-amniotic, fetal intrathoracic, and intraperitoneal pressure. However, further data are warranted to clarify the association between the extent of pressure and the effect on the fetus and to establish the selection criteria for fetal and neonatal surgeries.

Conflicts of Interest

The authors declare that there are no conflicts of interest regarding the publication of the article.

TABLE 1: Results and literature review of intra-amniotic and fetal intrathoracic and intraperitoneal pressures.

Case	Diagnosis	GA at measurement (weeks)	Intra-amniotic pressure (mmHg)			Intrathoracic pressure (mmHg)			Intraperitoneal pressure (mmHg)		
			Before R	After R/baseline[a]	With UC	Before R	After R	With UC	Before R	After R	With UC
1	Polyhydramnios	22	16	9	29						
2	Chylous ascites polyhydramnios	38							18	14	32
3	Chylothorax	22			20–22	30	19				
Our control cases	Amniocentesis for chromosome analysis	16		10, 10							
		18		10, 13							
Yamamoto et al. 2007	Chylothorax polyhydramnios	31	21	Baseline[a]		39				Baseline[a] 2.5 (1.4–3.6)	
Nicolini et al. 1989	Intrauterine transfusion										
		16		2.2–9.3							
		18		2.2–9.5							
		20		2.3–9.6							
		22		2.3–9.7							
		24		2.3–9.7							
Fisk et al. 1992		26		2.3–9.8							
		28		2.4–10.1							
		30		2.5–10.6							
		32		2.8–11.5							
		34		3.2–13.1							

GA, gestational age; R, removal of amniotic fluid; UC, uterine contraction; baseline[a], baseline pressure not related to amnioreduction.

Authors' Contributions

All authors have significantly contributed and are in agreement with the content of the manuscript.

Acknowledgments

The authors thank Takeshi Iwase and Hiroshi Soejima for their help in the measurement of pressures.

References

[1] R. Caldeyro-Barcia and J. J. Poseiro, "Physiology of the uterine contraction," *Clinical Obstetrics and Gynecology*, vol. 3, no. 2, pp. 386–410, 1960.

[2] R. C. Young, "Mechanotransduction mechanisms for coordinating uterine contractions in human labor," *Reproduction*, vol. 152, no. 2, pp. R51–R61, 2016.

[3] I. G. Sideris and K. H. Nicolaides, "Amniotic fluid pressure during pregnancy," *Fetal Diagnosis and Therapy*, vol. 5, no. 2, pp. 104–108, 1991.

[4] N. M. Fisk, D. Ronderos-Dumit, Y. Tannirandorn, U. Nicolini, D. Talbert, and C. H. Rodeck, "Normal amniotic pressure throughout gestation," *BJOG: An International Journal of Obstetrics & Gynaecology*, vol. 99, no. 1, pp. 18–22, 1992.

[5] M. Yamamoto, A. Insunza, J. Carrillo, L. A. Caicedo, E. Paiva, and Y. Ville, "Intrathoracic pressure in congenital chylothorax: Keystone for the rationale of thoracoamniotic shunting?" *Fetal Diagnosis and Therapy*, vol. 22, no. 3, pp. 169–171, 2007.

[6] U. Nicolini, D. G. Talbert, N. M. Fisk, and C. H. Rodeck, "Pathophysiology of pressure changes during intrauterine transfusion," *American Journal of Obstetrics & Gynecology*, vol. 160, no. 5, pp. 1139–1145, 1989.

[7] M. Sinding, D. A. Peters, J. B. Frøkjær, O. B. Christiansen, N. Uldbjerg, and A. Sørensen, "Reduced placental oxygenation during subclinical uterine contractions as assessed by BOLD MRI," *Placenta*, vol. 39, pp. 16–20, 2016.

[8] M. C. Moran, C. Mulcahy, G. Zombori, J. Ryan, P. Downey, and F. M. McAuliffe, "Placental volume, vasculature and calcification in pregnancies complicated by pre-eclampsia and intrauterine growth restriction," *European Journal of Obstetrics & Gynecology and Reproductive Biology*, vol. 195, pp. 12–17, 2015.

[9] H. Li, S. Gudmundsson, and P. Olofsson, "Acute centralization of blood flow in compromised human fetuses evoked by uterine contractions," *Early Human Development*, vol. 82, no. 11, pp. 747–752, 2006.

[10] Y. Takahashi, S. Iwagaki, Y. Nakagawa, I. Kawabata, and T. Tamaya, "Uterine contractions increase fetal heart preload," *Ultrasound in Obstetrics & Gynecology*, vol. 22, no. 1, pp. 53–56, 2003.

[11] P. Haider, R. Korejo, and S. Jafarey, "Fetal ascites as a cause of dystocia in labour.," *Journal of the Pakistan Medical Association*, vol. 41, no. 8, pp. 195–197, 1991.

[12] Y. Takahashi, I. Kawabata, M. Sumie et al., "Thoracoamniotic shunting for fetal pleural effusions using a double-basket shunt," *Prenatal Diagnosis*, vol. 32, no. 13, pp. 1282–1287, 2012.

[13] J. N. Wilson, J. B. Grow, C. V. Demong, A. E. Prevedel, J. C. Owens, and W. K. Hamilton, "Central venous pressure in optimal blood volume maintenance," *Survey of Anesthesiology*, vol. 85, pp. 563–578, 1964.

[14] A. Barbeito and J. B. Mark, "Arterial and Central Venous Pressure Monitoring," *Anesthesiology Clinics of North America*, vol. 24, no. 4, pp. 717–735, 2006.

3

Elevated CA 125 in a CASE of Leaking Endometrioma

Svetha Rao [ID],[1] Supuni Kapurubandara,[2] and Anbu Anpalagan[2]

[1]*Liverpool Hospital, Australia*
[2]*Westmead Hospital, Australia*

Correspondence should be addressed to Svetha Rao; svetharao1@gmail.com

Academic Editor: Maria Grazia Porpora

Extremely elevated CA 125, usually suggestive of ovarian malignancy, can be found in physiological or benign conditions such as endometriosis. We present a case of an extremely elevated serum CA 125 level in a patient with stage four endometriosis and bilateral unruptured ovarian endometriomas, with evidence of leakage unilaterally. To avoid costly and unnecessarily invasive tests and procedures it is important to consider the differential diagnosis of endometriosis and/or leaking endometrioma in patients with a profoundly elevated CA 125 level.

1. Introduction

The cancer antigen (CA) 125 is a high molecular weight glycoprotein, which originates from coelomic epithelium, which is expressed by normal tissues such as the endometrium, peritoneum, pericardium, and epithelial ovarian carcinomas (EOCs) [1]. It is most commonly used as a biomarker for EOC for the purposes of diagnosis, monitoring of disease progression, and response to treatment [2]. CA 125 also has an important role in differentiating benign and malignant pelvic masses, especially preoperatively, as higher CA 125 levels are considered to correlate with a higher probability of malignancy [2]. However, serum CA 125 levels can be elevated in other malignancies as well as various physiological and benign conditions such as endometriosis, uterine fibroids, pelvic inflammatory disease, early pregnancy, and normal menstruation [2, 3]. The positive predictive value of CA 125 for ovarian cancer is high among postmenopausal women (96%) [4] but is associated with a lower specificity among premenopausal women given the various benign conditions that can lead to elevated CA 125 levels [2]. Therefore, benign conditions such as endometriosis should be considered as differential diagnoses in the context of an elevated CA 125 level, especially among premenopausal women. Profoundly raised CA 125 in the absence of malignancy is rare; we review the literature regarding similar cases to help guide assessment and management of such patients.

2. Case Presentation

A 27-year-old nulliparous woman presented to the emergency department complaining of abdominal pain on the background of chronic pelvic pain.

On admission, an enlarged right ovary 150cc in volume with a cyst measuring 6.5cm and low internal echoes was demonstrated on pelvic ultrasound. Abdominopelvic computed tomography (CT) scan also demonstrated a 6.5cm dense right ovarian cyst with a moderate volume of free fluid and no evidence of appendicitis. Tumour markers taken at the time of acute presentation demonstrated a serum CA 125 level of 8142 U/ml (reference range: <35 U/ml) which had significantly increased from 115 U/ml when performed 12 months prior. Serum alpha fetoprotein (AFP) and human chorionic gonadotropin (hCG) levels were both <2 U/ml.

She was referred to the gynaecology clinic at Westmead hospital for further urgent review and management. An ultrasound scan for deep infiltrating endometriosis (DIE) verified the presence of a right ovarian cyst (6.3 x 5.0 x 4.4cm) with bowel adherent to the posterior aspect of the uterus. A gynaecological oncological opinion was sought at this time in light of the significantly raised CA 125 recommending a repeat level in 2 weeks on the provisional diagnosis of endometriosis after reviewing the ultrasound images and patients history of initial presentation. Repeat measurement of serum CA 125 level taken two weeks from her initial

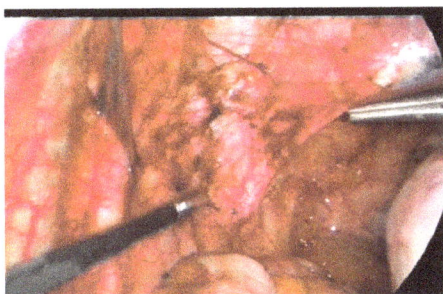

FIGURE 1: **Intraoperative images of widespread endometriotic deposits**, suggestive of leaking endometrioma.

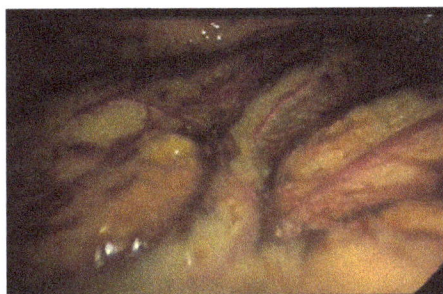

FIGURE 2: **Intraoperative images of widespread endometriotic deposits**, suggestive of leaking endometrioma.

presentation demonstrated a lower but still significantly elevated level of 2038 U/ml (day 12). Serum carcinoembryonic antigen (CEA) and CA 19.9 were <2 U/ml and 430 U/ml (reference range: <37 U/ml), respectively.

A multidisciplinary discussion with a gynaecologist oncologist was conducted to determine further management. Based on the images and decreasing serum CA 125 level an endometriotic leak from an ovarian endometrioma was considered most likely, with ovarian malignancy being the main differential and unlikely diagnosis.

At laparoscopy on day 58, stage four endometriosis and bilateral unruptured ovarian endometriomas, with features suggestive of leakage unilaterally, were revealed. Widespread endometriotic deposits were found at the upper and anterior abdominal wall, omentum, and bilateral uterosacral ligaments, likely secondary to leaking endometrioma (Figures 1 and 2). Laparoscopic excision of endometriosis, bilateral ureterolysis, bilateral excision of endometrioma, and insertion of a Mirena© intrauterine device were performed.

Histopathological examination confirmed the diagnosis of endometrioma. The patient recovered uneventfully and was discharged on the third postoperative day. At the third postoperative week the patient remained in a stable condition and routine follow-up with the general practitioner was recommended.

3. Discussion

CA 125 was first identified as an ovarian cancer antigen in 1981 [19] and later developed as a biomarker for EOC when serum levels > 35 U/ml were found in over 80% of patients with EOC but only 1% of healthy women [4]. The positive predictive value of CA 125 (> 95 IU/ml) for ovarian cancer is high among postmenopausal women (96%) [4] and is associated with a high sensitivity and specificity, of 69-97% and 81-93%, respectively [20]. While most commonly used in EOC, serum CA 125 levels can be elevated in other malignancies and various physiological and benign conditions including endometriosis [2, 3]. Consequently, CA 125 is associated with a poorer specificity among premenopausal women given the various benign conditions that can lead to an elevated CA 125 level [2, 21] and a physiologic serum half-life of approximately 6 days [22]. Routine CA 125 level is therefore not recommended in all premenopausal women with a simple appearing ovarian cyst [23].

Patients with endometriosis often do not have CA 125 levels > 100 U/ml [13, 16]. Still, endometriosis is one of the most common benign conditions associated with elevated serum CA 125 [14]. CA 125 has been extensively studied as a biomarker for endometriosis, with two meta-analyses concluding it has limited utility as a diagnostic marker for endometriosis given its low sensitivity (20-50%) [1, 24, 25]. This is supported by international guidelines for endometriosis which do not recommend the measurement of serum CA 125 level as part of routine diagnostic work-up [26]. The relationship between elevated CA 125 levels and endometriosis has been well established in the literature, with levels reflecting both the severity and the progression of the disease [3, 27, 28]. Elevated serum CA 125 levels are often related to ovarian endometriomas and endometriosis of higher severity such as stages three and four [3, 14, 23, 29]. CA 125 levels have also been shown to decrease following both medical and surgical treatment of endometriosis [10, 29].

Extremely elevated CA 125 levels have been reported in the presence of both ruptured [5, 7, 9, 10, 12, 30] and unruptured endometriomas [13–18] (Tables 1 and 2). The highest CA 125 level reported in proven endometriosis is 9537 U/ml following acute rupture of an endometrioma [7]. In the present case, we report an extremely elevated serum CA 125 level of 8142 U/ml in a patient found to have stage four endometriosis, bilateral unruptured ovarian endometriomas with evidence of leakage unilaterally, and widespread endometriotic deposits when viewed intraoperatively. The previous highest CA 125 level in the context of an unruptured endometrioma was 7900 U/ml [16]. This carries significant clinical importance as an elevated CA 125, especially in the presence of a pelvic mass, can mimic and raise suspicion of a malignant process leading to unnecessarily invasive procedures [15, 30]. Education of the patient regarding the significance of an elevated *tumour* marker in the absence of a malignant tumour is of prime importance, with sensitivity to the potential emotional distress such words can impose. The decision to manage as a benign gynaecological condition compared to a potentially malignant case should be discussed.

There are multiple theories behind elevated serum CA 125 levels in endometriosis. The fluid within an endometriotic cyst [or endometrioma] is thought to be rich in CA 125 with concentrations reported to be > 10000 U/ml [31]. Following

TABLE 1: Summary of cases of ruptured endometrioma with elevated CA 125 levels†.

Author & Year	Type of study and number of patients (n)	CA-125 level (IU/ml)	Clinical presentation	Imaging findings	Operative intervention / Management
Johansson J et al. (1998) [5]	Case report n = 1	9300	Abdominal pain	USS: Rt homogeneous ovarian 7x10cm	Laparotomy, Excision of endometrioma
Kashyap RJ. (1999) [6]	Case report n = 1	6114	Abdominal pain, Nausea	USS: 11 cm complex cyst	Laparotomy, Rt oophorectomy
Kurata, H et al. (2002) [7]	Case report n = 1	9537	Abdominal pain	USS: homogenous bilateral ovarian cysts, FF in pelvis MRI: ovarian masses, bloody liquid with T1-high signal and T2-low signal	Laparoscopy, enucelation of cysts
Cengiz et al. (2012) [8]	Case report n = 1	174.87	Abdominal pain, Nausea	USS: Lt heterogenous adnexal mass 6x8cm, FF in pelvis	Laparoscopy, Enucleation of cyst
A.K. Rani et al. (2012) [9]	Case report n = 1	9391	Abdominal pain	USS: Rt homogenous adnexal mass 10.5x7cm, moderate ascites CT: b/l adnexal mass, minimal ascites, nil lymphadenopathy	Laparotomy, excision of endometrioma
Duran M et al. (2013) [10]	Case report n = 1	2556	Pelvic and Abdominal pain, Dysuria	USS & CT: Lt heterogenous adnexal mass 5x5cm	Laparoscopy, Excision of endometrioma
Dereli et al. (2014) [11]	Case report n = 1	143.72	Bilateral pelvic masses	USS: hypoechoic bilateral adnexal masses	Laparoscopy, Rt adnexectomy, Lt cystectomy
X. Dai et al. (2015) [12]	Retrospective cohort n = 43	797.89 ± 1106.52	Abdominal pain, Pelvic mass, Asymptomatic	-	Laparoscopy/ Laparotomy

USS: ultrasound; CT: computerised tomography; MRI: magnetic resonance imaging; FF: free fluid; PoD: pouch of Douglas.
†In all cases reviewed endometrioma was confirmed histologically.

leakage of endometriotic fluid, from an endometrioma, this fluid will subsequently cover peritoneal surfaces which may be absorbed into the peripheral circulation and cause peritoneal inflammation, resulting in an elevated CA 125 level [7, 12, 16, 32, 33]. Given the increase in peritoneal fluid in the presence of mild endometriosis and the presence of higher levels of CA 125 in peritoneal fluid compared to corresponding serum levels [34], this could also contribute to elevated serum CA 125 measurements.

The reason for high CA 125 concentrations in cyst fluid compared to serum levels is attributed to the thick wall of the endometriotic cyst preventing large CA 125 glycoprotein molecules from diffusing out of the cyst and reaching systemic circulation; however, this inhibition of CA 125 molecules is not believed to be absolute [14, 35].

Elevated serum CA 125 levels in endometriosis are also attributed to a higher surface area of endometrial tissue such as endometriotic cysts [9], deep infiltrating endometriotic nodules, adhesions [25], and the stage of disease [13]. In our case leakage of CA 125 rich cystic fluid into the peritoneal cavity in combination with stage four endometriosis and bilateral endometriomas could explain the extremely elevated serum CA 125 level of 8142 U/ml, which had dramatically rose from 115 U/ml one year prior as well as the subsequent level of 2038 U/ml two weeks later. Concurrent menstruation has been shown to cause up to three-fold increase in CA 125 level among women with endometriosis [28]. While this could have impacted the initial level in this case, it does not account for a persistently elevated CA 125 two weeks later.

TABLE 2: Summary of cases of unruptured endometrioma with elevated CA 125 levels†.

Author & Year	Type of study and number of patients [n]	CA-125 level [IU/ml]	Clinical presentation	Imaging findings	Operative intervention / Management
Yilmazer M et al. (2003) [13]	Case report n = 1	1741.8	Abdominal pain, Bilateral adnexal masses	USS & CT: bilateral adnexal cystic masses	Laparoscopy, B/L cystectomy
Shiau C-S et al. (2003) [14]	Case report n = 1	6310	Pelvic mass, Abdominal pain, Nausea	USS & CT: homogenous Lt adnexal cystic mass 75mm	Laparotomy, Enucleation & excision of cyst
Atabekoglu C et al. (2003) [15]	Case report n = 1	3890	Abdominal pain, Dysmenorrhea	CT: right cystic ovarian mass of 12x10 cm	Laparotomy, Rt adnexectomy
Kahraman K et al. (2007) [16]	Case report n = 1	7900	Adnexal mass	USS & MRI: homogeneous Lt adnexal cystic mass	Laparoscopy, Cystectomy, U/L salpingectomy
Hosseini, M et al. (2009) [17]	Case report n = 1	2000	Abdominal pain, Dysmenorrhea	USS: bilateral ovarian cystic masses	Laparotomy, B/L cystectomy
Peker N et al. (2013) [18]	Case report n = 1	1061	Pelvic mass	USS: homogenous left ovarian cystic mass, FF at PoD	Laparotomy, Enucleation of cyst

USS: ultrasound; CT: computerised tomography; MRI: magnetic resonance imaging; FF: free fluid; PoD: pouch of Douglas
†In all cases reviewed endometrioma was confirmed histologically.

While there have been several reports of elevated serum CA 125 levels in both ruptured and unruptured endometriomas, the present case reports a rare finding of an extremely elevated serum CA 125 level in the context of bilateral endometriomas, with evidence of leakage unilaterally. This case demonstrates that serum CA 125 levels can be extremely elevated due to an unruptured leaking endometrioma and highlights the importance of considering the differential diagnosis of endometriosis and or endometrioma in patients with an elevated CA 125, when suspecting ovarian carcinoma as the cause of an adnexal mass.

Consent

Patient has given written informed consent for this case to be published in a medical journal.

References

[1] V. Nisenblat, P. M. Bossuyt, R. Shaikh, C. Farquhar, V. Jordan, C. S. Scheffers et al., "Blood biomarkers for the non-invasive diagnosis of endometriosis," *Cochrane Database of Systematic Reviews*, no. 5, 2016.

[2] R. C. Bast Jr., D. Badgwell, Z. Lu et al., "New tumor markers: CA125 and beyond," *International Journal of Gynecological Cancer*, vol. 15, Suppl 3, no. 6, pp. 274–281, 2005.

[3] R. L. Barbieri, J. M. Niloff, R. C. Bast Jr., E. Scaetzl, R. W. Kistner, and R. C. Knapp, "Elevated serum concentrations of CA-125 in patients with advanced endometriosis," *Fertility and Sterility*, vol. 45, pp. 630–634, 1986.

[4] C. M. Boyer, R. C. Knapp, and R. C. Bast Jr., "Biology and immunology," in *Practical Gynecologic Oncology*, J. S. Berek and N. F. Hacker, Eds., pp. 89-90, Williams & Wilkins, Baltimore, MD, USA, 2nd edition, 1994.

[5] J. Johansson, M. Santala, and A. Kauppila, "Explosive rise of serum CA 125 following the rupture of ovarian endometrioma," *Human Reproduction*, vol. 13, pp. 3503-3504, 1998.

[6] R. J. Kashyap, "Extremely elevated serum CA125 due to endometriosis," *The Australian & New Zealand Journal of Obstetrics & Gynaecology*, vol. 139, pp. 269-270, 1999.

[7] H. Kurata, M. Sasaki, H. Kase, Y. Yamamoto, Y. Aoki, and K. Tanaka, "Elevated serum CA125 and CA19-9 due to the spontaneous rupture of ovarian endometrioma," *European Journal of Obstetrics, Gynecology, and Reproductive Biology*, vol. 105, no. 1, pp. 75-76, 2002.

[8] H. Cengiz, Ş. Yıldız, L. Yaşar, M. Ekin, and C. Kaya, "Extremely elevated serum CA125 and CA19-9 levels following the rupture of ovarian endometrioma: a case report," *Gaziantep Medical Journal*, vol. 18, no. 3, pp. 189-190, 2012.

[9] A. K. Rani and D. Kapoor, "Ruptured ovarian endometrioma with an extreme rise in serum CA 125 level - A case report: Ovarian endometrioma with very high CA-125 level," *Gynecologic Oncology Reports*, vol. 2, no. 3, pp. 100-101, 2012.

[10] M. Duran, A. Kosus, N. Kosus, C. Duvan, and H. Kafali, "Treatment of ruptured ovarian endometrioma with extremely high CA 125, moderately high CA 19-9 and CA 15-3 Level," *Journal of Clinical and Analytical Medicine*, vol. 4, no. 3, pp. 299-300, 2013.

[11] L. Dereli, U. Solmaz, E. Mat, N. Peker, A. Dogan, and B. Yildirim, "Huge endometrioma with severe ascites mimicking ovarian cancer," *Journal of Cases in Obstetrics & Gynecology*, vol. 1, no. 3, pp. 49-50, 2014.

[12] X. Dai, C. Jin, Y. Hu et al., "High CA-125 and CA19-9 levels in spontaneous ruptured ovarian endometriomas," *Clinica Chimica Acta*, vol. 450, pp. 362–365, 2015.

[13] M. Yilmazer, M. Sonmezer, M. Gungor, V. Fenkci, and S. Cevrioglu, "Unusually elevated serum carbohydrate antigen 125 (CA125) and CA19-9 levels as a result of unruptured bilateral endometrioma," *Australian and New Zealand Journal of Obstetrics and Gynaecology*, vol. 43, no. 4, pp. 329-330, 2003.

[14] C. S. Shiau, M. Y. Chang, C. H. Chiang, C. C. Hsieh, and T. T. Hsieh, "Ovarian endometrioma associated with very high serum CA-125 levels," *Chang Gung Medical Journal*, vol. 26, no. 9, pp. 695–699, 2003.

[15] C. S. Atabekoglu, M. Sönmezer, B. Aydinuraz, and I. Dünder, "Extremely elevated CA 125 level due to an unruptured large endometrioma," *European Journal of Obstetrics, Gynecology, and Reproductive Biology*, vol. 110, no. 1, pp. 105-106, 2003.

[16] K. Kahraman, I. Ozguven, M. Gungor, and C. S. Atabekoglu, "Extremely elevated serum CA-125 level as a result of unruptured unilateral endometrioma: the highest value reported," *Fertility and Sterility*, vol. 88, no. 4, pp. e15–e17, 2007.

[17] M. A. Hosseini, A. Aleyasin, S. Khodaverdi, A. Mahdavi, and Z. Najmi, "Extra-ordinary High CA-125 and CA19-9 Serum levels in an ovarian endometrioma: case report," *Journal of Family Planning and Reproductive Health Care*, vol. 3, no. 2, pp. 67–70, 2009.

[18] N. Peker, A. Demir, and O. Bige, "Endometrioma mimicking ovarian cancer with unusual high levels of serum CA 125 and CA 19-9," *Basic and Clinical Sciences*, vol. 2, pp. 170–173, 2013.

[19] R. C. Bast Jr., M. Feeney, H. Lazarus, L. M. Nadler, R. B. Colvin, and R. C. Knapp, "Reactivity of a monoclonal antibody with human ovarian carcinoma," *The Journal of Clinical Investigation*, vol. 68, no. 5, pp. 1331–1337, 1981.

[20] E. R. Myers, L. A. Bastian, L. J. Havrilesky, S. L. Kulasingam, M. S. Terplan, K. E. Cline et al., "Management of adnexal mass," *Evidence Report/Technology Assessment*, vol. 130, pp. 1–145, 2006.

[21] T. A. D. Timmerman, T. Bourne, E. Ferrazzi, L. Ameye, M. L. Konstantinovic et al., "Logistic regression model to distinguish between the benign and malignant adnexal mass before surgery: a multicenter study by the international ovarian tumor analysis group," *Journal of Clinical Oncology*, vol. 23, pp. 8794–8801, 2005.

[22] G. J. Rustin, R. C. Bast, G. Kelloff, J. Barrett, S. Carter, P. Nisen et al., "Use of CA-125 in clinical trial evaluation of new therapeutic drugs for ovarian cancer," *Clinical Cancer Research*, vol. 10, pp. 3919–3926, 2004.

[23] RCOG, "Management of Suspected Ovarian Masses in Premenopausal Women (Green-top Guideline No. 62)," 2011.

[24] B. W. Mol, N. Bayram, J. G. Lijmer, M. A. Wiegerinck, M. Y. Bongers, F. van der Veen et al., "The performance of CA-125 measurement in the detection of endometriosis: a meta-analysis," *Fertility and Sterility*, vol. 70, pp. 1101–1108, 1998.

[25] Y.-M. Cheng, S.-T. Wang, and C.-Y. Chou, "Serum CA-125 in preoperative patients at high risk for endometriosis," *Obstetrics & Gynecology*, vol. 99, no. 3, pp. 375–380, 2002.

[26] Gynecologists TACoOa, "Practice bulletin no. 114: management of endometriosis," *Obstetrics and Gynecology*, vol. 116, no. 1, pp. 223–236, 2010.

[27] M. D. Hornstein, B. L. Harlow, P. P. Thomas, and J. H. Check, "Use of a new CA125 assay in the diagnosis of endometriosis," *Human Reproduction*, vol. 10, pp. 932–934, 1995.

[28] E. Donald, M. D. Pittaway, and J. A. Fazyez, "Serum CA-125 antigen levels increase during menses," *American Journal of Obstetrics & Gynecology*, vol. 156, no. 1, pp. 75-76, 1987.

[29] I. Jacobs and R. C. Bast Jr., "The CA 125 tumour-associated antigen: a review of the literature," *Human Reproduction*, vol. 4, no. 1, pp. 1–12, 1989.

[30] P. Uharček, M. Mlyncek, and J. Ravinger, "Elevation of serum CA 125 and D-Dimer levels associated with rupture of ovarian endometrioma," *The International Journal of Biological Markers*, vol. 22, no. 3, pp. 203–205, 2007.

[31] P. R. Koninckx, M. Muyldermans, P. Moerman, C. Meuleman, J. Deprest, and F. Cornillie, "CA 125 concentrations in ovarian 'chocolate' cyst fluid can differentiate an endometriotic cyst from a cystic corpus luteum," *Human Reproduction*, vol. 7, no. 9, pp. 1314–1317, 1992.

[32] B. J. Park, T. E. Kim, and Y. W. Kim, "Massive peritoneal fluid and markedly elevated serum CA125 and CA19-9 levels associated with an ovarian endometrioma," *The Journal of Obstetrics and Gynaecology Research*, vol. 35, p. 935, 2009.

[33] V. F. Amaral, R. A. Ferriani, M. F. Sa et al., "Positive correlation between serum and peritoneal fluid CA-125 levels in women with pelvic endometriosis," *Sa~o Paulo Medical Journal*, vol. 124, pp. 223–227, 2006.

[34] A. Barbati, M. M. Anceschi, G. C. Di Renzo, and E. V. Cosmi, "CA 125 in peritoneal fluid: reliable values at high dilutions," *Obstetrics and gynecology*, vol. 79, no. 6, pp. 1011–1015, 1992.

[35] P. R. Koninckx, L. Riittinen, M. Seppala, and F. J. Cornillie, "CA-125 and placental protein 14 concentrations in plasma and peritoneal fluid of women with deeply infiltrating pelvic endometriosis," *Fertility and Sterility*, vol. 57, pp. 523–530, 1992.

4

Lipschütz Genital Ulceration as Initial Manifestation of Primary Sjögren's Syndrome

Filipa de Castro Coelho ⓘ,[1] **Maria Amaral,**[2] **Lúcia Correia** ⓘ,[3] **Maria João Nunes Campos,**[4] **Tereza Paula,**[4] **Augusta Borges,**[2] **and Jorge Borrego**[4]

[1]*Gynecology Department, Hospital Dr. Nélio Mendonça, Serviço de Saúde da Região Autónoma da Madeira, EPE, Funchal, Portugal*
[2]*Internal Medicine Department, Maternidade Dr. Alfredo da Costa, Centro Hospitalar Lisboa Central, Lisboa, Portugal*
[3]*Gynecology Department, Instituto Português de Oncologia de Lisboa Francisco Gentil, EPE, Lisboa, Portugal*
[4]*Gynecology Department, Maternidade Dr. Alfredo da Costa, Centro Hospitalar Lisboa Central, Lisboa, Portugal*

Correspondence should be addressed to Filipa de Castro Coelho; filipacastrocoelho@gmail.com

Academic Editor: Massimo Origoni

Genital ulcers are challenging to any clinician and causes transcend many specialties. Skin ulceration in patients with primary Sjögren's syndrome is infrequent but an established feature of cutaneous involvement. Although gynecological symptoms, such as vulvovaginal dryness, dyspareunia, and pruritus, are common in women with primary Sjögren's syndrome, patients affected by vulvar ulcers are unknown. We describe an exceptional case of necrotic aphthous-type vulvar ulceration as initial presentation of primary Sjögren's syndrome that was possibly triggered by an infectious agent. Successful healing was achieved with oral corticosteroids, despite some loss of labia *minora* and labia *majora* as sequelae of the necrotizing process. Reactive acute genital ulcers (Lipschütz ulcers) should be considered as a possible manifestation of many autoimmune/inflammatory disorders, beyond the classic associations such as Behçet's syndrome or Crohn's disease.

1. Introduction

Primary Sjögren's syndrome (pSS) is an autoimmune inflammatory disorder, with a higher incidence in female patients. Extraglandular manifestations may result from lymphocytic infiltration, generation of pathogenic autoantibodies-mediated mechanisms, or vasculitis [1]. Cutaneous vasculitis is generally thought of as being palpable purpura, but other infrequent types of lesions can occur, such as ulcers or ischemic lesions [1, 2]. Vascular findings of pSS often occur on the legs, although a perivascular lymphocytic infiltrate has been observed in the underlying vaginal stroma of women with Sjögren's syndrome (SS) [3].

Cutaneous disorders serve as a reflex of systemic involvement. Autoimmune conditions can be triggered by infectious agents, which can also determine its clinical manifestations [4]. Lipschütz ulcers (LUs) or reactive nonsexually related acute genital ulcers (RNSAGU) are often described as a clinical sign of an immune response to an underlying infection.

LU's and pSS's pathogenesis share common infectious triggers across literature [4, 5]. Thus, a role for infection in both conditions is suggested. We present a case of a woman with Lipschütz genital ulceration as initial manifestation of pSS in the context of an infectious disease.

2. Case

A 26-year-old-woman, with history of labial herpes and asthmatic bronchitis, presented with bilateral retroocular pain, odynophagia, fever, vaginal discomfort and vulvar ulcers. The ulcers continued to progress despite treatment with nonsteroidal anti-inflammatory drugs and valacyclovir, prescribed at the primary healthcare site. Two days later, after initial consultation at our emergency room, she was admitted immediately at the Vulvar Clinic of our institution, with increasing vulvar pain, without other symptoms. Physical examination of the vulva showed extended vulvar oedema

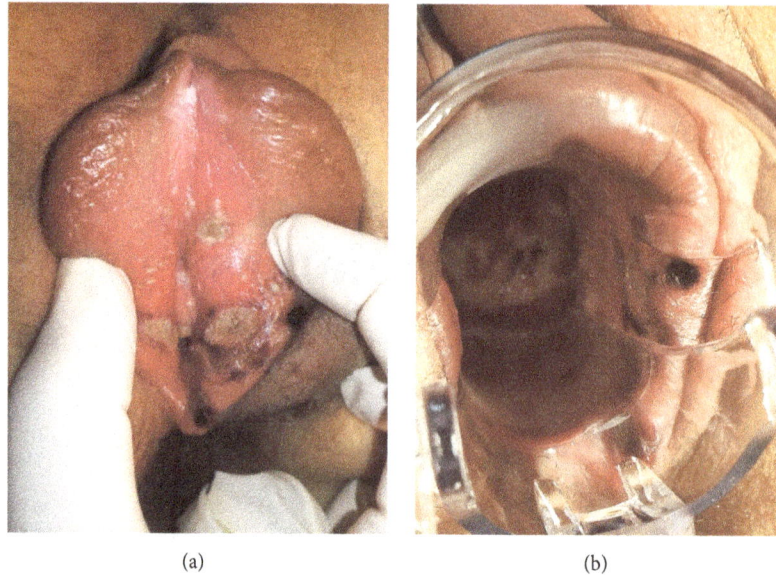

(a)   (b)

FIGURE 1: (a) Vulvar swelling and shallow "kissing" ulcers with necrotic debris and sharply demarcated borders, 2 mm-20 mm diameter, on labia minora and majora. (b) Ulcers on the bilateral labia, lower vagina, and cervix.

and *kissing pattern* ulcers on labia *minora* and majora, vagina and cervix (Figure 1). Inguinal lymph nodes were also bilaterally swollen. The patient denied the use of other medications and sexual activity in more than 6 months. First blood tests only showed C-reactive protein 12.35 mg/dL (normal: <0.5 mg/dL). Serologies for herpes virus 1 and 2, Ebstein-Barr virus (EBV; IgG+), cytomegalovirus, *mycoplasma pneumoniae*, parvovirus B19, toxoplasmosis, rubella, hepatitis, human immunodeficiency virus, and syphilis (using the Venereal Disease Research Laboratory test) were negative. After this, a multidisciplinary approach was performed. When directly asked, she complained about mild eye dryness and she often felt a discomfort of dry mouth. There was no familial history of autoimmune diseases, but her father had some episodes of oral aphthosis. Immunological examination was positive for rheumatoid factor (RF – 22.3 UI; normal: <15 UI), anti-nuclear antibodies [ANA (speckled, titer 1:320)] and antibodies to SSA/Ro (SSA 3+/ Ro52KD 3+)—initial screening step of ANA by indirect immunofluorescence on HEp-2 cells (*Euroimmun®, Germany*); autoantibodies confirmation assay by line immunoblot (*ANA profile 3 - Euroimmun®, Germany*)—antibodies detected on strips were evaluated semiquantitatively (negative, 1+, 2++, and 3+++). Anti-SSB/La, anti-RNP, anti-Sm, anti-dsDNA, antineutrophil cytoplasmic, anticardiolipin, and anti-beta(2)-glycoprotein1 antibodies were negative. Serum C3 level was 1.79 g/L (normal: 0.9-1.8 g/L) and C4 level was 0.31 g/L (0.1-0.4 g/L). Immunoglobulins (IgG, IgM, IgA) were measured and a high IgG level was found (20.50 g /L; normal: 7-16 g/L). Erythrocyte sedimentation rate was also high (45 mm/h; normal: <16 mm/h). Lupus anticoagulant and HLA-B27 were both negative. Ophthalmological evaluation was refused by the patient. Labial salivary gland (LSG) biopsy revealed focal lymphocytic sialadenitis (FLS), with a focus score (FS) =1 (per 4 mm2) obtained by four LSGs (3-5 mm). No other histopathological features were reported. The patient

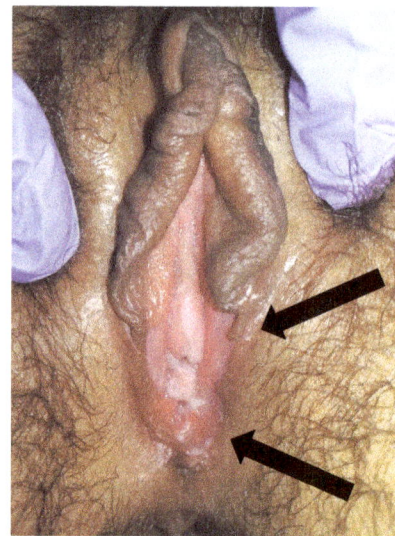

FIGURE 2: Complete resolution of the vulvar lesions with partial loss of left labia *minora* and *majora* (black arrows).

was diagnosed as having pSS on the basis of dry eyes and dry mouth, positive anti-SSA/Ro antibody, and typical histopathologic abnormalities on LSG biopsy. Prednisolone 20 mg/day was prescribed and vulvar healing appeared within 2 weeks with partial loss of left labia (Figure 2).

3. Discussion

pSS occurs in a primary form not associated with other well-defined autoimmune disease. Current consensus classification criteria for pSS by American College of Rheumatology and the European League Against Rheumatism (EULAR) set this diagnosis in our patient who meets the inclusion criteria (sicca symptoms) and has a score ≥4 based on anti-SSA/Ro antibody positivity and FLS (each scoring 3) [2].

A LSG biopsy is considered positive if minor salivary glands demonstrate FLS, with a FS of 1 or more (defined as several lymphocytic foci, containing more than 50 lymphocytes per 4 mm2 of glandular tissue) [6, 7]. Experts recommendations also propose to obtain a minimum of four LSGs, unless these are small (2 mm). [7] We have adopted this standardised consensus guidance for the use of LSG histopathology in the classification of pSS. FLS cannot be attributed when morphologic patterns of chronic inflammation such as nonspecific chronic sialadenitis and sclerosing chronic sialadenitis occur in LSG biopsy specimens [6–8]. Our histopathological assessment did not find these patterns. A FS count of 1 was present and this reflects SS autoimmunity [6]. We opted not to perform imaging tests. Future modifications of the present-day criteria may arise with the adoption of new diagnostic tests, such as salivary gland ultrasonography or the use of magnetic resonance imaging for a more precise, noninvasive diagnostic approach to SS. Yet, EULAR consensus guidance reinforces LSG as a key marker of pSS [2, 7, 8]. And further validation studies are required before imaging modalities are included in a new set of classification criteria for pSS [7, 8].

This chronic autoimmune inflammatory disorder yields multiple clinical expressions, including exocrine gland involvement and extraglandular disease features. Among extraglandular manifestations, cutaneous vasculitis may manifest as ulcers [1, 2]. Compared to the patients without vasculitis, affected patients had a higher prevalence of positive ANA, anti-Ro/SS-A antibodies, and RF [1, 2]. These were findings in our patient.

LUs, *ulcus vulvae acutum* and RNSAGU, are synonymous of a distinct aphthous-type ulcers classified either as an idiopathic process or as secondary to other diseases such as Crohn's, Behçet's, and various infectious conditions [9, 10]. The precise aetiology and pathogenesis remain unclear; however, LUs are described as a result from an exuberant immune response to an infection [5, 10]. Most cases do not have an identifiable pathogen [5, 10]. Reactive acute genital ulcers present with fever, malaise and inguinal lymphadenopathy, resembling our patient. The main vulvar symptom is pain, sometimes with characteristic "kissing pattern" and notable oedema of labia. Necrosis is a complication previously described [10]. LUs are typically located on labia *minora*, but our patient also had lesions on the labia *majora*, lower vagina and cervix. Time to full healing was coincident with previous reports [5]. Retrospective studies emphasized that LUs should not be seen as a young virginal women exclusive vulvar dermatoses [5, 10]. It is mandatory the exclusion of sexually and nonsexually infections, drug reactions and autoimmune/inflammatory conditions, including Crohn's and Behçet's disease [5, 9, 10]. The authors could not find any report regarding pSS as a systemic illness to exclude. Treatment is supportive, but if a systemic disease is suspected, the multidisciplinary approach is appropriate, and treatment should be targeted to the specific etiology.

Similar to LUs, the underlying cause of pSS remains obscure. Infectious agents (viruses, bacteria, parasites, and fungi) are thought to trigger inflammation, autoantibody production and immune-mediated tissue injury [1]. LU's and pSS's pathogenesis has its focus in the genetics–autoimmunity–infection triad across scientific literature. Recent studies have reemphasized the role of molecular mimicry in which genetically predisposed individuals may make immune responses to self-antigens by immune mistake. This model has been applied to several pathogens, with the EBV being the paradigmatic example, but the spectrum of possible microorganisms is getting wider [1, 4, 5]. In this report, an infectious cause well-grounded on clinical and laboratory findings (without an aetiological diagnosis) was identified as the probable trigger for the final diagnosis of Sjögren's syndrome-associated Lipschütz genital ulceration.

Dyspareunia, vulvovaginal dryness and pruritus are common symptoms in pSS women [3]. To our knowledge, there are no previous reports describing acute vulvar ulcers as a cutaneous manifestation of pSS. The wide diversity of cutaneous processes, both vasculitic and nonvasculitic, observed in pSS patients, suggests that skin involvement in this condition reflects systemic involvement and manifests itself in different clinical forms [1, 2].

Vaginal ulcers completely resolved with oral prednisolone, but partial loss of left labia was observed. SS may be a predisposing factor for the impaired healing process [11].

No genital biopsies were performed for three main reasons: there was no suspicion of intraepithelial neoplasia or cancer; cervical, vaginal and vulvar histopathology on pSS women is nonspecific; biopsy is not mandatory for cutaneous involvement in pSS [2, 3].

An analysis of 33 cases identified autoimmune phenomena in 18,2% women with LUs [5]. Close follow-up is recommended to confirm healing and to rule out progression to systemic disease [10]. The described case report shows LUs as a clinical sign of pSS, due to an overexpressed immune response to infection on the presence of a predisposing autoimmune background. Even in cases with documented infection, LU's should be considered as a possible manifestation of many autoimmune/inflammatory disorders, beyond the classic associations such as Behçet's syndrome or Crohn's disease. This can only be achieved with a broad multidisciplinary approach toward individualized care for patients with acute genital ulcers.

Abbreviations

ANA: Anti-nuclear antibodies
EBV: Ebstein-Barr virus
EULAR: European League Against Rheumatism
FLS: Focal lymphocytic sialadenitis
FS: Focus score
IgG: Immunoglobulin G
LSG: Labial salivary gland
LUs: Lipschütz ulcers
pSS: Primary Sjögren's syndrome
RF: Rheumatoid factor
RNSAGU: Reactive nonsexually related acute genital ulcers
SS: Sjögren's syndrome.

Consent

A signed written consent was obtained from the patient.

Authors' Contributions

All authors listed on submitted manuscript have read and agreed to its content and meet the authorship requirements as detailed.

References

[1] R. I. Fox and A. Y. Liu, "Sjögren's syndrome in dermatology," *Clinics in Dermatology*, vol. 24, no. 5, pp. 393–413, 2006.

[2] M. Ramos-Casals, P. Brito-Zerón, R. Seror et al., "Characterization of systemic disease in primary Sjögren's syndrome: EULAR-SS Task Force recommendations for articular, cutaneous, pulmonary and renal involvements," *Rheumatology*, vol. 54, pp. 2230–2238, 2015.

[3] S. M. Bongi, M. Orlandi, A. De Magnis et al., "Women with primary sjögren syndrome and with Non-Sjögren Sicca syndrome show similar vulvar histopathologic and immunohistochemical changes," *International Journal of Gynecological Pathology*, vol. 35, no. 6, pp. 585–592, 2016.

[4] S. Kivity, N. Agmon-Levin, M. Blank, and Y. Shoenfeld, "Infections and autoimmunity—friends or foes?" *Trends in Immunology*, vol. 30, no. 8, pp. 409–414, 2009.

[5] P. Vieira-Baptista, J. Lima-Silva, J. Beires, and J. Martinez-De-Oliveira, "Lipschütz ulcers: Should we rethink this? an analysis of 33 cases," *European Journal of Obstetrics & Gynecology and Reproductive Biology*, vol. 198, pp. 149–152, 2016.

[6] T. E. Daniels, D. Cox, C. H. Shiboski et al., "Associations between salivary gland histopathologic diagnoses and phenotypic features of Sjögren's syndrome among 1,726 registry participants," *Arthritis & Rheumatology*, vol. 63, no. 7, pp. 2021–2030, 2011.

[7] B. A. Fisher, R. Jonsson, T. Daniels et al., "Standardisation of labial salivary gland histopathology in clinical trials in primary Sjögren's syndrome," *Annals of the Rheumatic Diseases*, vol. 76, no. 7, pp. 1161–1168, 2017.

[8] P. Brito-Zerón, E. Theander, C. Baldini et al., "Early diagnosis of primary Sjögren's syndrome: EULAR-SS task force clinical recommendations," *Expert Review of Clinical Immunology*, vol. 12, no. 2, pp. 137–156, 2016.

[9] P. J. Lynch, M. Moyal-Barracco, J. Scurry, and C. Stockdale, "2011 ISSVD terminology and classification of vulvar dermatological disorders: An approach to clinical diagnosis," *Journal of Lower Genital Tract Disease*, vol. 16, no. 4, pp. 339–344, 2012.

[10] J. S. Lehman, A. J. Bruce, D. A. Wetter, S. B. Ferguson, and R. S. Rogers III, "Reactive nonsexually related acute genital ulcers: Review of cases evaluated at Mayo Clinic," *Journal of the American Academy of Dermatology*, vol. 63, no. 1, pp. 44–51, 2010.

[11] K. Beksac, M. Turgal, D. Basaran, O. Aran, and M. S. Beksac, "Vaginoperineal fistula as a complication of perianal surgery in a patient with sjögren's syndrome: a case report," *Case Reports in Rheumatology*, vol. 2014, Article ID 359605, 3 pages, 2014.

5

MRA Mapping and Selective Embolization of a Large Uterine Cavity Pseudoaneurysm at 20 Weeks of Gestation

Jean V. Storey ⓘ,[1] Timothy B. Dinh,[2] Deirdre M. McCullough,[1] Steven H. Craig,[2] and Christian L. Carlson[2]

[1]Department of Obstetrics and Gynecology, Brooke Army Medical Center, 3551 Roger Brooke Drive, Fort Sam Houston, San Antonio, TX 78234, USA
[2]Department of Radiology, Brooke Army Medical Center, 3551 Roger Brooke Drive, Fort Sam Houston, San Antonio, TX 78234, USA

Correspondence should be addressed to Jean V. Storey; jean.v.storey.mil@mail.mil

Academic Editor: Akihisa Fujimoto

Antepartum uterine cavity pseudoaneurysm rupture can cause massive hemorrhage with high maternal and fetal mortality risk. Invasive placentation can predispose to vascular malformations. We present a novel use of macrocyclic intravenous contrast-enhanced magnetic resonance angiography for preprocedure planning followed by selective low radiation embolization of a uterine cavity pseudoaneurysm in the setting of invasive placentation at 20 weeks of gestation. To our knowledge, this is the first reported case of uterine cavity pseudoaneurysm successfully mapped with MRA and treated with embolization at 20 weeks of gestation.

1. Introduction

Uterine surgery can predispose to future pregnancy complications to include abnormal placentation and vascular lesions such as arteriovenous malformations and fistulas and pseudoaneurysms [1, 2]. Hormonal and hemodynamic changes also play a role in development of vascular lesions in pregnancy [3]. Vascular lesions may present with life-threatening hemorrhage. Low patient risk and relatively low cost make ultrasound the screening method of choice with contrast angiography used for problem solving, treatment planning, and therapeutic intervention [1, 4]. Historically, treatment required hysterectomy, but arterial embolization currently offers a less invasive, fertility-sparing treatment option with a low complication rate [1, 5]. We report a novel use of dynamic IV contrast-enhanced magnetic resonance angiography (MRA) for further characterization and treatment planning/mapping of a uterine cavity pseudoaneurysm in a 20-week gravid female followed by low radiation embolization of feeding arteries, resulting in successful maternal and fetal outcome.

2. Case Presentation

A 35-year-old gravida 4 para 3 with a history of three previous cesarean deliveries presented at 16 weeks 6 days of gestation for follow-up ultrasound of perigestational hemorrhage seen at 10 weeks and 4 days. A large uterine cavity pseudoaneurysm measuring 4.2 × 3.8 × 3.7 cm and appearing to arise from abnormal placentation at the previous cesarean scar was identified (Figure 1). Repeat ultrasound six days later revealed a normal active fetus in breech position compressing the pseudoaneurysm upon contact. An unenhanced MRI one week later confirmed a 4 cm hypointense lesion projecting into the lower right uterine cavity at the inferior margin of the placenta (Figures 2 and 3). Management options were discussed to include conservative imaging observation versus embolization. Due to high maternal mortality risk from spontaneous hemorrhage, elective termination was also discussed but was rejected by the patient.

A novel use of dynamic time-resolved contrast-enhanced MRA utilizing a functional MR urography protocol™ was performed for enhanced characterization of feeding arteries

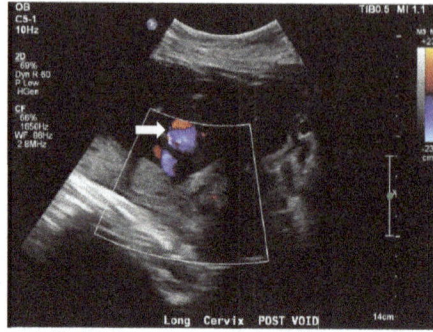

FIGURE 1: Follow-up ultrasound at 16 weeks and 6 days of gestation reveals a vascular malformation (arrow) at the lower uterine segment with swirling flow within the malformation consistent with a pseudoaneurysm.

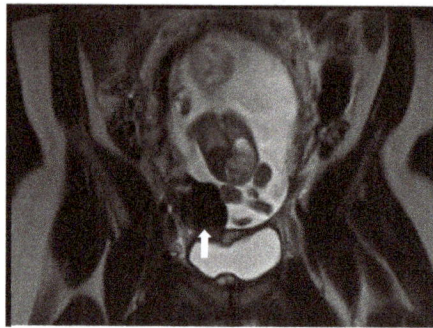

FIGURE 2: Coronal T2-weighted image of the pelvis at 18 weeks of gestation demonstrates a hypointense round structure (arrow) at the lower uterine segment infringing upon (and invaginating into) the gestational cavity. Fetal knee abuts and deforms the lesion.

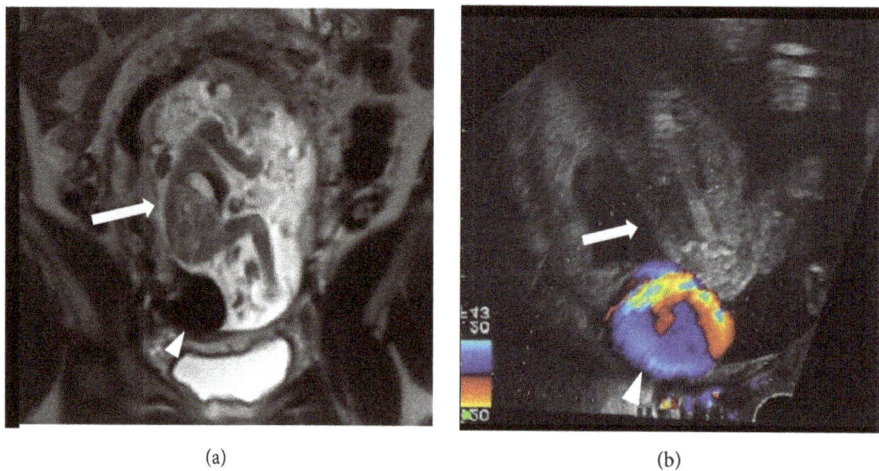

(a)   (b)

FIGURE 3: Maternal coronal (sagittal fetal) T2-weighted image of the pelvis (a) at 18 weeks of gestation with similar fetal positioning in relation to the lesion on ultrasound (b) as if the fetus (arrow) is sitting (or bouncing) on the lesion (arrowhead). Note the Yin/Yang swirling flow on color Doppler.

and treatment planning/mapping [6]. The specific MRA parameters utilized can be viewed in detail online at www.chop-fmru.com. Although not FDA-approved for a second trimester fetus, Gadobutrol® contrast agent was selected to reduce risk of gadolinium deposition. Gadobutrol is a macrocyclic agent that imparts strong chelation of the substrate to gadolinium. It reduces potential toxicity from free gadolinium and, at the time, was the only FDA-approved

agent for patients below 2 years of age (down to 37 weeks of gestation). Gadobutrol was dosed per the manufacturer's protocol with recommended weight-based dosing of 0.1–0.3 mmol/kg. Informed consent was obtained for this unique use of MRA at 20 weeks of gestation.

MRA revealed two suspected feeding vessels: a branch off the right ovarian artery parasitized to the uterine arcuate artery (Figure 4) and a branch off the right uterine artery

(a)   (b)

(c)

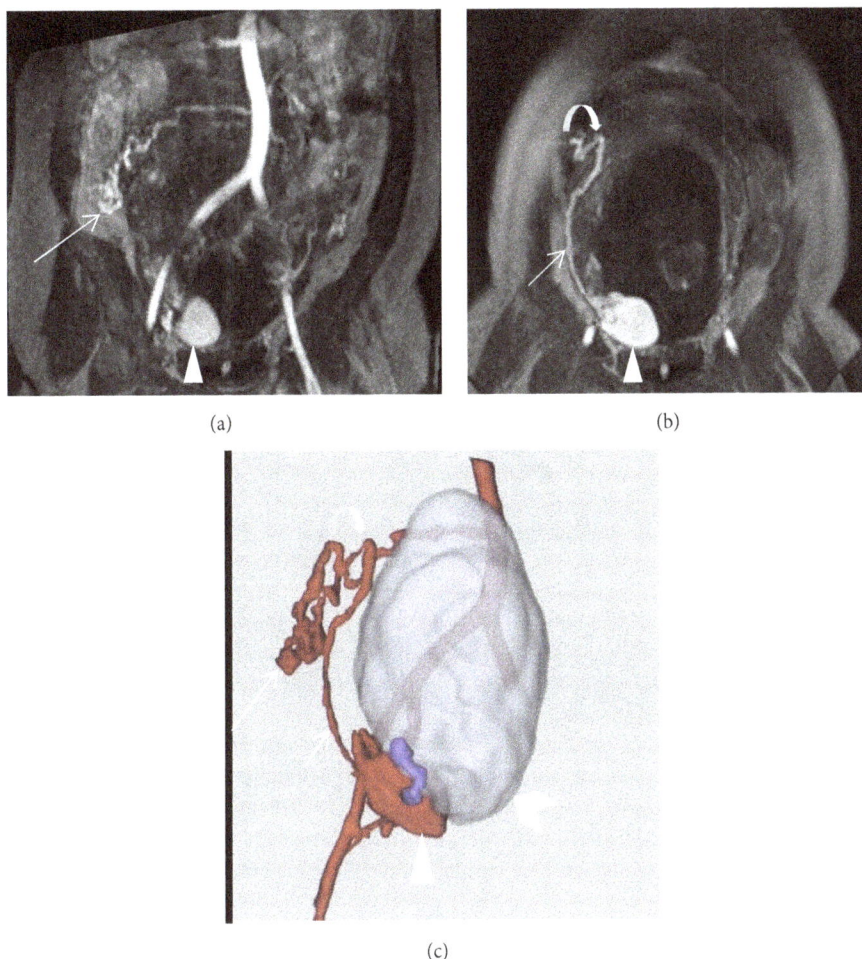

FIGURE 4: Coronal T1 MRA and 3D surface rendered reconstruction (Vital Images® postprocessing software) of the aberrant right ovarian artery branch feeder at 19 weeks of gestation. The proximal right ovarian artery originates from the aorta and courses into a tangle of vessels (long arrows) in the right abdomen ((a) and (c)) before penetrating the myometrium (curved arrows) ((b) and (c)) and extending caudally (short arrows) as an arcuate artery to the lesion. Pseudoaneurysm (arrowhead), uterine cavity (chevron), and aortoiliac vessels. Draining vein (blue).

parasitized to the uterine arcuate and radial arteries (Figure 5). The lesion now measured nearly 5 cm. Abnormal placentation was again suggested.

Fetal and maternal risks of embolization were reviewed with the patient who strongly desired intervention. A conventional arteriogram performed with iodinated contrast diluted 50/50 with normal saline demonstrated a prominent right ovarian artery with origin off the aorta at L2/3 as seen on MRA. Prominent hypogastric arteries were noted along with a subtle blush in the right pelvis suspicious for the target lesion. A right ovarian arteriogram revealed a prominent tortuous right ovarian artery similar to that seen on MRA (Figure 6). A more distal right ovarian arteriogram suggested a blush of contrast in the pelvis suggestive of the target lesion. The right ovarian artery was then embolized with coils (Figure 6). A right hypogastric arteriogram revealed a prominent right uterine artery and a large ovoid lesion opacifying with contrast consistent with the target lesion (Figure 6). The right uterine artery was then embolized. Postcoil imaging revealed no lesion opacification (Figure 6). In an effort to

reduce radiation dose to the fetus, all angiographic runs were performed without digital subtraction. The required 30.4 minutes of fluoroscopic time resulted in a total radiation dose of only 490 mGy.

Ultrasound interrogation the next morning revealed no flow within the lesion (Figure 7). Repeat ultrasound 24 hours later, however, showed recurrence of small blood flow into the lesion, with a significant decrease in lesion size to 3.3 cm, which remained stable prior to discharge 4 days later (Figure 8). Serial ultrasound examinations throughout the duration of the pregnancy demonstrated appropriate interval fetal growth. The pseudoaneurysm progressively decreased in size, measuring 1.4 × 2.0 cm just prior to delivery (Figure 9).

The patient presented with premature rupture of membranes at 33 weeks. Cervical changes and painful contractions necessitated an urgent prophylactic cesarean delivery 13 weeks after embolization. On attempt to deliver the placenta, it was adherent to the uterus, consistent with invasive placentation. The placenta was left in situ and a supracervical hysterectomy was performed. The patient was discharged on

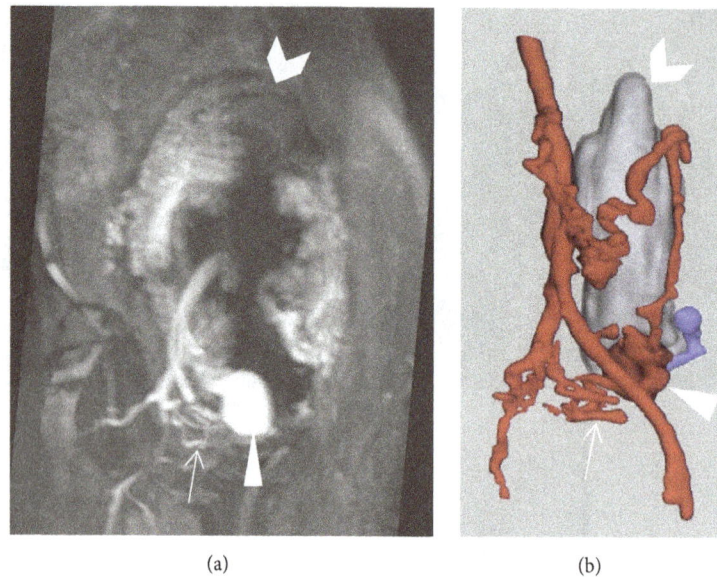

(a)   (b)

FIGURE 5: (a) Sagittal oblique reconstruction of T1 MRA and 3D surface rendered image (Vital Images postprocessing software) (b) of uterine artery feeder (arrows) to the pseudoaneurysm (arrowheads). Uterine cavity (chevrons).

postoperative day 3. The baby was admitted to the NICU secondary to prematurity and discharged home in stable condition at 19 days of life.

3. Discussion

Repeat cesarean delivery increases the risk of abnormal placentation and predisposes to vascular malformations [1, 2]. Hormonal and hemodynamic changes in pregnancy contribute to development of vascular lesions [3]. Pseudoaneurysms develop when trauma, degeneration, or necrosis causes a defect or weakening in the arterial wall through which blood escapes, forming a contained hematoma with or without a thin wall of adventitia and in continuity with the artery that supplies continuous blood flow. Absence of a three-layered arterial wall lining differentiates pseudoaneurysm from true aneurysm [1, 4]. We hypothesize that pseudoaneurysms can occur from invasive processes such as abnormal placentation at the cesarean scar, resulting in abnormal vasculature predisposing to pseudoaneurysm formation.

Research suggests that the initial insult in placenta accreta is a deciduomyometrial defect secondary to surgical scarring. The defect exposes myometrium and its vasculature to migrating trophoblasts, leading to morbidly adherent placenta and loss of the normal cleavage plane between the placenta and myometrium, resulting in excessive remodeling of myometrial arteries [2]. Likely a secondary complication of invasive placentation, our pseudoaneurysm arose at the site of uterine cesarean scar and bulged into the uterine cavity with parasitized, remodeled feeding vessels traversing the myometrium and placenta. The initial perigestational hemorrhage may have been the first signal of abnormal placentation and vascular insult.

Rupture of uterine arterial pseudoaneurysms may cause sudden vaginal hemorrhage unresponsive to typical interventions [1]. Ultrasound is an effective screening modality for pseudoaneurysm and typically reveals an anechoic cyst on grey scale, characteristic "Yin/Yang" or swirling color flow pattern, and bidirectional waveform on duplex Doppler. Most pseudoaneurysms will increase in size over time and eventually rupture with risk of rupture proportional to size and hydrostatic pressure [3]. Pregnancy is a hyperdynamic state, with up to 20% of maternal cardiac output being directed toward the uterus, increasing the risk of pseudoaneurysm formation and rupture [7]. A pseudoaneurysm extending into the intrauterine cavity without a source of tamponade is especially dangerous and hemorrhagic shock can quickly develop with exsanguination into the uterine cavity.

Rebarber et al. reported the first case of bilateral uterine artery embolization at 20 weeks of gestation in 2009 for treatment of an 8 cm lower uterine segment arteriovenous malformation with a successful pregnancy outcome [8]. Ours is the first second trimester case of uterine cavity pseudoaneurysm reported with successful selective unilateral embolization. No immediate postprocedure fetal or maternal complications were encountered. Complete disappearance was noted immediately after the procedure, with partial recurrence observed at 36 hours after embolization. This recurrence was thought to be secondary to the remarkable collateral blood flow of the uterus. Preservation of this collateral blood flow was an important consideration in planning the procedure. The decision was made to proceed with coil rather than particle embolization as particle embolization would have caused more distal embolization, potentially leading to necrosis and vascular compromise of the placenta and poorer fetal outcome.

Lesion overall size significantly decreased from 5.0 cm before the procedure to 2.0 cm just prior to delivery. This

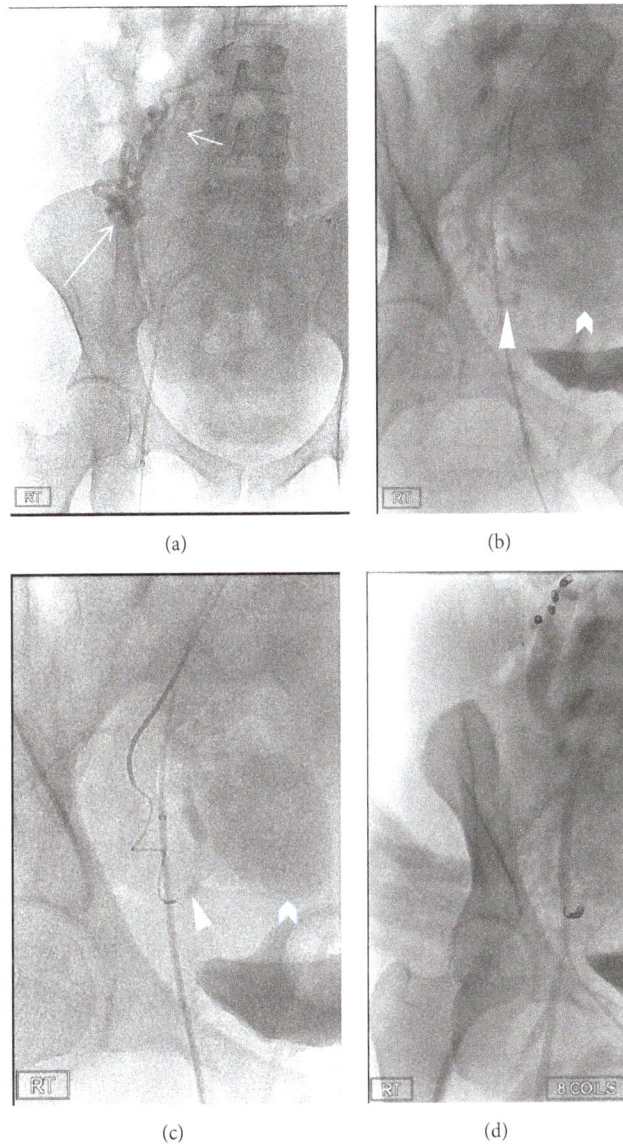

FIGURE 6: Interventional fluoroscopic images. (a) Tortuous right ovarian artery off the aorta (long arrow) with perforating branch into the myometrium (short arrow). Faint blush of pseudoaneurysm on real-time imaging (not shown). (b) Selected right hypogastric artery showing uterine branch (arrowhead) leading to faint oval blush of pseudoaneurysm (chevron). (c) Subselected uterine artery feeder (arrowhead) and pseudoaneurysm blush (chevron). (d) Postcoiling images of parasitized right ovarian and uterine arteries without flow to the target lesion.

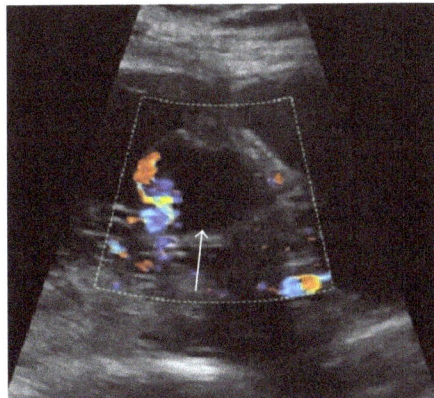

FIGURE 7: Postprocedure ultrasound the next morning demonstrates significantly reduced flow within the pseudoaneurysm (arrow).

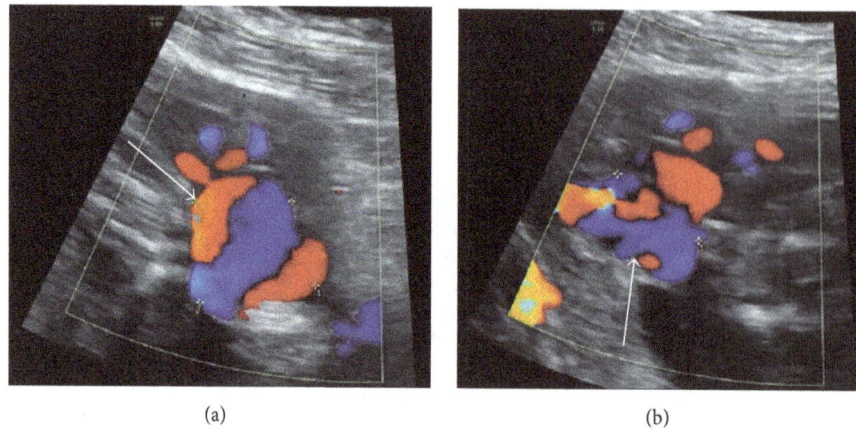

(a)   (b)

FIGURE 8: Transverse (a) and longitudinal (b) ultrasound two days after procedure reveal return of flow to the lesion, however, with significant reduction in lesion size to 3.3 cm (arrows) form 5 cm before embolization.

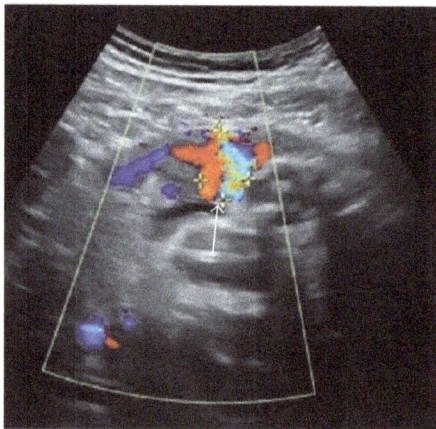

FIGURE 9: Final ultrasound image taken prior to delivery demonstrates persistence of the aneurysm, although it was significantly reduced in size to 2.0 cm (arrow).

preserve fertility. Preembolization mapping with MRA may help reduce fluoroscopy time and radiation dose at embolization. Future cases of antepartum uterine cavity vascular lesions may benefit from MRA followed by low dose selective embolization.

Disclosure

The views expressed are those of the authors and do not reflect the official views or policy of the Department of Defense.

Acknowledgments

The article's processing charges are funded by the Graduate Medical Education Office at Brooke Army Medical Center.

progressive decrease in size throughout the remainder of the pregnancy was felt to significantly decrease the risk of rupture and associated complications. At the time of initial recurrence, the benefits of further embolization were considered. However, the potential benefit did not outweigh the risk of additional fetal and maternal exposure to radiation and iodinated contrast. Tighter collimation during the embolization could have reduced the radiation dose further. However, the dose of radiation was very low for this complex procedure and was achieved by performing the procedure without digital subtraction, further decreasing radiation dose.

This case demonstrates that dynamic MRA with judicious use of gadolinium may be safe and can aid in characterization and treatment planning of antepartum uterine cavity vascular lesions without radiation to the fetus. This case also demonstrates that low radiation selective embolization is an appropriate and effective treatment option for high-risk antepartum uterine cavity vascular lesions as an alternative to pregnancy termination and surgical intervention when patients desire to maintain an ongoing pregnancy and/or

References

[1] J. H. Kwon and G. S. Kim, "Obstetric iatrogenic arterial injuries of the uterus: Diagnosis with US and treatment with transcatheter arterial embolization," *RadioGraphics*, vol. 22, no. 1, pp. 35–46, 2002.

[2] E. Jauniaux and D. Jurkovic, "Placenta accreta: pathogenesis of a 20th century iatrogenic uterine disease," *Placenta*, vol. 33, no. 4, pp. 244–251, 2012.

[3] W. Henrich, I. Fuchs, A. Luttkus, S. Hauptmann, and J. W. Dudenhausen, "Pseudoaneurysm of the uterine artery after cesarean delivery: Sonographic diagnosis and treatment," *Journal of Ultrasound in Medicine*, vol. 21, no. 12, pp. 1431–1434, 2002.

[4] P. Bouchet, P. Chabrot, M. Fontarensky, A. Delabaere, M. Bonnin, and D. Gallot, "Pitfalls in diagnosis of uterine artery pseudoaneurysm after Cesarean section," *Ultrasound in Obstetrics & Gynecology*, vol. 40, no. 4, pp. 481–483, 2012.

[5] S. Vedantham, S. C. Goodwin, B. McLucas, and G. Mohr, "Uterine artery embolization: An underused method of controlling pelvic hemorrhage," *American Journal of Obstetrics & Gynecology*, vol. 176, no. 4, pp. 938–948, 1997.

[6] D. Khrichenko and K. Darge, "Functional analysis in MR urography - Made simple," *Pediatric Radiology*, vol. 40, no. 2, pp. 182–199, 2010.

[7] F. G. Cunningham, K. J. Leveno, S. L. Bloom, J. C. Hauth, D. J. Rouse, and C. Y. Spong, *Williams Obstetrics*, McGraw Hill, New York city, NY, USA, 23rd edition, 2010.

[8] A. Rebarber, N. S. Fox, D. A. Eckstein, R. A. Lookstein, and D. H. Saltzman, "Successful bilateral uterine artery embolization during an ongoing pregnancy," *Obstetrics & Gynecology*, vol. 113, no. 2, pp. 554–556, 2009.

6

Uterine Prolapse in Pregnancy: Two Cases Report and Literature Review

Chunyan Zeng,[1] Feng Yang,[2] Chunhua Wu,[1] Junlin Zhu,[2]
Xiaoming Guan ⓘ,[3] and Juan Liu ⓘ[1]

[1]Key Laboratory for Major Obstetric Diseases of Guangdong Province, Key Laboratory of Reproduction and Genetics of Guangdong Higher Education Institutes, Department of Obstetrics and Gynecology, The Third Affiliated Hospital of Guangzhou Medical University, No. 63 Duobao Road, Liwan District, Guangzhou, Guangdong 510150, China
[2]Department of Ultrasound Medicine, Laboratory of Ultrasound Molecular Imaging, The Third Affiliated Hospital of Guangzhou Medical University, No. 63 Duobao Road, Liwan District, Guangzhou, Guangdong 510150, China
[3]Division of Minimally Invasive Gynecologic Surgery, Department of Obstetrics and Gynecology, Baylor College of Medicine, 6651 Main Street, 10th Floor, Houston, Texas 77030, USA

Correspondence should be addressed to Juan Liu; liujuan90011@163.com

Academic Editor: Kyousuke Takeuchi

Uterine prolapse complicating pregnancy is rare. Two cases are presented here: one patient had uterine prolapse at both her second and third pregnancy, and the other developed only once prolapse during pregnancy. This report will analyze etiology, clinical characteristics, complication, and treatment of uterine prolapse in pregnancy. Routine gynecologic examination should be carried out during pregnancy. If uterine prolapse occurred, conservative treatment could be used to prolong the gestational period as far as possible. Vaginal delivery is possible, but caesarean section seems a better alternative when prolapsed uterus cannot resolve during childbirth.

1. Introduction

Uterine prolapse is the descent of the uterus and cervix down the vaginal canal toward the introitus. Uterine prolapse during pregnancy is a rare event with incidence of one in 10000-15000 pregnancies, but this may be highly risky [1]. It can cause antepartum, intrapartum, and puerperal complication. Only a few cases of uterine prolapse during pregnancy have been reported and the efficiency of management varies from a conservative approach to laparoscopic treatment. We report two cases that simply benefit from a conservative management.

2. Presentation of Cases

2.1. Case 1. A 27-year-old Chinese woman, gravida 3, para 2, body mass index (BMI) 17.20 kg/m^2, visited our clinic with eight-week pregnancy in a prolapsed uterus on 4th of September 2013. Pelvic examination revealed stage 3 pelvic organ prolapse (POP), with point C as the leading edge using the Pelvic Organ Prolapse Quantification (POPQ) examination (Aa+3, Ap+3, Ba+6, Bp+6, C+6, D+2, gh 4.5, pb 2, tvl 9). Her prolapsed uterus could be restored to pelvic cavity within bed rest. It was more serious while standing or walking. Hospitalization was recommended for this pregnant woman, but she refused and she waited at home for delivery.

Her previous pregnant record was as follows: a dead female baby was induced at the 30th week of gestation during her first vaginal delivery in 2003, puerperium was uneventful, and two days after delivery, she was discharged in good health. She had her second vaginal delivery, after 38^{+3}rd week of gestation and seven-hour labor in 2007; a 2800 g alive baby boy was delivered, with Apgar scores of 10/10. Pelvic examination revealed stage 3 POP using the POPQ examination (Aa+3, Ap+3, Ba+6, Bp+6, C+6, D+2, gh 4.5, pb 2, tvl 9) at the 36^{+3}rd week of gestation in her second pregnancy. No special examination or treatment was executed before and after childbirth. However, the prolapsed vaginal mass was spontaneously restored after childbirth.

The woman presented to our hospital again with premature rupture of membrane (PROM) in labor at 39^{+6}th week of gestation with an irrestorable uterine prolapse for 8 months on the 8th of May 2014. Pelvic examination revealed stage 4 POP using the POPQ examination (Aa+3, Ap+3, Ba+9, Bp+9, C+9, D+5, gh 4.5, pb 2, tvl 9) and it revealed that prolapsed uterus was in size of 20×20 cm, pink, hyperaemic, and edematous but not ulcerated. The cervical canal did not subside, internal orifice of cervix did not open, amnionic vesicle has been broken, and regular contraction was seen. A series of transabdominal ultrasonographic examinations showed a normally developing fetus in the longitudinal position in the uterine cavity, isthmus uteri was 64 mm and it was partially extruded outside the vulva which was protruding from the perineum about 64×68 mm, and the boundary was still clear, and with cervical oedema. Emergency caesarean delivery was decided and an alive boy baby weighting 2480 g, with Apgar scores of 10/10, was delivered. We used Magnesium Sulfate Solution to nurse the prolapsed uterus. Three days postpartum, the prolapsed uterus was in size of 10×10 cm. On the seventh day postpartum, the prolapsed uterus was in size of 7×5 cm, and it was restored inside the pelvic cavity after manual reposition. Pelvic floor three-dimensional ultrasound indicated that residual urine was 40 ml, cervical length was 5.6 cm and internal orifice cervix was dilated, bladder neck displacement was 15 mm, posterior angle of bladder was 180 degree, and hiatus of levator antimuscle was 32 cm^2. She was discharged on the eighth days postpartum. A telephone postpartum follow-up on the 14th day showed that there was no lump prolapse when the patient was standing or walking. But when the abdominal pressure increased, such as when squatting and defecating, prolapsed vaginal mass could be palpable, with size of 2 cm × 1 cm. 42 days after childbirth, she refused regular postpartum examinations for personal reasons.

2.2. Case 2. A 33-year-old Chinese woman, gravida 2, para 1, BMI 20.70 kg/m^2, noticed a protrusion in size of 2 × 1 cm from her vagina at 13th week of gestation in 2015. Her first pregnancy resulted in one uncomplicated spontaneous vaginal delivery in 2009; the newly-born baby weighted 3000 g. There was neither history of pelvic trauma or prolapse, nor any stress incontinence during or after the first pregnancy.

The protrusion was not sensible while resting but rather palpable after moving. She visited our outpatient clinic at her 15th week of gestation in 2015 and complained worsened uterine prolapse. Pelvic examination revealed stage 3 POP, with point C as the leading edge using the POPQ examination (Aa+3, Ap+3, Ba+6, Bp+6, C+6, D+1, gh 5, pb 1, tvl 10). A no. 5 ring pessary in size of 7×7 cm (see Figure 1) was applied to keep the uterus inside the pelvic cavity after manual reposition. The gravid uterus persisted in the abdominal cavity after removing at the 30th week of gestation because it became larger. An alive healthy baby boy of 2680 g was delivered after four-hour labor at 39+3 week's gestation on

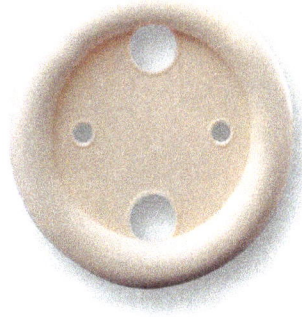

FIGURE 1: Ring pessary.

the 5th of October 2015. She was discharged three days postpartum with complete resolution of the uterine prolapse. A follow-up postpartum examination after 42 days revealed evidence of uterine prolapse and a no. 3 ring pessary in size of 5×5 cm has been applied to keep the uterus inside the pelvic cavity after manual reposition until now. At the time of reporting, pelvic examination of this woman revealed stage 3 POP, with point C as the leading edge using the POPQ examination (Aa-2, Ap-2, Ba-1, Bp-1, C+2, D-3, gh 5, pb 1, tvl 10). Pelvic floor four-dimensional ultrasound indicated that bladder neck mobility was slightly increasing, posterior wall of the bladder was slightly bulged, and anterior vaginal wall was slightly prolapsed in anterior compartment. Stage 2 uterus prolapse was seen in middle compartment, the levator animuscle was not broken, and hiatus of levator animuscle was normal in posterior compartment (see Figure 2). Follow-up is on-going.

3. Discussion

Uterine prolapse is a common case in nonpregnant older women; however, uterine prolapse complicating pregnancy is a rare event, which either exists before or has an acute onset during pregnancy.

The etiology of uterine prolapse during pregnancy is probably multifactorial. Parity, malnutrition, race, vaginal delivery, short interval between consecutive pregnancies, increased strain on the support of the uterus, physiologic change of pregnancy causing cervical elongation, hypertrophy and relaxation of the support ligament, and previous medical record of prolapse are among the most common risk factors [2]. Uterovaginal prolapse is more common in white and Hispanic women compared to women of African or Asian descent [3, 4].

POP presenting before pregnancy is less common and often resolves during pregnancy, but recurs after delivery [5–7]. Acute onset of POP in pregnancy is more common; it is usually firstly noted in the third trimester [5] and disappears after labor and delivery [8]. This might be due to a different aetiology compared with prepregnancy POP. This type of prolapse is most frequently caused by a history of trauma to the pelvic floor or congenital disorder that weakens the

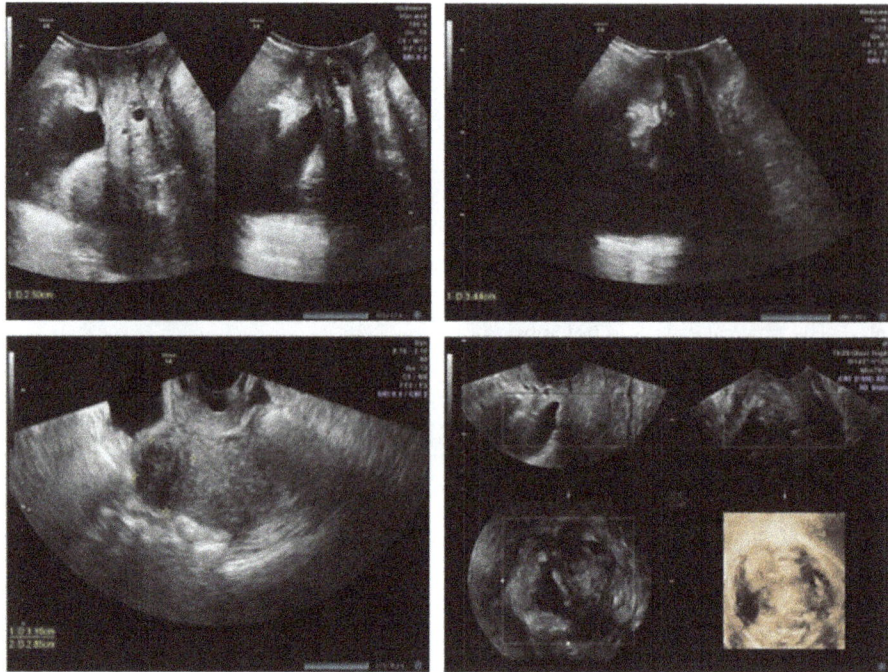

FIGURE 2: Pelvic floor four-dimensional ultrasound of Case 2. Pelvic floor four-dimensional ultrasound indicated that residual urine was 0 ml, thickness of detrusor was normal, internal orifice of urethra was closed, posterior angle of bladder was intact, and there was no dark area of liquid and scattered point of calcification around urethra in quiescent condition. CDFI revealed that sparse color flow signals were seen around the urethra, the bladder neck was 19 mm above the pubic symphysis, the uterus was 17 mm above the pubic symphysis, and ampulla portion of rectum was located at the pubic symphysis. Bladder neck displacement was 15 mm, bladder neck was located 9 mm below the pubic symphysis, posterior angle of bladder was intact, the uterus was 35 mm below the pubic symphysis, ampulla portion of rectum was located at the pubic symphysis, rectocele was not seen, and anal sphincter was complete in Valsalva.

pelvic floor support. Prolapse developing in pregnancy is more likely to be due to an escalation of the physiological changes in pregnancy which lead to weakening of pelvic organ support [9]. Pregnancy itself may have triggered the prolapse. Increased cortisol and progesterone levels during pregnancy may contribute to the uterine relaxation. Damage to the genitourinary supports from repeated pregnancies and labor are the most important predisposing factors in POP. During childbirth, the pelvic floor is extended due to direct pressure of the fetal presenting part and maternal pressure effects. Decline in the elevator antimuscle tone is caused either by denervation or by direct muscle trauma, and hence resulting in an open urogenital hiatus, which, combining with the functional and anatomic alterations in the muscles and nerves of the pelvic floor, contribute to the development of POP. This would explain why the prolapse almost always recurs or persists in patients with prepregnancy prolapse, but spontaneously resolves in those developing during pregnancy. It would also explain the possible protective effect of a caesarean section in patients with acute onset of POP in pregnancy and not in those with prepregnancy POP [10].

The two patients in this report are multiparous women. Uterine prolapse during pregnancy most frequently occurs in multiparous women. None of the two patients in this report had uterine prolapse during the first pregnancy, but they had it in their second, even third pregnancy. Mant et al. [11] reported that women with twice vaginal deliveries have four times higher risk of prolapse compared to nulliparous women. Erata et al. [12] reported that the relative risk of developing uterine prolapse was 2.48 (95 % confidence interval [CI], 0.69–9.38) in women who had given birth to one child and increased to 4.58 (95 % CI, 1.64–13.77), 8.4 (95 %CI, 2.84–26.44), and 11.75 (95 % CI, 3.84–38.48) in women who had delivered 2, 3, or >3 children, respectively, compared with nulliparous women.

Uterine prolapse in pregnancy can cause antepartum, intrapartum, and puerperal complication. Antepartum complications include preterm labor, abortion, urinary tract infection, acute urinary retention, and even maternal death. The main intrapartum complications include inability to attain adequate cervical dilatation, as well as cervical laceration, obstructive labor, hysterorrhexis at the lower segment of the uterus, fetal death, and maternal morbidity. Puerperal infection and postpartum hemorrhage due to uterine inertia are common consequences of POP after delivery [13]. Similar to other case reports, our patients had antepartum complication of PROM, but we did not observe any intrapartum or puerperal complication. Moreover, Lau and Rijhsinghani [14] used Magnesium Solution to prevent cervical dystocia and lacerations for a prolapsed cervix which is edematous.

We use Magnesium Sulfate Solution to nurse the prolapsed uterus postpartum in Case 1; the mechanism proposed may be due to osmotic diuretic properties of magnesium.

Successful pregnancy outcome requires individualized treatment with respect to patient's wishes, gestation, and severity of prolapse. Obstetrician should consider the above-mentioned possible complications. The management varies from a conservative approach to laparoscopic treatment. Conservative management with genital hygiene and bed rest in a moderately Trendelenburg position to enable prolapse replacement should be considered as the foremost treatment option. These precautions protect the cervix from trauma desiccation and reduce the incidence of preterm labor. Case 1 had successful pregnancy outcome because of bed rest. This again demonstrated that bed rest in a moderately Trendelenburg position is a practical management strategy.

Continual use of a pessary is recommended, which should not be removed until the onset of labor [6, 7]. A no. 5 ring pessary was applied to keep the uterus inside the pelvis after manual reposition and protect the prolapsed cervix in Case 2. The patient was managed with close follow-up on an outpatient basis. The gravid uterus persisted in the abdominal cavity because it became larger, and the pessary was removed at the 30th week of gestation. In 1949, Klawans and Kanter [15] advised continual use of the Smith-Hodge pessary throughout the pregnancy for women with late occurrence of prolapse. Vaginal pessaries can be obtained and applied easily. Vaginal discharge, odor, mucosal erosion and abrasions of vagina, and urinary retention are common complications of vaginal pessaries [16]. For this patient, we did not encounter any of these complications. Different types of vaginal pessary have been used, but this management was reported as unsuccessful in literature since pessaries frequently fell out after a few days. Contrary to the literature, our case was managed successfully with a pessary. The ring pessary and its size perfectly fitted the patient. The patient was taught how to use the pessary and she performed the procedure perfectly. Thus, selection of pessary shape and its size and the patient's congruity to the treatment are the basis of success of this management.

When conservative management fails and prolonged bed rest is impossible, laparoscopic uterine suspension may be another treatment choice during early pregnancy. However, this procedure should be performed with experienced hands since several failed laparoscopic uterine suspension cases have been reported [17].

The method of delivery should be individualized according to the patients' preferences, status of cervix uteri, and labor progression. A vaginal delivery can be expected. Nonetheless, according to our experience, an elective caesarean section near term could be a valid and safe delivery option when the prolapsed uterus cannot be restored. Patient in Case 2 already had a favorable ripened cervix and the prolapsed uterus has already been in the pelvic cavity when she was referred to our hospital at 39+3 week's gestation. We did not have to insist on a caesarean section, so the patients ended with vaginal delivery. However, considering cervical dystocia, which results in inability to attain adequate

cervical dilatation, in addition to obstructive labor, as well as cervical laceration and a predisposition to rupture of the lower uterine segment, emergency caesarean section was performed to avoid the above-mentioned intrapartum complication in Case 1.

Follow-up is necessary, pelvic floor four-dimensional ultrasound can clearly show the spatial relationship of anterior, middle, and posterior compartments in pelvic cavity, and pelvic examination and pelvic floor four-dimensional ultrasound may be a valid method for follow-up.

4. Conclusion

Obstetricians as well as all involved caregivers should be aware of this rare phenomenon, as early diagnosis is crucial for a safe gestation. Conservative treatment of these patients throughout pregnancy can lead to an uneventful, normal, spontaneous delivery. Management of uterine prolapse in pregnancy during labor should be individualized depending on the severity of the prolapse, gestational age, parity, and patient's preference.

Acknowledgments

This study was supported by National Natural Science Foundation of China (Grant no. 81671440). The authors alone are responsible for the content and writing of this article.

References

[1] D. De Vita and S. Giordano, "Two successful natural pregnancies in a patient with severe uterine prolapse: A case report," *Journal of Medical Case Reports*, vol. 5, p. 459, 2011.

[2] C. M. Tarnay and C. H. Dorr, *Current Obstetric And Gynecology Diagnosis and Treatment*, A. H. DeCherney and L. Nathan, Eds., Lange Medical/McGraw-Hill, New York, NY, USA, 2003.

[3] S. A. Obed, "Pelvic Relaxation," in *Comprehensive Gynaecology in the Tropics*, E. Y. Kwawukume and E. E. Emuveyan, Eds., pp. 138–146, Science & Education, Accra, Ghana, 2005.

[4] H. A. Ugboma, A. O. Okpani, and S. E. Anya, "Genital prolapse in Port Harcourt, Nigeria," *Nigerian Journal of Medicine*, vol. 13, no. 2, pp. 124–129, 2004.

[5] E. R. Horowitz, Y. Yogev, M. Hod, and B. Kaplan, "Prolapse and elongation of the cervix during pregnancy," *International Journal of Gynecology and Obstetrics*, vol. 77, no. 2, pp. 147-148, 2002.

[6] P. S. Hill, "Uterine prolapse complicating pregnancy. A case report," *The Journal of Reproductive Medicine*, vol. 29, no. 8, pp. 631–633, 1984.

[7] H. L. Brown, "Cervical prolapse complicating pregnancy," *Journal of the National Medical Association*, vol. 89, pp. 346–348, 1997.

[8] L. Guariglia, B. Carducci, A. Botta, S. Ferrazzani, and A. Caruso, "Uterine prolapse in pregnancy," *Gynecologic and Obstetric Investigation*, vol. 60, no. 4, pp. 192–194, 2005.

[9] A. L. O'Boyle, J. D. O'Boyle, B. Calhoun, and G. D. Davis, "Pelvic organ support in pregnancy and postpartum," *International Urogynecology Journal*, vol. 16, no. 1, pp. 69–72, 2005.

[10] Z. Rusavy, L. Bombieri, and R. M. Freeman, "Procidentia in pregnancy: a systematic review and recommendations for practice," *International Urogynecology Journal and Pelvic Floor Dysfunction*, vol. 26, no. 8, pp. 1103–1109, 2015.

[11] B. Cingillioglu, M. Kulhan, and Y. Yildirim, "Extensive uterine prolapse during active labor: A case report," *International Urogynecology Journal*, vol. 21, no. 11, pp. 1433-1434, 2010.

[12] Y. E. Erata, B. Kilic, S. Güçlü, U. Saygili, and T. Uslu, "Risk factors for pelvic surgery," *Archives of Gynecology and Obstetrics*, vol. 267, no. 1, pp. 14–18, 2002.

[13] P. Tsikouras, A. Dafopoulos, N. Vrachnis et al., "Uterine prolapse in pregnancy: Risk factors, complications and management," *The Journal of Maternal-Fetal and Neonatal Medicine*, vol. 27, no. 3, pp. 297–302, 2014.

[14] S. Lau and A. Rijhsinghani, "Extensive cervical prolapse during labor: a case report," *The Journal of Reproductive Medicine*, vol. 53, no. 1, pp. 67–69, 2008.

[15] A. H. Klawans and A. E. Kanter, "Prolapse of the uterus and pregnancy," *American Journal of Obstetrics & Gynecology*, vol. 57, no. 5, pp. 939–946, 1949.

[16] P. J. Sulak, "Nonsurgical correction of defects, the use of vaginal support devices," in *Te Linde's Operative Gynecology*, pp. 1082-1083, 8th edition, 1997.

[17] T. Matsumoto, M. Nishi, M. Yokota, and M. Ito, "Laparoscopic treatment of uterine prolapse during pregnancy," *Obstetrics & Gynecology*, vol. 93, no. 5, p. 849, 1999.

7

Epithelial Ovarian Carcinoma Associated with Metastases to Central Nervous System: Two Case Reports

Yasuyuki Kawagoe (ID),[1] Tetsuo Nakayama,[1] Satoshi Matuzawa,[1] Kazuko Fukushima,[1] Junji Onishi,[1] Yuichiro Sato,[2] Kimihiro Nagai,[3] and Hiroshi Sameshima (ID)[1]

[1]Department of Obstetrics and Gynecology, Faculty of Medicine, University of Miyazaki, 5200 Kihara, Kiyotake, Miyazaki 889-1692, Japan
[2]Department of Diagnostic Pathology, University of Miyazaki Hospital, Faculty of Medicine, University of Miyazaki, 5200 Kihara, Kiyotake, Miyazaki 889-1692, Japan
[3]Department of Palliative Care, Miyazaki Medical Association Hospital, 738-1 Funado, Shinbeppu, Miyazaki City, Miyazaki 889-0834, Japan

Correspondence should be addressed to Yasuyuki Kawagoe; yasuyuki_kawagoe@med.miyazaki-u.ac.jp

Academic Editor: Kyousuke Takeuchi

We experienced two rare cases of metastases to the central nervous system (cerebral and leptomeningeal metastases) from primary epithelial ovarian carcinoma. The first case was a 55-year-old woman who developed carcinomatous meningitis while on chemotherapy for ovarian cancer stage IIIC. Cytological analysis confirmed carcinomatous cells of ovarian origin in the cerebrospinal fluid. Magnetic resonance imaging demonstrated abnormal hyperintensity in the cerebral sulci on fluid attenuated inversion recovery (FLAIR) sequence with enhanced gadolinium indicating leptomeningeal metastases. Her consciousness rapidly declined and she died 42 days after diagnosis. The second case was a 63-year-old woman who underwent surgery for ovarian cancer and who was diagnosed as stage IA. Thirty-eight months after surgery, she developed weakness of the left hand and headaches. A CT scan revealed metastases to the right cerebrum and she was treated with surgical resection followed by radiotherapy. Five months after resection, she developed ileus caused by multiple relapses in the pelvis. Despite chemotherapy, her performance status declined and she died nine months after the resection. Both cases were rare because the first case was isolated leptomeningeal metastases, and the second case was confirmed relapse site in the cerebrum due to neurological symptoms despite her early clinical stage.

1. Introduction

In Japan, 9,804 cases of ovarian carcinoma and 4,758 disease-related deaths annually were reported in 2009 [1]. Almost half of the cases were higher than stage III at initial diagnosis, which usually results in a poor prognosis. Metastases from primary epithelial ovarian carcinoma usually occurs in the abdomen, lungs, and lymph nodes, but metastasis to the central nervous system (CNS) is rare. Advancements in the therapy of ovarian cancer have improved the patient response rate and prolonged the survival period. However, it has also increased the incidence of CNS metastases, which usually develop after long-term treatment. In this report, we describe two types of metastases to the CNS, cerebral and leptomeningeal metastases, from epithelial ovarian carcinoma.

2. Case Presentation

A 55-year-old Japanese woman, gravida 2 para 2, underwent surgery for a tumor in the left ovary (11×13×12 cm). Laparotomy revealed the swelling of both ovaries, rectum involvement, and peritoneal dissemination from the pelvic cavity to the upper abdominal cavity. She underwent a hysterectomy, bilateral salpingo-oophorectomy, omentectomy, and low-anterior resection of the rectum, which resulted in suboptimal surgery. Histological diagnosis confirmed high-grade serous carcinoma in the adnexal mass and peritoneal biopsy. She was diagnosed as stage IIIC ovarian cancer according to the International Federation of Gynecology and Obstetrics (FIGO) classification. Six cycles of adjuvant chemotherapy combining paclitaxel (180 mg/m^2) and

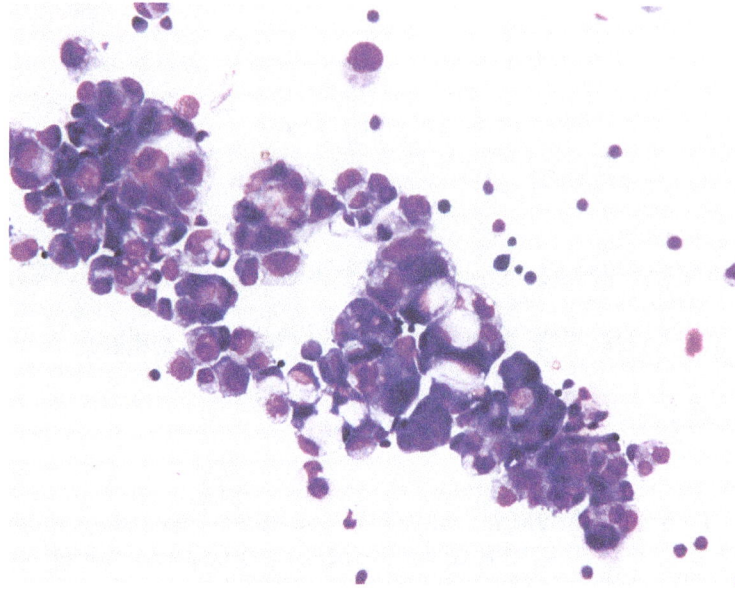

FIGURE 1: Numerous atypical epithelial clusters were present in the CSF. These atypical cells have eccentric large hyperchromatic nuclei and scant cytoplasm. Some cells show vacuolar changes.

carboplatin (area under the curve (AUC) = 5) were administrated every 3 weeks, and her serum levels of CA125 decreased to normal. Thirteen months after the end of therapy, the same regimen plus bevacizumab was added because relapse sites were confirmed in the pelvis and also her CA-125 levels were elevated. After three cycles of chemotherapy, the regimen was changed to doxorubicin ($60 \, mg/m^2$) because of progressive disease. She developed dizziness, back pain, and severe headaches without neurologic signs after two cycles of the therapy, at forty-three months after the primary surgery. After hospitalization, physical and neurological examination showed normal results and no parenchymal lesion was detected on a contrast-enhanced CT scan of the cranium. Diagnostic lumbar puncture was performed the next day, which revealed carcinomatous cells of ovary origin in the cerebrospinal fluid (CSF) (Figure 1). Magnetic resonance imaging (MRI) demonstrated abnormal hyperintensity in the cerebral sulci, mainly in the left lateral, occipital lobes, and folia in the cerebellar hemispheres and vermis on FLAIR with enhancement after gadolinium injection (Figure 2). On the basis of these results, she was diagnosed with carcinomatous meningitis. High-dose corticosteroid therapy was begun, although systemic or intrathecal chemotherapy was not added because of her poor performance status. Her general condition and consciousness declined rapidly and she died forty-two days after the diagnosis. An autopsy was not performed.

The second case was a 63-year-old Japanese woman, gravida 2 para 2, with a history of hysterectomy because of fibroids at 45 years of age. A partially solid cystic tumor (5×4×6 cm) was detected in the pelvis at a private clinic. She was referred to our hospital for surgery. Her serum CA125 and CA19-9 levels were not elevated before surgery. Laparotomy revealed a tumor in the left ovary, and she was diagnosed as adenocarcinoma by frozen section without peritoneal

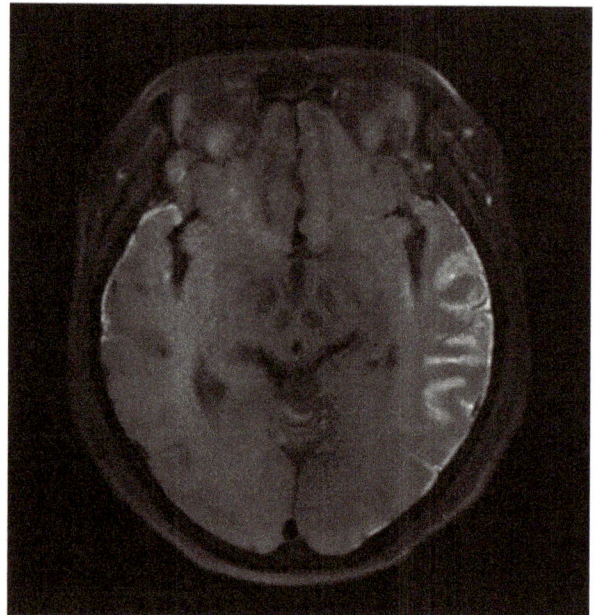

FIGURE 2: Cranial-enhanced MRI T1-weighted images reveal abnormal linear hyperintensity mainly on the left lateral lobe.

lesions. The capsule of the tumor was intact and ascites was scanty. We performed bilateral salpingo-oophorectomy and omentectomy, resulting in compete surgery. Cytology of ascites was negative and the final pathological examination showed mucinous carcinoma limited to the left ovary (FIGO stage IA). After the surgery, she was followed up every 3–6 months at the outpatient department. After thirty-eight uneventful months, she developed headaches, dizziness, memory problems, and weakness of her left arm. A solitary

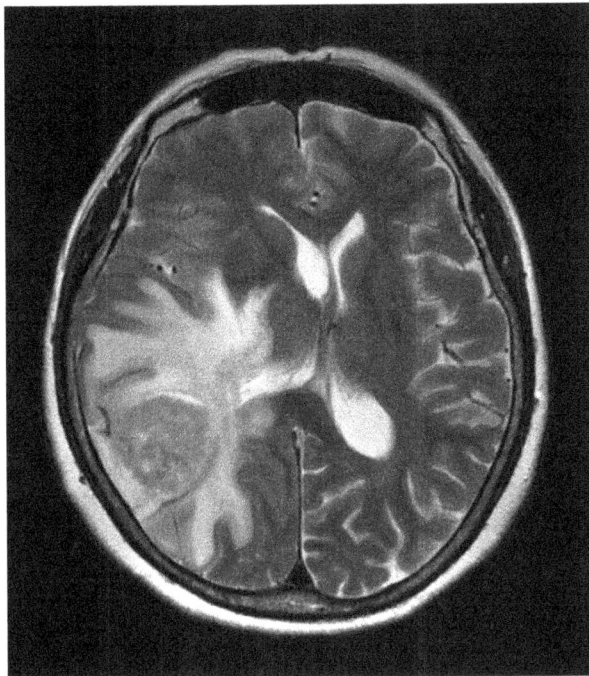

FIGURE 3: Axial T2-weighted brain MRI scan shows a solitary metastatic lesion in the right temporal lobe with brain edema.

tumor was found in the right lateral lobe (diameter 3 cm) on cranial MRI and a suspected relapse of the ovarian carcinoma was determined (Figure 3). She underwent surgical resection of the cerebral lesion and pathological examination confirmed metastatic disease. Gamma-knife radiosurgery followed (49 Gy) without further chemotherapy. Four months after the brain surgery, she presented with nausea and vomiting caused by ileus. A CT scan revealed multiple recurrent tumors in the pelvic cavity. She underwent laparotomy, but we could not resect these multiple recurrent lesions, and colectomy was done to improve ileus. Postoperatively, we used chemotherapy combining paclitaxel (180 mg/m^2) and carboplatin (AUC=5). Despite the therapy, she was diagnosed as a progressive disease after three cycles. At the same time, her performance status declined gradually without intracranial relapse and neurological symptoms. She succumbed to abdominal involvement nine months after resection of the cerebral lesion and no autopsy was performed.

3. Discussion

Herein, we report two rare cases of CNS metastases from ovarian carcinoma. The first case was leptomeningeal metastases with no obvious parenchymal lesions, and the second case was solitary brain metastases with neurological symptoms as the first manifestation of relapse in the cerebrum regardless of her early clinical staging. CNS metastases observed in stages III and IV account for about 86% of cases whereas stage I accounts for only 9–10% [2, 3].

Brain metastases from the lung, breast, renal, and colorectal carcinoma and melanoma are common and occur in up to 40% of cases [4, 5], whereas leptomeningeal metastases are commonly seen in melanoma, lung, and breast carcinoma in 3–5% of cases [6]. The incidence of metastases from epithelial ovarian carcinoma to the brain parenchyma and leptomeninges is 0.9–3.3% [7–11] and 0.06% [12], respectively, indicating their rarity. Recent studies reported an increase in the incidence of metastases during the past decade. Chiang et al. reported a single institutional study where the incidence of metastases was increased from 0.18% (1995–1999) to 2.12% (2005–2009) [3]. The main reasons for this increase might be improvements in brain imaging and treatment for local relapse.

Almost 90% of CNS metastases develop an average of 25 months after the initial treatment [2]. Nasu et al. recently reported that CNS metastases from ovarian carcinoma had a statistically better prognosis than those from corpus and cervical carcinoma [2]. The median survival time was 12.5 months for ovarian cancer and 6.2 and 4.8 months for corpus and cervical cancer, respectively. Therefore, despite its poor prognosis, a prompt diagnosis of CNS metastases might provide an opportunity for appropriate treatment and palliative care.

The most common site of metastasis in the CNS is the cerebral hemisphere (75%) followed by the cerebellum (11%) and meninges (7.3%) [13]. Symptoms of CNS metastases from ovarian carcinoma were confirmed in approximately 90% of patients at diagnosis [2, 14]. A headache is the most common symptom seen in 40–50% of patients, which results from brain edema and/or hydrocephalus [15]. Other symptoms such as confusion, dizziness, decreased mental status, consciousness disturbance, general weakness, ataxia, and neurological motor deficits are also observed depending on the location of the metastases.

Symptoms of leptomeningeal metastases without parenchymal lesions are caused by increased intracranial pressure and meningeal irritation. The most common symptoms are headache and seizures. Gait difficulties from weakness or ataxia, memory problems, incontinence, and sensory abnormalities are sometimes reported, although classic cerebral signs such as hemiparesis and aphasia are less common. Cases with symptoms such as deafness, vertigo, facial weakness, and blindness as a first manifestation were also previously reported [16–18]. Both our cases showed headache and other neurological signs, while localized neurological signs were confirmed in the cerebral metastases case. Symptoms of cranial nerves were not observed in our cases.

Diagnosis of brain metastases is usually based on imaging techniques, but the diagnosis of carcinomatous meningitis can be difficult. The first step of the examination is a detailed check of neurological findings. After the physical examination, a computed tomography (CT) scan is used to detect metastatic lesions and rule out cerebrovascular events. MRI imaging is the most useful tool for the diagnosis of brain lesions as well as leptomeningeal metastases showing nodular subarachnoid enhancement after gadolinium injection. These findings were reported in 75–90% of patients whose cerebrospinal fluid (CSF) cytology was positive [19, 20]. The optimal test for a definitive diagnosis of leptomeningeal metastases is the detection of cancer cells in the CSF. However, the sensitivity of this method is low; for the first sample it is approximately 45%–75% [21, 22], although repetition of a sample three times can improve the sensitivity to 90% or more [22]. The sensitivities of MRI with gadolinium enhancement and enhanced CT scanning for the diagnosis of carcinomatous meningitis are approximately 70% and 30%, respectively [23–25]. Our first case was positive for MRI imaging and CSF examination at the first sampling. These findings allowed a prompt diagnosis, but also indicated severe meningitis. Serum CA125 levels are a useful biomarker to diagnose the relapse of epithelial ovarian carcinoma. However, it is of limited value for the detection of CNS metastases because it is impermeable to the blood-brain barrier. Anupol et al. reported that ten of 15 patients (66.6%) with brain metastases from ovarian carcinoma had elevated serum CA125 levels [26]. In our cases, the first case had already shown an elevated CA125 level because of other multiple relapses and the second case was negative for CA125 levels throughout the clinical course. Therefore, we were unable to use CA125 levels as a manifestation of brain metastases.

The mechanism of CNS metastases might involve vasculopathy or direct vascular obliteration by cancer cells, while that of leptomeningeal metastases remains the subject of investigation. It is suspected that cancer cells may reach the leptomeninges through hematogenous spread, direct invasion from parenchymal lesions, or spread along the perineurium from cranial or spinal nerves. After the cancer cells reach the subarachnoid space, they spread to the meninges directly through the CSF. Our leptomeningeal metastases case had multiple intra-abdominal relapses mainly in the pelvis with no evidence of liver, lung, or parenchymal lesions. We speculate the path of spread might be from spinal cord lesions. Although she had back pain, indicating spinal symptoms, we did not perform MRI of the spine.

The type and amount of CNS metastases were 42% for single lesions, 55% for multiple parenchymal lesions, and 3% for leptomeningeal disease [27]. To date, no clinical trials have been initiated for CNS metastases from ovarian carcinoma because of its rarity. Surgical resection, whole-brain radiotherapy, systemic chemotherapy, and gamma knife stereotactic radiosurgery alone or in combination have been used, dependent on the patient's condition and the metastatic sites in the brain. In a review article, Piura et al. reported that a significantly better survival was observed for multimodal therapy compared with whole-brain radiotherapy alone [27]. Cohen et al. also reported that surgical resection of solitary ovarian cancer metastases followed by whole-brain radiotherapy resulted in better survival compared with radiotherapy alone [7]. A limited meta-analysis recommended surgical resection followed by radiation therapy for patients with a solitary lesion and well-controlled relapse sites. In our case, cranial surgery followed by radiation therapy was performed because of the solitary lesion. Her neurological symptoms were improved remarkably even after the pelvic relapses were confirmed. These therapies were effective at improving her neurological symptoms without adverse effects.

The goal of treatment for leptomeningeal metastases is mainly the palliation of symptoms. The median interval between initial diagnosis and detection of leptomeningeal metastases was 26 months and its prognosis is extremely poor with a median survival ranging from 1.8 to 5.7 months [28]. In a clinical review, 67% of patients died within two months after the diagnosis [29]. Treatments are usually based on experiences with other carcinomas, because of its rarity. Chemotherapy and radiotherapy have been used; most cases were treated with intrathecal chemotherapy using methotrexate, with or without whole-brain radiation therapy. In some reports, treatment with intrathecal methotrexate succeeded in prolonging the survival period from 6 to 18 months [30–33]. Regarding our case, we had no chance to treat with methotrexate for palliation as her condition declined rapidly after the diagnosis.

4. Conclusion

In conclusion, CNS metastases from epithelial ovarian carcinoma have become a critical issue for clinicians, especially in patients receiving long-term chemotherapy. Currently, routine brain imaging is not recommended during the follow-up period for epithelial ovarian carcinoma. Clinicians should consider metastases to the CNS whenever a cancer patient shows neurological symptoms or behavioral changes. If a prompt diagnosis is made, it might lead to a better prognosis and the early initiation of palliative care, which should be beneficial.

Acknowledgments

We thank Edanz Group (http://www.edanzediting.com/ac) for editing a draft of this manuscript.

References

[1] M. Hori, T. Matsuda, A. Shibata, K. Katanoda, T. Sobue, and H. Nishimoto, "Cancer incidence and incidence rates in Japan in 2009: a study of 32 population-based cancer registries for the Monitoring of Cancer Incidence in Japan (MCIJ) project," *Japanese Journal of Clinical Oncology*, vol. 45, no. 9, pp. 884–891, 2015.

[2] K. Nasu, T. Satoh, S. Nishio et al., "Clinicopathologic features of brain metastases from gynecologic malignancies: a retrospective study of 139 cases (KCOG-G1001s trial)," *Gynecologic Oncology*, vol. 128, no. 2, pp. 198–203, 2013.

[3] Y. Chiang, J. Qiu, C. Chang et al., "Brain metastases from epithelial ovarian carcinoma: evaluation of prognosis and managements — A Taiwanese Gynecologic Oncology Group (TGOG) Study," *Gynecologic Oncology*, vol. 125, no. 1, pp. 37–41, 2012.

[4] R. R. Langley and I. J. Fidler, "The seed and soil hypothesis revisited—the role of tumor-stroma interactions in metastasis to different organs," *International Journal of Cancer*, vol. 128, no. 11, pp. 2527–2535, 2011.

[5] L. J. Schouten, J. Rutten, H. A. M. Huveneers, and A. Twijnstra, "Incidence of brain metastases in a cohort of patients with carcinoma of the breast, colon, kidney, and lung and melanoma," *Cancer*, vol. 94, no. 10, pp. 2698–2705, 2002.

[6] B. Gleissner and M. C. Chamberlain, "Neoplastic meningitis," *The Lancet Neurology*, vol. 5, no. 5, pp. 443–452, 2006.

[7] Z. R. Cohen, D. Suki, and J. S. Weinberg, "Brain metastases in patients with ovarian carcinoma: pPrognostic factors and outcome," *Journal of Neuro-Oncology*, vol. 66, no. 3, pp. 313–325, 2004.

[8] G. C. Rodriguez, J. T. Soper, A. Berchuck et al., "Improved palliation of cerebral metastases in epithelial ovarian cancer using a combined modality approach including radiation therapy, chemotherapy, and surgery," *Journal of Clinical Oncology*, vol. 10, no. 10, pp. 1553–1560, 1992.

[9] G. H. Barker, J. Orledge, and E. Wiltshaw, "Involvement of the central nervous system in patients with ovarian carcinoma," *BJOG: An International Journal of Obstetrics and Gynaecology*, vol. 88, no. 7, pp. 690–694, 1981.

[10] J. P. Geisler and H. E. Geisler, "Brain metastases in epithelial ovarian carcinoma," *Gynecologic Oncology*, vol. 57, no. 2, pp. 246–249, 1995.

[11] P. D. LeRoux, M. S. Berger, J. P. Elliott et al., "Cerebral metastases from ovarian carcinoma," *Cancer*, vol. 67, pp. 2194–2199, 1991.

[12] S. Yust-Katz, S. Mathis, and M. D. Groves, "Leptomeningeal metastases from genitourinary cancer: the University of Texas MD Anderson Cancer Center experience," *Medical Oncology*, vol. 30, no. 1, article 429, 2013.

[13] L. Kumar, S. Barge, A. K. Mahapatra et al., "Central nervous system metastases from primary epithelial ovarian cancer," *Cancer Control*, vol. 10, no. 3, pp. 244–253, 2003.

[14] G. M. Gressel, L. S. Lundsberg, G. Altwerger et al., "Factors Predictive of Improved Survival in Patients with Brain Metastases from Gynecologic Cancer: A Single Institution Retrospective Study of 47 Cases and Review of the Literature," *International Journal of Gynecological Cancer*, vol. 25, no. 9, pp. 1711–1716, 2015.

[15] D. Pectasides, M. Pectasides, and T. Economopoulos, "Brain metastases from epithelial ovarian cancer: a review of the literature," *The Oncologist*, vol. 11, no. 3, pp. 252–260, 2006.

[16] R. Vitaliani, M. Spinazzi, A. R. Del Mistro, R. Manara, B. Tavolato, and D. M. Bonifati, "Subacute onset of deafness and vertigo in a patient with leptomeningeal metastasis from ovarian cancer," *Neurological Sciences*, vol. 30, no. 1, pp. 65–67, 2009.

[17] M. Krupa and K. Byun, "Leptomeningeal carcinomatosis and bilateral internal auditory canal metastases from ovarian carcinoma," *Radiology Case Reports*, vol. 12, no. 2, pp. 386–390, 2017.

[18] J. Levy, M. Marcus, I. Shelef, and T. Lifshitz, "Acute bilateral blindness in meningeal carcinomatosis," *Eye*, vol. 18, no. 2, pp. 206–208, 2004.

[19] C. R. A. S. De Azevedo, M. R. S. Cruz, L. T. D. Chinen et al., "Meningeal carcinomatosis in breast cancer: Prognostic factors and outcome," *Journal of Neuro-Oncology*, vol. 104, no. 2, pp. 565–572, 2011.

[20] J. M. Gomori, N. Heching, and T. Siegal, "Leptomeningeal metastases: Evaluation by gadolinium enhanced spinal magnetic resonance imaging," *Journal of Neuro-Oncology*, vol. 36, no. 1, pp. 55–60, 1998.

[21] W. R. Wasserstrom, J. P. Glass, and J. B. Posner, "Diagnosis and treatment of leptomeningeal metastases from solid tumors: Experience with 90 patients," *Cancer*, vol. 49, no. 4, pp. 759–772, 1982.

[22] T. Leal, J. E. Chang, M. Mehta, and H. I. Robins, "Leptomeningeal metastasis: challenges in diagnosis and treatment," *Current Cancer Therapy Reviews*, vol. 7, no. 4, pp. 319–327, 2011.

[23] M. C. Chamberlain, "Neoplastic meningitis," *The Oncologist*, vol. 13, no. 9, pp. 967–977, 2008.

[24] G. C. Jayson and A. Howell, "Carcinomatous meningitis in solid tumours," *Annals of Oncology*, vol. 7, no. 8, pp. 773–786, 1996.

[25] N. Pavlidis, "The diagnostic and therapeutic management of leptomeningeal carcinomatosis," *Annals of Oncology*, vol. 15, no. 4, pp. iv285–iv291, 2004.

[26] N. Anupol, S. Ghamande, K. Odunsi, D. Driscoll, and S. Lele, "Evaluation of prognostic factors and treatment modalities in ovarian cancer patients with brain metastases," *Gynecologic Oncology*, vol. 85, no. 3, pp. 487–492, 2002.

[27] E. Piura and B. Piura, "Brain Metastases from Ovarian Carcinoma," *ISRN Oncology*, vol. 2011, Article ID 527453, 13 pages, 2011.

[28] W. T. Sause, J. Crowley, H. J. Eyre et al., "Whole brain irradiation and intrathecal Methotrexate in the treatment of solid tumor leptomeningeal metastases — A Southwest Oncology Group study," *Journal of Neuro-Oncology*, vol. 6, no. 2, pp. 107–112, 1988.

[29] E. Miller, I. Dy, and T. Herzog, "Leptomeningeal carcinomatosis from ovarian cancer," *Medical Oncology*, vol. 29, no. 3, pp. 2010–2015, 2012.

[30] A. N. Gordon, J. J. Kavanagh Jr., J. T. Wharton, F. N. Rutledge, E. A. M. T. Obbens, and G. P. Bodey Sr., "Successful treatment of leptomeningeal relapse of epithelial ovarian cancer," *Gynecologic Oncology*, vol. 18, no. 1, pp. 119–124, 1984.

[31] H. Ohta, R. Koyama, T. Nagai, Y. Hirayama, S. Saito, and A. Yonesaka, "Meningeal carcinomatosis from an ovarian primary with complete response to adjuvant chemotherapy after cranial irradiation," *International Journal of Clinical Oncology*, vol. 6, no. 3, pp. 157–162, 2001.

[32] H. Yamakawa, H. Ariga, A. Enomoto, S. Netsu, Y. Suzuki, and R. Konno, "Meningeal dissemination from an ovarian carcinoma with effective response to intrathecal chemotherapy," *International Journal of Clinical Oncology*, vol. 14, no. 5, pp. 447–451, 2009.

[33] Y. Goto, N. Katsumata, S. Nakai et al., "Leptomeningeal metastasis from ovarian carcinoma successfully treated by the intraventricular administration of methotrexate," *International Journal of Clinical Oncology*, vol. 13, no. 6, pp. 555–558, 2008.

8

A Case of Macrolide-Refractory *Mycoplasma pneumoniae* Pneumonia in Pregnancy Treated with Garenoxacin

Yoko Matsuda,[1] Yoshitsugu Chigusa,[1] Eiji Kondoh,[1] Isao Ito,[2]
Yusuke Ueda,[1] and Masaki Mandai[1]

[1]*Department of Gynecology and Obstetrics, Kyoto University, 54 Shogoin Kawahara-cho, Sakyo-ku, Kyoto 606-8507, Japan*
[2]*Department of Respiratory Medicine, Kyoto University, 54 Shogoin Kawahara-cho, Sakyo-ku, Kyoto 606-8507, Japan*

Correspondence should be addressed to Yoshitsugu Chigusa; chigusa@kuhp.kyoto-u.ac.jp

Academic Editor: Erich Cosmi

Pneumonia in pregnancy is associated with adverse maternal and foetal outcomes, and intensive treatment with appropriate antibiotics is essential. However, cases caused by pathogens that are resistant to antibiotics suitable for the developing foetus are challenging. We herein report a case of macrolide-refractory *Mycoplasma pneumoniae* pneumonia in pregnancy. A 40-year-old multigravida with twin pregnancy complained of cough and fever at 13 weeks of gestation and was diagnosed with pneumonia. Even though empiric treatment with ceftriaxone and oral azithromycin was started, her condition deteriorated rapidly. The findings of chest computed tomography suggested *Mycoplasma pneumoniae* pneumonia. Since azithromycin did not work, this strain was considered to be macrolide-refractory. Garenoxacin, an oral quinolone, was selected and was dramatically effective. The use of quinolone could be justified with the emergence of drug-resistant bacterial/atypical pneumonia and in the maternal life-threatening condition.

1. Introduction

Pneumonia in pregnant women can become severe and is the most common nonobstetric infection contributing to maternal mortality in the peripartum period. In the recent years, concern has arisen regarding pathogens of pneumonia which are resistant to the initial empiric treatment such as β-lactam antibiotics. The treatment strategy of drug-resistant pneumonia is challenging, especially in pregnant patients, because several kinds of promising antibiotics are considered to be avoided in pregnancy. Here, we describe a case of macrolide-refractory *Mycoplasma pneumoniae* pneumonia at 13 weeks of gestation. The administration of Garenoxacin, an oral quinolone antibiotic, dramatically ameliorated severe cough, dyspnoea, and fever, and the patient recovered quickly. To the best of our knowledge, this is the first case in which Garenoxacin was administered to a pregnant woman. We also discuss the rationale and safety of quinolone usage in pregnancy based on the relevant literatures.

2. Case Report

A 40-year-old female, gravida 3, para 1, with an unremarkable past medical history conceived with in vitro fertilization. At 12 weeks and 5 days of gestation, she was referred to our hospital with the diagnosis of dichorionic diamniotic twin pregnancy. She complained of slight general fatigue and anorexia. Two days later, at 13 weeks and 0 days of gestation, she visited us again with a complaint of unproductive cough and fever. Regarding the obstetrical examination, she had no abnormal findings. Her vaginal secretions were yellowish, and her cervix was closed. Transvaginal ultrasound showed 5 cm of cervical length and normal heart beats of two foetuses. Her vital signs were as follows: body temperature, 38.1°C, pulse, 102 beats per minute, blood pressure, 101/67 mmHg, SpO_2, 93% (room air), and respiratory rate, 25 per minute. The laboratory data are shown in Table 1. Although she had persistent cough, her chest auscultation findings were subtle; only weak inspiratory wheeze was appreciated. Even though

TABLE 1: The laboratory data of the case.

WBC	7,500	/μL
Hb	12	g/dL
Ht	33.3	%
PLT	21.1×10^4	/μL
AST	14	IU/L
ALT	5	IU/L
LDH	170	IU/L
ALP	136	IU/L
TP	7	g/dL
Alb	3.2	g/dL
T-bil	1.2	mg/dL
Cre	0.43	mg/dL
BUN	7	mg/dL
CK	23	IU/L
Glu	88	mg/dL
AMY	43	IU/L
Na	133	mEq/L
K	3.4	mEq/L
Cl	98	mEq/L
CRP	8.8	mg/dL

Streptococcus pneumoniae urinary antigen test was negative, the chest X-ray revealed infiltrate with bronchial tram lines in right lower lobe (Figure 1(a)). Therefore, pneumonia was suspected and empiric therapy was commenced with 1 g of ceftriaxone every 12 hours and single administration of 2 g of oral azithromycin in order to cover both bacterial and nonbacterial pathogens of community-acquired pneumonia. Nasal oxygenation was also employed to keep her SpO$_2$ above 95%. Despite the antibiotic therapy for 72 hours, her fever was not alleviated, and she remained with cough and dyspnoea and deteriorated rapidly. The chest computed tomography (CT) revealed airspace consolidation, ground-glass opacity, centrilobular nodules, and thickening of the bronchial walls (Figures 1(b) and 1(c)), which are distinctive features of the CT findings of *Mycoplasma pneumoniae* pneumonia [1]. Combined with the fact that azithromycin did not work, macrolide-resistant *Mycoplasma pneumoniae* pneumonia was suspected. Thus, after consultation with a chest physician, oral administration of 400 mg of Garenoxacin every 24 hours was started at 13 weeks and 3 days of gestation. Shortly after Garenoxacin administration, dyspnoea dramatically ameliorated, and fever began to subside within 24 hours. She took Garenoxacin for seven days and was discharged from the hospital at 14 weeks and 6 days of gestation. Eventually, she was diagnosed with *Mycoplasma pneumoniae* pneumonia based on the serological test; *Mycoplasma* particle agglutination titres increased from 1 : 80 to 1 : 2,560 (32 times) in seven days. The subsequent pregnancy course was uneventful; because the first foetus presented as breech, she delivered twins by caesarean section at 37 weeks and 5 days of gestation. The twin male babies weighed 2402 g and 2404 g, respectively, and had no abnormal findings. There were no signs of infection, either.

3. Discussion

Pneumonia is a relatively uncommon complication of pregnancy arising in 0.78 to 2.7 per 1,000 deliveries. The most common aetiological agents of pneumonia in pregnancy are typical bacterial pathogens, such as *Streptococcus pneumoniae* and *Haemophilus influenzae*. Additionally, atypical bacterial pathogens, including *Mycoplasma pneumoniae*, *Chlamydia pneumoniae*, and *Legionella pneumophilia*, are also identified. Although antibiotic therapy has advanced, pneumonia in pregnancy can be associated with considerable maternal mortality and morbidity [2]. A change in maternal cellular immunity, namely, immunosuppression caused by pregnancy or maternal physiologic changes such as a decrease in the functional residual capacity of lungs, may be related to an unfavourable course of pneumonia in pregnant women. Furthermore, pneumonia during gestation is associated with adverse pregnancy outcomes. Preterm labour is one of the most notable complications of pneumonia in pregnancy. The incidence of preterm labour reportedly has reached almost 44%, and, for preterm births, this figure is 36% [3]. Another recent population-based study revealed that the adjusted odds ratio for preterm birth in pregnant women with pneumonia was 1.71; moreover, the figures for low birth weight and small size for gestational age were 1.73 and 1.35, respectively [4]. Thus, pneumonia in pregnancy should be treated promptly and intensively using appropriate antibiotics.

Mycoplasma pneumoniae pneumonia is one of the common community-acquired respiratory tract infections and prevails among school-aged children and young adults [5]. Unfortunately, as far as we have searched, the exact incidence of *Mycoplasma pneumoniae* pneumonia in pregnant women is unknown. The major clinical manifestations are cough, fever, dyspnoea, and hypoxia. Generally, *Mycoplasma pneumoniae* pneumonia is treated using macrolides, and fulminant cases are relatively rare. However, the emergence and prevalence of macrolide-resistant strains have been a pressing challenge. The macrolide-resistance rates in adults are dramatically different from area to area: 3.5 to 13% in America, 0 to 10% in Europe, 3.3% in Oceania, 90 to 100% in Asia, and 56 to 89% in Japan [6]. The precise reason why this rate is very high in Asia, including Japan, is currently unknown. A plausible speculation is that macrolide-resistance *Mycoplasma* pneumonia was detected in Japan for the first time in the world [7], and the number of prescriptions of macrolide agents is high in China and Japan [8]. Importantly, macrolide-resistance strains are isolated more frequently from adolescent and paediatric patients than from adults; therefore, in adults, Japanese guiding principle still recommends macrolide for the treatment of *Mycoplasma pneumoniae* pneumonia. Meanwhile, a change of antibiotics to second-line drugs is also recommended if the fever does not subside in 48–72 h from macrolide administration [9].

In the case of macrolide-resistance in nonpregnant adult patients, tetracyclines or quinolones should be employed for the treatment of *Mycoplasma pneumoniae* pneumonia [9]. Because tetracycline exposure in utero causes congenital defects and permanent discolouration of bones and teeth, it

(a)

(b)

(c)

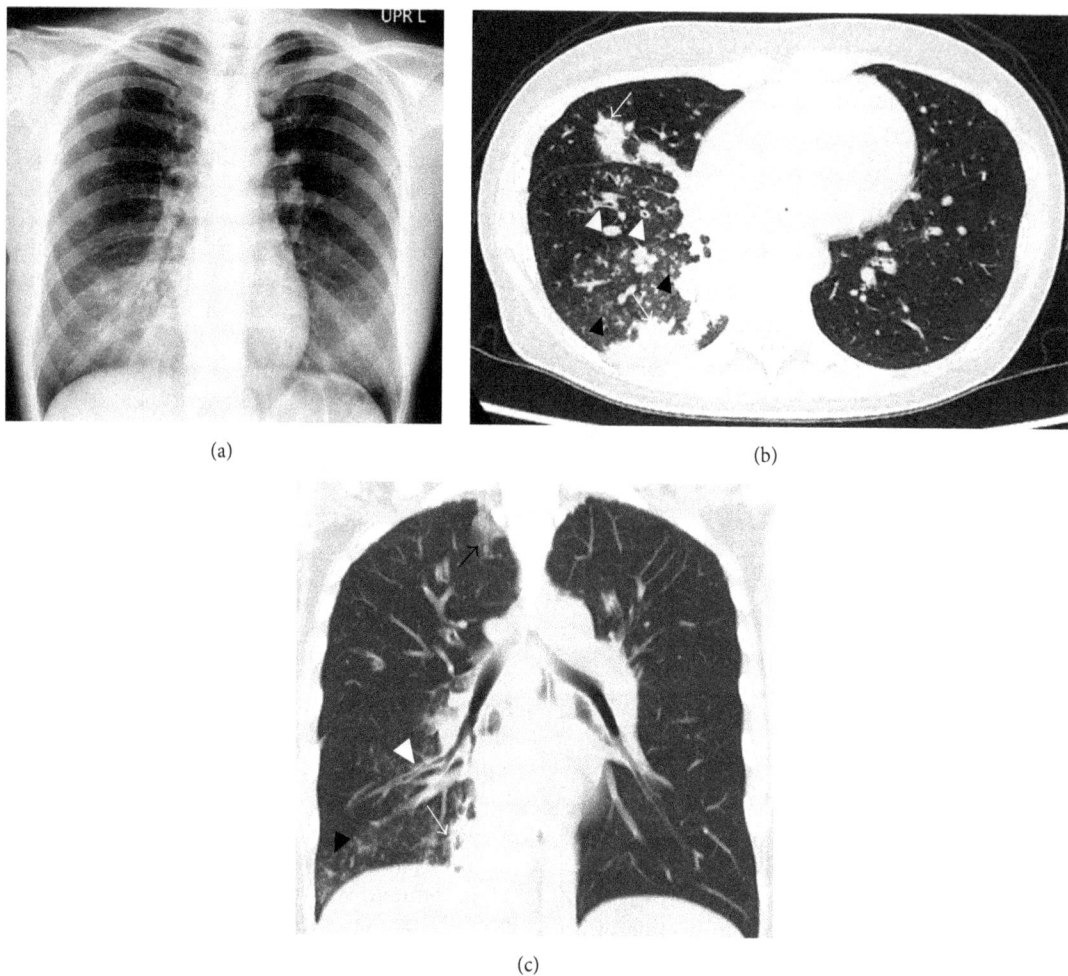

FIGURE 1: Chest radiography (a), axial view (b), and coronal view (c) of chest computed tomography (CT) images of the case. The chest X-ray showed a high-density area in right lower lobe. The chest CT revealed airspace consolidations (white arrows), thickening of bronchial walls (white triangles), and numerous centrilobular nodules (black triangles). The coronal view showed ground-glass opacity in the right upper lobe (black arrow).

should be avoided in pregnancy. Quinolones are a class of broad-spectrum antimicrobial agents that act by inhibiting bacterial DNA gyrase. Basically, definitive evidence for the teratogenic effect of quinolones has not thus far been shown. Instead, postnatal exposure to quinolones in juvenile mice and dogs caused arthropathy [10]. Thus, quinolones have been considered to be contraindicated, in principal, for pregnant women, although cartilage degeneration has not been reported in human neonate and children. In contrast, clinical data have been accumulated for decades that suggest the relative safety of quinolones in pregnancy.

The cohort study conducted by the European Network of Teratology Information Service reported that no clear adverse reactions, including birth defects, were revealed due to in utero exposure to quinolones [11]. Bar-Oz et al. conducted a meta-analysis and concluded that the use of quinolones during the first trimester of pregnancy did not appear to represent an increased risk of major malformations, preterm birth, or low birth weight [10]. Furthermore, according to the observational cohort study by Padberg et al., an increased

risk of spontaneous abortion or major birth defects was not detected after intrauterine fluoroquinolone exposure [12].

Garenoxacin is a comparatively new oral quinolone that has a broad spectrum of antibacterial activities and shows the best antimycoplasmal activity among quinolones [13]. Additionally, according to the manufacturer's report, teratogenicity of Garenoxacin was not detected in rats or rabbits. Currently, the use of Garenoxacin in pregnancy is contraindicated despite insufficient clinical data. In the present case, however, the condition of the patient was deteriorating rapidly, and both maternal mortality and foetal mortality were concerned. Furthermore, the patient's gestational age, 13 weeks, was past the period of organogenesis. Consequently, after close consultation with the chest physician and patient, she fully understood the concerns about Garenoxacin usage in pregnancy and gave her written consent. Then, Garenoxacin was selected in expectation of definite effect.

In summary, we described a case of macrolide-refractory *Mycoplasma pneumoniae* pneumonia in pregnancy, in which administration of the oral quinolone, Garenoxacin, was highly effective. Although the use of quinolones has long been avoided in pregnancy, it can be justified with the emergence of drug-resistant bacterial pneumonia and in maternal life-threatening conditions.

Consent

Written informed consent was obtained from the patient for publication of this case report and accompanying images.

References

[1] I. Ito, T. Ishida, K. Togashi et al., "Differentiation of bacterial and non-bacterial community-acquired pneumonia by thin-section computed tomography," *European Journal of Radiology*, vol. 72, no. 3, pp. 388–395, 2009.

[2] W. H. Goodnight and D. E. Soper, "Pneumonia in pregnancy," *Critical Care Medicine*, vol. 33, supplement 10, pp. S390–S397, 2005.

[3] N. E. Madinger, J. S. Greenspoon, and A. Gray Ellrodt, "Pneumonia during pregnancy: Has modern technology improved maternal and fetal outcome?" *American Journal of Obstetrics & Gynecology*, vol. 161, no. 3, pp. 657–662, 1989.

[4] Y. Chen, J. Keller, I. Wang, C. Lin, and H. Lin, "Pneumonia and pregnancy outcomes: a nationwide population-based study," *American Journal of Obstetrics & Gynecology*, vol. 207, no. 4, pp. 288.e1–288.e7, 2012.

[5] I. Ito, T. Ishida, M. Osawa et al., "Culturally verified Mycoplasma pneumoniae pneumonia in Japan: a long-term observation from 1979–99," *Epidemiology and Infection*, vol. 127, no. 2, pp. 365–367, 2001.

[6] S. Pereyre, J. Goret, and C. Bébéar, "Mycoplasma pneumoniae: current knowledge on macrolide resistance and treatment," *Frontiers in Microbiology*, vol. 7, p. 974, 2016.

[7] N. Okazaki, M. Narita, S. Yamada et al., "Characteristics of macrolide-resistant Mycoplasma pneumoniae strains isolated from patients and induced with erythromycin in vitro," *Microbiol Immunol*, vol. 45, no. 8, pp. 617–620, 2001.

[8] T. Tanaka, T. Oishi, I. Miyata et al., " Macrolide-Resistant ," *Emerging Infectious Diseases*, vol. 23, no. 10, pp. 1703–1706, 2017.

[9] "The Committee of Japanese Society of Mycoplasmology SK, Tadashi Ishida, Koichi Izumikawa, Satoshi Iwata, Jun-ichi Kadota, Hiroshi Tanaka, Mitsuo Narita, Naoyuki Miyashita, Hidehiro Watanabe," Guiding principles for treating Mycoplasma pneumoniae pneumonia, 2014.

[10] B. Bar-Oz, ME. Moretti, R. Boskovic, L. O'Brien, and G. Koren, "The safety of quinolones—a meta-analysis of pregnancy outcomes," *European Journal of Obstetrics & Gynecology and Reproductive Biology*, vol. 143, no. 2, pp. 75–78, 2009.

[11] C. Schaefer, E. Amoura-Elefant, T. Vial et al., "Pregnancy outcome after prenatal quinolone exposure: Evaluation of a case registry of the European Network of Teratology Information Services (ENTIS)," *European Journal of Obstetrics & Gynecology and Reproductive Biology*, vol. 69, no. 2, pp. 83–89, 1996.

[12] S. Padberg, E. Wacker, R. Meister et al., "Observational cohort study of pregnancy outcome after first-trimester exposure to fluoroquinolones," *Antimicrobial Agents and Chemotherapy*, vol. 58, no. 8, pp. 4392–4398, 2014.

[13] N. Miyashita, H. Akaike, H. Teranishi, K. Ouchi, and N. Okimoto, "Macrolide-resistant mycoplasma pneumoniae pneumonia in adolescents and adults: clinical findings, drug susceptibility, and therapeutic efficacy," *Antimicrobial Agents and Chemotherapy*, vol. 57, no. 10, pp. 5181–5185, 2013.

9

Successful Pregnancy Outcome after Open Strassman Metroplasty for Bicornuate Uterus

Edgar Gulavi ⓘ,[1] **Steve Kyende Mutiso,**[1]
Charles Mariara Muriuki,[2] **and Abraham Mukaindo Mwaniki**[3]

[1]*Obstetrics and Gynecology, Aga Khan University Hospital, Nairobi, Kenya*
[2]*Kijabe Mission Hospital, Kiambu, Kenya*
[3]*Aga Khan University Hospital, Nairobi, Kenya*

Correspondence should be addressed to Edgar Gulavi; edgargulavi@gmail.com

Academic Editor: Maria Grazia Porpora

Introduction. Müllerian duct anomalies represent a group of congenital malformations that result from failure to complete bilateral paramesonephric duct elongation, fusion, canalization, or septal resorption. These anomalies are rare in the general population with a bicornuate or didelphys uterus being among the common ones. Bicornuate uterine malformations are of clinical significance due to their adverse reproductive outcomes. Metroplasty has been shown to improve reproductive outcomes of bicornuate uterine malformations. We document a case of bicornuate uterus that was managed with Strassman metroplasty and a subsequent successful pregnancy outcome. *Case.* A Black African lady was seen with a history of six prior miscarriages. Her diagnostic workup revealed a bicornuate uterus for which she had a Strassman metroplasty performed. She later conceived and was followed up to term with a successful live birth. *Conclusion.* Strassman metroplasty is a rare procedure in Sub-Saharan Africa and this case seeks to add to the body of knowledge on surgical management of Müllerian duct anomalies specifically bicornuate uterus in this region. This case report aims to increase the awareness of Müllerian duct abnormalities specifically bicornuate uterus in cases of recurrent miscarriages and highlight the diagnostic strategies to investigate and to demonstrate management options in low resource settings.

1. Introduction

Müllerian duct anomalies represent a group of congenital malformations that result from failure to complete bilateral paramesonephric duct elongation, fusion, canalization, or septal resorption [1]. These anomalies can be classified according to the American Society of Reproductive Medicine (ASRM) as segmental Müllerian hypoplasia or agenesis (Group I), unicornuate uterus (Group II), uterine didelphys (Group III), bicornuate uterus (Group IV), septate uterus (Group V), arcuate uterus (Group VI), and diethylstilbestrol related anomalies (Group VII) [2].

The prevalence of these malformations in general population is approximately 5%. It is 5–10% in those suffering from recurrent miscarriages and greater than one in four in women with late pregnancy losses and preterm deliveries [3]. Among the Müllerian duct anomalies, bicornuate and didelphic uteri are the more common forms, with a prevalence of 25 and 11%, respectively. Moreover, they are associated with recurrent first and second trimester miscarriages as well as higher rates of preterm delivery [3].

Bicornuate uterus is caused by incomplete fusion of the Müllerian ducts. It is characterized by two separate but communicating endometrial cavities and a single uterine cervix. Failed fusion may extend to the cervix resulting in a complete bicornuate uterus or may be partial, causing a milder abnormality. Pregnancy outcomes in patients with these anomalies are not favorable. Previous reports have demonstrated that those with bicornuate uterus have higher rates of miscarriages and preterm delivery [36% and 23%, respectively] [3–5]. The clinical presentation of bicornuate uterus includes menstrual dysfunction, primary infertility, recurrent miscarriages, preterm deliveries, and late pregnancy losses. A multidisciplinary approach is recommended in the management of patients diagnosed with Müllerian duct anomalies with input from a psychologist, an endocrinologist, and consultant gynecologist adept at such cases. With that in mind, surgical intervention remains the standard of care for those with Müllerian duct anomalies suffering from recurrent pregnancy loss or poor pregnancy outcomes [4]. Strassman metroplasty is the standard surgical procedure for correction of bicornuate uteri [5]. Paul Strassman in 1907 reported the first surgical correction for the double uterus by performing an anterior colpotomy in a patient with 8 pregnancy losses [5].

Uterine malformations are rare occurrences worldwide and surgical management of these cases is not well documented in Sub-Saharan Africa perhaps due to challenges in diagnosis or treatment. We present a case of a patient with a bicornuate uterus that was surgically managed with open Strassman metroplasty with a successful subsequent pregnancy.

2. Case

2.1. Patient Information. A 35-year-old para 0+6 Black African lady presented with a history of five first and one second trimester recurrent pregnancy losses. In addition, she had a nine-year history of irregular heavy bleeding associated with dysmenorrhea.

Her menarche was at 17 years of age with regular painful cycles that lasted 10 days. She was not on any contraceptive method and did not report any dyspareunia or urinary symptoms. Her first miscarriage occurred 11 years and was surgically managed by dilatation and curettage. Subsequently she noted changes in her menstrual cycle. Her menstrual cycle became irregular with a heavy flow for 10 days associated with severe dysmenorrhea and bowel symptoms of bloating and diarrhea. She used tranexamic acid one gram three times a day during her menses for the heavy prolonged periods and Mefenamic Acid 500 milligrams three times a day for the dysmenorrhea with reported relief of the symptoms.

2.2. Clinical Findings. The physical examination was unremarkable except for mild tenderness in the suprapubic region; she had grossly normal external genitalia and normal looking cervix.

2.3. Diagnostic Assessment. Her initial hormonal profile was as follows:

FSH: 4.5 IU/m (3.1-7.9 IU/L)

LH: 10 IU/L (1-18 IU/L)

She had a recent pap smear one year ago that was normal.

Transabdominal and transvaginal (TVS) scans had shown separate right and left cornu with multiple cysts in the peripheral ovarian parenchyma features suggestive of bicornuate uterus and polycystic ovaries (Figure 1). She also had a hysterosalpingogram (HSG) that was reported to have a uterus opacified with banana configuration oriented to

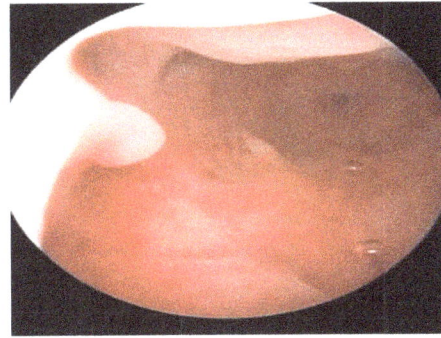

FIGURE 1: Hysteroscopy findings.

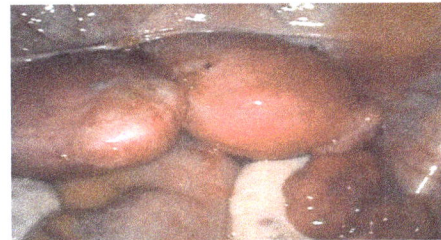

FIGURE 2: Laparoscopy findings.

the right with no delineation of fallopian tubes, findings suggestive of a unicornuate uterus.

Her past medical history was not significant. She was recently divorced, a condition she attributed to her history of several miscarriages in the context of an African cultural expectation of siring children.

She was subsequently scheduled her for hysteroscopy and diagnostic laparoscopy. She also gave consent for possible open Strassmans metroplasty.

2.4. Therapeutic Intervention. On hysteroscopy, a normal looking endometrium was visualized with a right sided tubal ostia and a small tubal ostia on the left that did not appear patent (Figure 1). Laparoscopically, a bicornuate uterus was found (Figure 2) with associated endometriosis at the vesicouterine fold. Open metroplasty was done (Figures 3 and 4). A fundal transverse incision was made and dissection done to the level of the endometrium after injection of subserosal vasopressin. Apposition of the two horns was done and the uterus sutured in layers (Figures 3 and 4). A copper intrauterine device was left in situ to separate the uterine walls and possibly reduce the chances of uterine synechiae though the evidence for this practice is still not conclusive. In addition, endometriotic deposits discovered at the vesico uterine fold were ablated.

2.5. Follow-Up and Outcomes. She had an unremarkable follow-up after surgery with no complications reported.

A HSG 6 months after surgery revealed unification of the uterine horns but both tubes were not delineated.

Patient was lost to follow-up but two years later she presented having conceived spontaneously and a TVS revealed

TABLE 1: Antenatal profile.

Profile	Value
Hemoglobin	11.5 g/dl
Blood group	A+
Hepatitis BsAg	Negative
VDRL	Negative
HIV	Negative

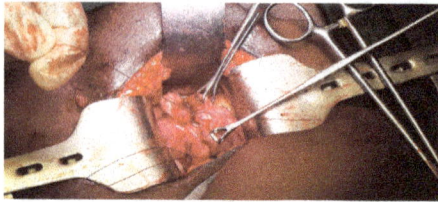

FIGURE 3: Ongoing metroplasty.

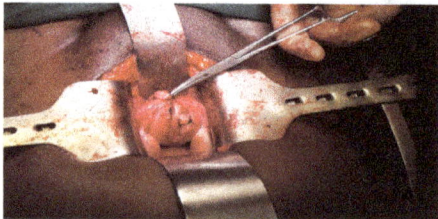

FIGURE 4: After metroplasty.

a single intrauterine pregnancy at 13 weeks. Her antenatal workup was as highlighted in Table 1.

She was subsequently followed up at the antenatal clinic and had no concerns till 33 weeks when she presented with a history of lower abdominal pain worsening over the past few weeks and right sided fundal tenderness pain score of seven out of ten on the pain assessment scale. The main concern at the time of assessment was possible uterine rupture. She did not have any features suggestive of bowel obstruction as she was passing stool and bowel sounds were present. She had a normal NST and an obstetric ultrasound that was done showed a single intrauterine pregnancy with normal biophysical profile and no features of placental abruption or slower uterine segment site dehiscence. She had no other investigations done at this time. The pain was significant enough to warrant an admission for which she subsequently received antenatal steroids for lung maturity and opioid analgesia for pain relief. However, the pain did not completely resolve and she underwent a caesarean delivery at 33 weeks and 5 days due to persistent lower abdominal pain. The outcome was a live male infant with a birth weight of 1950 grams and APGAR of 9, 10, 10. There was no evidence of uterine rupture although she had venous congestion and massive varicose veins bilaterally at the cornual areas. The previous metroplasty scar was intact.

She had a resolution of the abdominal pain postoperatively and had an unremarkable postoperative recovery. She was discharged on the fifth postoperative day.

3. Discussion

Müllerian duct anomalies represent a group of congenital malformations that result from failure to complete bilateral duct elongation, fusion, canalization, or septal resorption [1].

Various classification schemes for female reproductive tract anomalies exist, but the most common classification was proposed by Buttram and Gibbons (1979) and adapted by the American Society for Reproductive Medicine (ASRM) (former American Fertility Society, 1988). Within this system, six groups are elucidated: segmental Müllerian hypoplasia or agenesis (Group I), unicornuate uterus (Group II), uterine didelphys (Group III), bicornuate uterus (Group IV), septate uterus (Group V), arcuate uterus (Group VI), and diethylstilbestrol related anomalies (Group VII) [2]. The case highlighted above of bicornuate uterus fell into Group IV ASRM classification.

Among the Müllerian duct anomalies, bicornuate and didelphic uteri are common forms, with the prevalence of 25 and 11%.

There are no specific risk factors highlighted in literature that predispose to these abnormalities. Uterine congenital anomalies have a heterogeneous genetic basis, with implications of Wilms tumour 1 gene (WT1), paired box gene 2 (Pax2), WNT2, pre-B-cell leukemia transcription factor 1 (PBX1), and homeobox (HOX) genes [6]. In the case highlighted above no risk factor was found.

Most cases are diagnosed during evaluation for obstetric or gynecologic conditions, but in the absence of symptoms, most anomalies remain undiagnosed [6]. In this particular case, a history of first and second trimester miscarriages as well as menstrual irregularities warranted clinical evaluation and investigation.

The question of whether Müllerian anomalies are significantly more often combined with endometriosis is a controversially discussed problem. Some publications described this association in patients with obstructive but not nonobstructive Müllerian anomalies or controls without Müllerian anomalies. It is well known that obstructive Müllerian anomalies are significantly more often associated with endometriosis, a disease with an adverse effect on fertility. The underlying pathophysiological mechanism could be the increased risk of retrograde menstruation [7, 8]. Radiologic discrimination of bicornuate uterus from the septate uterus and unicornuate uterus with a horn can be challenging as was in the case highlighted here where initial HSG was suggestive of a unicornuate uterus. However, it is important to distinguish them because septate uterus is easily treated with hysteroscopic septal resection. Widely diverging horns seen on HSG may suggest a bicornuate uterus. An intercornual angle greater than 105 degrees suggests bicornuate uterus, whereas one less than 75 degrees indicates a septate uterus [9]. However, MRI may be necessary to define fundal contour. With this, an intrafundal downward cleft measuring greater than or equal to 1 cm is indicative of bicornuate uterus, whereas a cleft depth < 1 cm indicates a septate uterus [9]. Use of 3D sonography also allows internal and external uterine assessment. Thus, sonography and HSG seem acceptable imaging techniques in the initial investigation. When the presumptive diagnosis is a septate uterus, laparoscopy may be performed for a definitive diagnosis and before hysteroscopic resection of the septum is initiated if in doubt. In this present case, HSG and TVS combined with findings from a hysteroscopy and laparoscopy were sufficient to make the diagnosis.

Surgical intervention through Strassman metroplasty provides an important decrease in the percentage of fetal loss (8-12%) compared to patients without surgical treatment (70-96%) [5]. Conventional transabdominal metroplasty seems to be a safe and efficient procedure in women with bicornuate uterine anomaly [5].

The actual benefit of metroplasty for a bicornuate uterus, however, has not been tested in a controlled clinical trial and metroplasty for now should be reserved for women in whom recurrent pregnancy loss occurs with no other identifiable cause [4].

In other centers, laparoscopic and hysteroscopy metroplasty has been shown to be a safe procedure and with all the additional benefits of minimally invasive surgery and it is a viable alternative to conventional open abdominal metroplasty [10]. Significant challenges exist in Sub-Saharan Africa in terms of access and skills in laparoscopic surgery which pose a significant drawback to the possibility of laparoscopic metroplasty and this case highlights this [10, 11].

All patients with Müllerian agenesis should be offered counseling and encouraged to connect with peer support groups where available. The psychological effect of the diagnosis of Müllerian agenesis cannot be underestimated. Many patients experience anxiety and depression, question their female identity, and grieve their infertility. These patients struggle with how to share their conditions with family members, peers, and romantic partners. Several cultural issues also come into play in the African setting with stigma directed to women who have had miscarriages and those with challenges getting children. This is an aspect of care that should be considered in cultural contexts similar to this case.

There is a paucity of data demonstrating reproductive success after metroplasty in cases of bicornuate uterus in Sub-Saharan Africa. In Kenya, not much work on management of Müllerian anomalies has been reported or published in recent years. This case report aims to increase the awareness of Müllerian duct abnormalities more specifically bicornuate uterus in cases of recurrent miscarriages, highlighting the diagnostic strategies to investigate and to demonstrate management options in low resource settings.

References

[1] C. G. Zorlu, H. Yalçin, M. Ugur, S. Özden, S. Kara-Soysal, and O. Gökmen, "Reproductive outcome after metroplasty," *International Journal of Gynecology and Obstetrics*, vol. 55, no. 1, pp. 45–48, 1996.

[2] American Fertility Society, "The American Fertility Society classifications of adnexal adhesions, distal tubal occlusion, tubal occlusion secondary to tubal ligation, tubal pregnancies, Mullerian anomalies and intrauterine adhesions," *Fertility and Sterility*, vol. 49, no. 6, pp. 944–955, 1988.

[3] D. E. Lolis, M. Paschopoulos, G. Makrydimas, K. Zikopoulos, A. Sotiriadis, and E. Paraskevaidis, "Reproductive outcome after strassman metroplasty in women with a bicornuate uterus," *Obstetrics, Gynaecology and Reproductive Medicine*, vol. 50, no. 5, pp. 297–301, 2005.

[4] M. Sugiura-Ogasawara, B. L. Lin, K. Aoki et al., "Does surgery improve live birth rates in patients with recurrent miscarriage caused by uterine anomalies?" *Journal of Obstetrics & Gynaecology*, vol. 35, no. 2, pp. 155–158, 2015.

[5] R. Tomasz, M. Marta, and B. Aleksandra, "Clinical effectiveness of Strassman operation in the treatment of bicornuate uterus," *Ginekologia Polska*, vol. 80, no. 2, pp. 88–92, 2009.

[6] M. Takagi, H. Yagi, R. Fukuzawa, S. Narumi, and T. Hasegawa, "Syndromic disorder of sex development due to a novel hemizygous mutation in the carboxyl-terminal domain of ATRX," *Human Genome Variation*, vol. 4, p. 17012, 2017.

[7] E. Chu, B. Tjaden, D. Grainger, and L. Frazier, "P-447," *Fertility and Sterility*, vol. 86, no. 3, p. S301, 2006.

[8] L. C. Giudice and L. C. Kao, "Endometriosis," *The Lancet*, vol. 364, no. 9447, pp. 1789–1799, 2004.

[9] K. L. Reuter, D. C. Daly, and S. M. Cohen, "Septate versus bicornuate uteri: Errors in imaging diagnosis," *Radiology*, vol. 172, no. 3, pp. 749–752, 1989.

[10] E. Khalifa, J. P. Toner, and H. W. Jones Jr., "The role of abdominal metroplasty in the era of operative hysteroscopy," *Surgery, Gynecology and Obstetrics*, vol. 176, no. 3, pp. 208–212, 1993.

[11] Z. Papp, G. Mezei, M. Gávai, P. Hupuczi, and J. Urbancsek, "Reproductive performance after transabdominal metroplasty: A review of 157 consecutive cases," *Obstetrics, Gynaecology and Reproductive Medicine*, vol. 51, no. 7, pp. 544–552, 2006.

10

Uterine Tumors Resembling Ovarian Sex Cord Tumors: Case Report of Rare Pathological and Clinical Entity

Rotem Sadeh,[1] Yakir Segev,[1] Meirav Schmidt,[1] Jacob Schendler,[2] Tamar Baruch,[2] and Ofer Lavie[1]

[1]*Division of Gynecology Oncology, Department of Obstetrics and Gynecology, Carmel Medical Center, Haifa, Israel*
[2]*Department of Pathology, Carmel Medical Center, Haifa, Israel*

Correspondence should be addressed to Yakir Segev; segevyakir@yahoo.com

Academic Editor: Yoshio Yoshida

Uterine tumors resembling ovarian sex cord tumors (UTROSCT) are rare uterine neoplasms. These tumors are usually benign, displaying a nodular or polypoid growth pattern; common occurrence is observed at the 4th to 6th decade of life. This entity is divided according to clinical behavior and pathological typical findings including different immunohistochemical staining. Traditionally type I tumors show a predominant endometrial stromal pattern with less than 50% ovarian sex cord component. This type has been shown to behave more aggressively with a decreased disease free survival period. Type II tumors, the classical UTROSCT, are less invasive but have the tendency to recur. We report a case of a 57-year-old patient presenting with postmenopausal bleeding. Hysteroscopic polypectomy showed the diagnosis of UTROSCT. This case presents a less morbid minimally invasive treatment plan and exemplifies that in patients where low malignant potential exists and their will is taken into consideration such management is both crucial and correct.

1. Introduction

Uterine tumors resembling ovarian sex cord tumor (UTROSCT) is an extremely rare type of uterine neoplasm and its clinical characteristics are not fully understood. To date, only 77 cases have been reported in the English literature [1–3]. Gomes et al. initially described the concept of sex cord differentiation in a uterine tumor and categorized them into two subtypes [3, 4]. The first type termed as endometrial stromal tumor with sex cord-like elements (ESTSCLE) largely resembles traditional endometrial stromal tumors. The second type is comprised of tumors entirely composed of elements resembling sex cord tumors of ovary and is named as UTROSCT [5].

This classification is critical due to the fact that the two types of tumors resemble each other histologically and yet differ significantly in terms of clinical behavior and genetic features, thus requiring different clinical approaches [6].

Since the initial report in 1976, a distinct separation between the two subtypes has been formed. Until recent years, this categorization was solemnly clinically based [1, 2].

Recently the classification has been reframed based on several immunohistochemical markers, including Calretinin, CD99, Inhibin, and Melan [7].

Type I ESTCLE shows a predominant endometrial stromal pattern, with usually less than 50% ovarian sex cord pattern. Such tumors typically express Calretinin immunohistochemical marker. This tumor also contains unique genetic features and a characteristic translocation. These findings are absent in Type II tumor [6].

Type I is known to have a significantly higher malignant potential and the outcome is contingent upon grade and stage of the underlying stromal neoplasm [1].

Type II also known as classical URTOSCT is considered to be of low malignant potential secondary to occasional recurrence, although they typically exhibit benign biological behavior. A positive Calretinin, as well as another positive staining by Inhibin, CD 99 or Melan A, is to be obtained in order to reach the diagnosis of this specific type [5, 8]. UTROSCT usually occurs in middle-aged women. Most patients present with abnormal uterine bleeding and/or

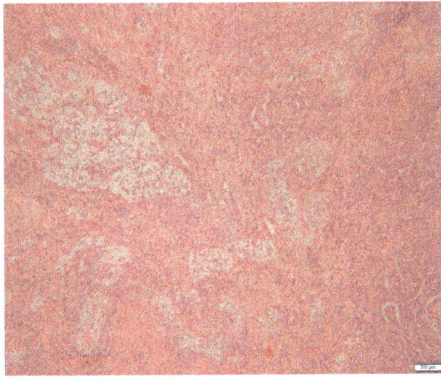

FIGURE 1: H&E microscopic image of the polyp which was composed of elements resembling ovarian sex cord tumors, including solid areas, glomeruloid structures, and small nests.

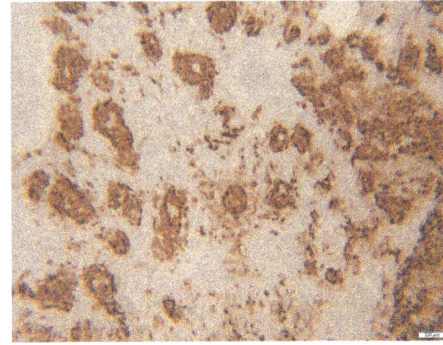

FIGURE 2: Immunohistochemistry of the tumor cells which were positive for Calretinin.

abdominal pain, along with an enlarged uterus or a palpable uterine mass [4]. Hysterectomy with or without bilateral salpingo-oophorectomy is the acceptable treatment for UTROSCT [6].

2. Case

A 57-year-old Caucasian woman presented with postmenopausal bleeding (PMB) and hot flushes was admitted to our department. Initial workup included physical examination and transvaginal sonography with no pathological findings.

Since the presenting symptom was PMB, an endometrial aspiration (pipelle) was performed and pathologic examination revealed syncytial metaplasia. Consequently, the patient experienced a few more episodes of bleeding; therefore hysteroscopy was performed revealing normal appearing endometrium with an endometrial polyp. Eventually, polypectomy was performed. On gross examination there was an elastic pale grey mass measuring 9 ∗ 8 ∗ 2.5 mm. On microscopic examination, fragments of uterine wall infiltrated by malignant nonpleomorphic tumor cells with pale chromatin small nucleoli minor variations in their round to oval nuclear contour and rare mitosis. The cytoplasm of tumor cells is mostly scant but some epithelioid cells with abundant foamy cytoplasm are seen. These neoplastic cells form different patterns of growth: ovarian sex cord tumors, including solid areas, glomeruloid structures, and small nests (Figure 1).

On immunohistochemistry tumor cells were positive for Calretinin (Figure 2), MART-1, Inhibin, CD 99, Desmin, Actin, Vimentin, and Pankeratin. Staining for EMA, Chromogranin, Synaptophysin, S100, CD30, CD31, CD34, CD117, Myf-4, A-FP, oct 3/4, and PLAP was all negative. Histopathological findings were consistent with uterine tumor resembling sex cord tumor.

Due to the rare histological result of the polypectomy a computerized tomography (CT) was done and showed no abnormality. No other imaging studies were performed.

Pathological results correlated with a neoplasm of low malignant potential (subtype 1). Taking into account the

patient's age and personal preference she underwent laparoscopic total abdominal hysterectomy and bilateral salpingo-oophorectomy without the additional omentectomy and regional lymph node dissection.

No further macroscopic abnormal finding was observed in the operative field. Upon final pathological review, the uterus showed an inactive endometrium with focal ulceration, fibrin, and giant cell reaction consistent with previous polypectomy. No residual tumor was documented. An unremarkable cervix and lower uterine segments were observed; furthermore bilateral ovaries with atrophic changes and inclusion cysts as well as bilateral benign fallopian tube were described. Today, three years after the initial treatment the patient is being followed up with no evidence of recurrence.

3. Discussion

We present here an additional case report of UTROSCT. It is of utmost importance to bring forward every such patient in order to reveal the unknown complexity of this intriguing entity.

UTROSCT are rare uterine neoplasms. The differential diagnosis includes leiomyoma, endometrial polyp, and malignant neoplasm of the uterus (endometrial carcinoma and sarcoma). The initial morphologic description in the literature failed to describe whether UTROSCT represents a variant within the spectrum of endometrial stromal tumors (ESTs), which may rarely exhibit areas of sex cord-like differentiation or whether it is a distinct uterine neoplasm unrelated to ESTs [7]. The neoplasm usually occurs in middle-aged women. Most patients present with abnormal uterine bleeding and/or abdominal pain, along with an enlarged uterus or a palpable uterine mass [3]. It is now understood relatively clear that two main subtypes exist. Type I tumors which show a predominant endometrial stromal pattern with less than 50% focal ovarian sex cord component. This subtype has been tagged as ESTSCLE. These tumors also typically present cytogenetic findings which are unique to stromal tumors and are not found in the classical URTOSCT. In ESTSCLE fusion of two novel genes (JAZF1 and JJAZ1) occurs, which is not observed in UTROSCT, emphasizing that UTROSCT is another entity than ESTSCLE; however, the origin of UTROSCT remains uncertain [9]. Furthermore, it has been shown that this type has a more aggressive behavior and statistically a decreased disease free survival. Type II tumors also known as classical UTROSCT have well known histological criteria mentioned previously [5, 6]. These neoplasms present a mild clinical course and thus require a more conservative and less invasive treatment plan; nevertheless it is not unheard-of to observe recurrence even in this subtype [10]. There are no specific pathognomonic imaging findings, and the diagnosis is made exclusively on histopathologic examination. An array of architectural patterns has been introduced; these include plexiform cords, watered-silk, microfollicle, and diffuse patterns of growth [10, 11]. These findings suggest that UTROSCT may result from divergent differentiation in endometrial stromal tumors or represent a distinct group of uterine tumors with sex cord-like differentiation that are closer in histogenesis to ovarian sex cord stromal tumors [11, 12].

The most significant information from recently conducted studies concerns the immunophenotype of these lesions, especially of UTROSCT. Out of the plethora of the immunohistochemical stains, a panel of 4 stains, including Calretinin, Inhibin, CD99, and Melan A, seemed to be the most characteristic sex cord markers. Positivity for Calretinin and at least for one more of the other above-mentioned markers confirms the diagnosis of UTROSCT. Endometrial stromal tumors with sex cord-like elements, on the other hand, usually express only one of these sex cord markers, mostly Calretinin [5]. In our case report immunohistochemistry tumor cells were positive for 3 out of these four stains: Calretinin, Inhibin, and CD 99, which confirms the diagnosis. It is thus highly important to request these staining procedures in order to construct a modified custom maid treatment plan for each individual and his unique pathological findings.

Hysterectomy with or without bilateral salpingo-oophorectomy is usually the treatment for UTROSCT [2]. UTROSCT are associated with less aggressive behavior compared with ESTSCLEs, and given this fact there are no specific guidelines for the radicality of the surgical procedure, nor the need for adjuvant therapy [13].

The decision to remove the adnexa is based on the clinical status, tumor histological type, and the age of the patient. Our patient was 57 years old, with postmenopausal bleeding, and therefore, bilateral salpingectomy was performed. However, owing to the uncertain malignant potential of UTROSCT, while fertility sparing surgery in young patients could seem safe, the risks of recurrence are precipitating the need for close follow-up.

To date there are no recommendations for adjuvant chemotherapy or radiotherapy [13]. Although the prognosis of these tumors is usually favorable, we should keep in mind that these tumors may cause metastatic lesions due to malignant transformation [14]. Our patient, today, three years after treatment, is free of disease. Owing the late recurrences described in the literature, follow-up is recommended.

4. Conclusions

In this case report, a description of a patient with classical subtype UTROSCT was presented. We believe that the distinction between the two subtypes is fundamental for both gynecooncologists and the gynecopathologists in order to prevent overtreatment and supply adequate care for those rare patients.

This subclassification can be performed readily by requesting immunostaining in all subsequent pathological results. By doing so, treatment is proportionate and tailored on an individual basis. We also urge that the importance of bringing forward such similar cases in the future thus strengthens our clinical practice and management.

References

[1] A. A. Hashmi, N. Faridi, M. M. Edhi, and M. Khan, "Uterine tumor resembling ovarian sex cord tumor (UTROSCT), case report with literature review," *International Archives of Medicine*, p. 47, 2014.

[2] M. G. Uçar, T. T. Ilhan, A. Gül, C. Ugurluoglu, and Ç. Çelik, "Uterine tumour resembling ovarian sex cord tumour- A rare entity," *Journal of Clinical and Diagnostic Research*, vol. 10, no. 12, pp. QD05–QD07, 2016.

[3] J. R. Gomes, F. M. Carvalho, M. Abrão, and F. C. Maluf, "Uterine tumors resembling ovarian sex-cord tumor: A case-report and a review of literature," *Gynecologic Oncology Reports*, vol. 15, pp. 22–24, 2016.

[4] J. Sutak, D. Lazic, and J. E. Cullimore, "Uterine tumour resembling an ovarian sex cord tumour," *Journal of Clinical Pathology*, vol. 58, no. 8, pp. 888–890, 2005.

[5] E. A. Blake, T. B. Sheridan, K. L. Wang et al., "Clinical characteristics and outcomes of uterine tumors resembling ovarian sex-cord tumors (UTROSCT): a systematic review of literature," *European Journal of Obstetrics Gynecology and Reproductive Biology*, vol. 181, pp. 163–170, 2014.

[6] B. Czernobilsky, "Uterine tumors resembling ovarian sex cord tumors: an update," *International Journal of Gynecological Pathology*, vol. 27, no. 2, pp. 229–235, 2008.

[7] J. A. Irving, S. Carinelli, and J. Prat, "Uterine tumors resembling ovarian sex cord tumors are polyphenotypic neoplasms with true sex cord differentiation," *Modern Pathology*, vol. 19, no. 1, pp. 17–24, 2006.

[8] P. B. Clement and R. E. Scully, "Uterine tumors resembling ovarian sex-cord tumors: a clinicopathologic analysis of fourteen cases," *American Journal of Clinical Pathology*, vol. 66, no. 3, pp. 512–525, 1976.

[9] B. Hermsen, B. Fabrizio, B. Maaike et al., "Uterine Tumour Resembling Ovarian Sex Cord Tumour (UTROSCT): Experience with a Rare Disease. Two Case Reports and Overview of the Literature," *Obstetrics and Gynaecology Cases - Reviews*, vol. 2, no. 4, pp. 2377–9004, 2015.

[10] D. Pradhan and S. K. Mohanty, "Uterine tumors resembling ovarian sex cord tumors," *Archives of Pathology and Laboratory Medicine*, vol. 137, no. 12, pp. 1832–1836, 2013.

[11] M. Gupta, L. De Leval, M. Selig, E. Oliva, and G. P. Nielsen, "Uterine tumors resembling ovarian sex cord tumors: An ultrastructural analysis of 13 cases," *Ultrastructural Pathology*, vol. 34, no. 1, pp. 16–24, 2010.

[12] W. G. McCluggage, "Uterine tumours resembling ovarian sex cord tumours: immunohistochemical evidence for true sex cord differentiation.," *Histopathology*, vol. 34, no. 4, pp. 375-376, 1999.

[13] C.-Y. Liu, Y. Shen, J.-G. Zhao, and P.-P. Qu, "Clinical experience of uterine tumors resembling ovarian sex cord tumors: A clinicopathological analysis of 6 cases," *International Journal of Clinical and Experimental Pathology*, vol. 8, no. 4, pp. 4158–4164, 2015.

[14] K. Biermann, L. C. Heukamp, R. Büttner, and H. Zhou, "Uterine tumor resembling an ovarian sex cord tumor associated with metastasis," *International Journal of Gynecological Pathology*, vol. 27, no. 1, pp. 58–60, 2008.

11

Uterine Rupture after Laparoscopic Myomectomy in Two Cases: Real Complication or Malpractice?

Antonella Vimercati,[1] Vittoria Del Vecchio,[1] Annarosa Chincoli,[1] Antonio Malvasi,[2] and Ettore Cicinelli[1]

[1]*Department of Biomedical and Human Oncological Science (DIMO), 2nd Unit of Obstetrics and Gynaecology, University of Bari, Bari, Italy*
[2]*Santa Maria Hospital, GVM Care & Research, Bari, Italy*

Correspondence should be addressed to Vittoria Del Vecchio; vittoria.delvecchiomd@gmail.com

Academic Editor: Kyousuke Takeuchi

We describe two cases of uterine rupture in pregnancy after laparoscopic myomectomy and analyze all the aetiological factors involved in this circumstance according to the recent literature, focusing above all on the surgical procedures and the characteristics of the excised myomas. The two cases of uterine rupture in pregnancy following laparoscopic myomectomy occurred at 36 and 18 weeks of gestation, respectively. Both women had undergone laparoscopic multiple myomectomy and uterine rupture occurred along the isthmic myomectomy scars, despite the fact that compliance with all the recent technical surgical recommendations for the previous laparoscopic multiple myomectomy had been fully observed. In our cases we identified the isthmic localization, size of the excised myomas (≥4 cm), and individual characteristics of the healing process as possible risk factors for "a real complication." Larger studies and robust case-control analyses are needed to draw reliable conclusions; special care should be paid when performing laparoscopic myomectomy in women planning a later pregnancy.

1. Introduction

Uterine rupture in pregnancy is a rare and often catastrophic complication with a high incidence of fetal and maternal morbidity and mortality. The rate of uterine rupture is known to increase in patients with a history of uterine surgery, such as cesarean section and abdominal or laparoscopic myomectomy, but it can also occur in women with a native, unscarred uterus. Laparoscopic adenomyomectomies are widely performed to treat or palliate symptoms such as abnormal uterine bleeding, dysmenorrhea, pelvic and lower abdominal pain or discomfort, urinary bladder irritability, bowel dysfunction, subfertility, pregnancy complications, and pregnancy loss [1, 2]. The natural history of pregnancies following laparoscopic myomectomy is not well understood. It has been hypothesized that uterine rupture following laparoscopic myomectomy is the result of suboptimal healing, coupled with the relatively poor vascularisation of some parts of the uterus, predisposing those sites to weak scar formation after certain types of electrosurgery [3]. In comparison with abdominal myomectomy, the laparoscopic procedure is associated with less postoperative pain, a short hospital stay, and faster recovery time [4, 5]. The frequently reported complications of laparoscopic surgery generally arise due to failure to adequately suture myometrial defects, poor hemostasis with subsequent hematoma formation or excessive use of monopolar or bipolar electrosurgery, and hence devascularization of the myometrium, which can interfere with myometrial wound healing and increase the risk of rupture [6]. Uterine rupture refers to a complete separation of all the uterine layers [7] and of the overlying visceral peritoneum and is often associated with clinically significant paroxysmal pain, uterine bleeding, fetal distress, and even protrusion or expulsion of the fetus and/or placenta into the abdominal cavity. It entails the need for prompt cesarean delivery, uterine repair, or hysterectomy. From the time of diagnosis to delivery, generally only 10–37 minutes elapse before clinically significant fetal morbidity becomes inevitable. Fetal morbidity occurs as a result of catastrophic hemorrhage, fetal anoxia, or both. The diagnosis of uterine rupture is made by clinical observation and can be confirmed by ultrasound imaging. Several aetiological factors have been identified, and here we report our experience of two cases of uterine rupture after previous laparoscopic myomectomy, focusing on the characteristics of the surgery, and the type, localization, and size of the fibroids. In this regard, the new US classification of myomas, MUSA 2015 (morphological uterus sonographic assessment; [8, 9]) introduced to define and standardize US imaging of uterus fibroids, could be useful to better correlate the localization and characteristics of myoma before laparoscopy and reduce the risk of rupture in pregnancy. We considered the site of fibroids according to this classification as G0 = pedunculated intracavitary; G1 = submucosal < 50% intramural; G2 = submucosal $\geq$ 50% intramural; G3 = 100% intramural, but in contact with the endometrium; G4 = intramural; G5 = subserosal $\geq$ 50% intramural; G6 = subserosal < 50% intramural; G7 = subserosal pedunculated; G8 = other (e.g., cervical, parasitic).

2. Cases Presentation

In the last five years of our clinical and surgical activity 3800 cesarean deliveries (CS) have been performed and in 57 cases (1.5%) cesarean deliveries followed a laparoscopic myomectomy. We report the only two cases (3.5%) of uterine rupture that occurred among these 57 CS following laparoscopic myomectomy. The first case was a 31-year-old woman para 0/0/1/0 hospitalized for abdominal pain of sudden onset in the 34th week of gestation [10]. She had undergone laparoscopic multiple myomectomy 2 years earlier, when different types of myoma were excised: one intramural- (IM-) G4 myoma of the posterior wall of the uterus with a mean diameter (diam.) of 5 cm, one IM-G5 left isthmic myoma (diam. 3 cm), one IM-G4 on the fundus (diam. 3 cm), one subserosal- (SS-) G6 of the right wall (diam. 2 cm), and two IM-G4 of the anterior wall of the uterus (diam. 2 cm each one). At the first clinical examination, the findings were deep abdominal pain, dysuria, and a positive Giordano's sign on the right. Her blood pressure was 132/66 mmHg and heart rate 77 beats/min. She was afebrile and not pale. The fetus was alive at cardiotocographic evaluation. There were no palpable uterine contractions, although the patient was groaning with pain. The cervix was closed and there was no evidence of vaginal bleeding. We performed transabdominal 2D ultrasound that showed an alive intrauterine podalic fetus with normal Doppler flowmetry, oligohydramnios, and minimal intraperitoneal fluid; the patient complained of increasing pain on the left side of the abdomen, where ultrasound revealed the presence of a vascularised area whose venous and arterial flow seemed to be in continuity with the umbilical cord and had the same ultrasound characteristics (Figure 1(a)). This vascularised area was located outside the left wall of the uterus and was likely an early sign of uterine rupture (Figure 1(b)). The breach seemed to be 2 cm long on the left wall of the uterus, at the level of one of the previous laparoscopic myomectomy wounds. Continuous cardiotocographic assessment showed a normal fetal heartbeat and the

absence of uterine contractions, but the patient continued to complain of abdominal discomfort and started vomiting. An emergency laparotomy was performed. Surgical findings included a breach running horizontally through the entire anterior wall of the uterus (Figure 1(c)), a moderate quantity of hemoperitoneum, while the fetus had turned so that the left shoulder was facing the abdominal cavity. The baby was delivered alive with the placenta, and no emergency procedure was required. The tear was repaired and the hemoperitoneum drained. The patient made satisfactory clinical progress and was discharged home with a healthy baby on the fifth postoperative day; neonatal follow-up was regular.

The second case was a 37-year-old woman, para 0/0/0/0, at 18 weeks of gestation, referred for pregnancy termination due to fetal abnormalities. She, too, had undergone laparoscopic multiple myomectomy 3 years earlier, when two types of myomas were excised: an IM-G5 left isthmic myoma (4 cm) (Figure 2(a)) and a SS-G6 myoma on the fundus (5 cm).

Abortion was induced with vaginal prostaglandin suppositories. Three hours after the administration of the third suppository, the patient began to complain of deep, persistent abdominal pain. On examination, the abdomen was tender, the cervix 2 cm was dilated, and there was evidence of vaginal bleeding. Her blood pressure was 80/50 mmHg and heart rate 120 beats/min. Because of the increasing pain, not correlated with fetal expulsion, and of the worsening clinical conditions, we performed transabdominal 2D ultrasound that showed, inside the peritoneal cavity, herniation of the amniotic sac and fetus through the uterine wall along the previous isthmic laparoscopic myomectomy scar (Figure 2(b)).

The treatment team decided to proceed with laparotomy under general anesthesia. The entire amniotic sac containing the fetus protruded through uterine isthmic breach and about 800 mL hemoperitoneum was detected and drained. The amniotic fluid was clear and odor-free; the placenta was located on the fundus and removed. The tear was repaired in two layers and the patient was discharged 4 days later.

In both cases, the previous laparoscopic myomectomy recording was examined together with the surgeon. There had been no mistakes in the surgical technique related to uterine closure: multiple layer suturing (three-layer) had been performed, the electrosurgery (bipolar coagulation) was gentle, there was no excessive bleeding, and entry into the endometrial cavity had been avoided. Moreover, the two patients had suffered no postoperative complications such as hematoma or infections, which could have interfered with correct wound healing. Compliance with all the recent technical surgical recommendations had been observed.

In the remaining 55 cases of CS after a previous myomectomy, who had suffered no complications in the following pregnancy, the previous myoma was single in 20 cases with the following characteristics: 4 G2 (3 with a mean diameter > 4 cm; no case with an isthmic site); 6 G3 (2 with a mean diameter > 4 cm, 1 isthmic myoma with a diameter of 2 cm); 5 G4 (4 with a mean diameter > 4 cm and no case of isthmic myoma); and 5 G5 (all with a diameter > 5 cm and no case of isthmic myoma). In the other 35 cases of different-sized multiple myomas in various sites, only in one case was the

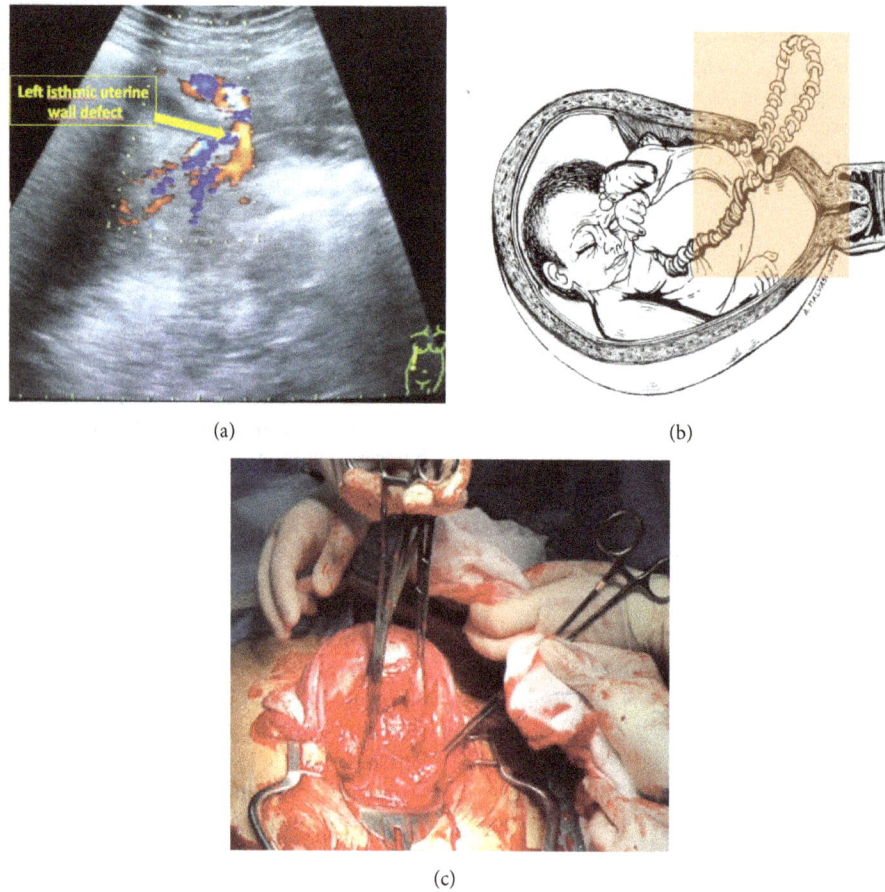

FIGURE 1: (a) 2D transabdominal US and color Doppler findings: a loop of umbilical cord was noted outside the uterus and running through the left isthmic uterine wall focal defect. (b) Graphic depiction of the loop of umbilical cord herniated outside the uterus through the left isthmic focal defect. (c) Macroscopic appearance of the uterine rupture at surgery.

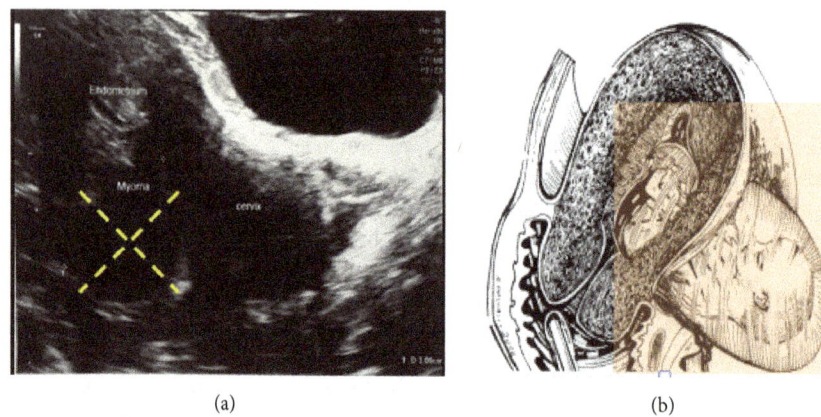

FIGURE 2: (a) 2D transvaginal ultrasound of the IM isthmic myoma type 5. (b) Graphic depiction of the herniated fetus through the isthmic defect on the previous myomectomy scar.

myoma, with a mean diameter of 1.5 cm, localized in the isthmic area. No statistically significant conclusions can be drawn due to the small sample size.

3. Discussion

Rupture of a pregnant uterus is one of the life-threatening complications encountered in obstetric practice. Although it may occur in an unscarred uterus, the most common cause of uterine rupture is splitting of a previous cesarean scar. Several aetiological factors may be responsible for rupture of the uterus, including previous cesarean section or laparotomic/laparoscopic adenomyomectomy, trauma, uterine overdistension, uterine anomalies, placenta percreta, and choriocarcinoma [11, 12]. Uterine rupture implies a defect in the uterine musculature, with extravasation of fetal parts and intra-amniotic contents into the peritoneal cavity [13, 14]. It is difficult to make a realistic estimation of the rate of uterine rupture after laparoscopic myomectomy. Several recent studies including large numbers of cases have reported on the efficacy of laparoscopic myomectomy: in a multicenter study, Sizzi et al. evaluated 2050 operations and reported 1 rupture among 386 pregnancies; Malzoni et al. evaluated 982 operations and reported no uterine ruptures [1]. In our experience there seems to be a higher prevalence of uterine rupture after previous laparoscopic myomectomy (3%) but it must be remembered that one of the two cases occurred during the induction of pregnancy termination, in a high risk condition. Our series is still too small for a realistic estimation of the risk.

Uterine rupture after laparoscopic myomectomy is one of the complications of the procedure. It depends on wound healing that can be affected by various factors such as the method and tools used for uterine incision, unsuccessful hemostasis and closing of the myometrial defect [15], the extent of local tissue destruction, the potential formation of infection or hematoma within the myometrium, gas pneumoperitoneum in laparoscopic procedures, and, finally, the individual characteristics of the healing process related to the production of growth factors or excess collagen deposition [6]. Meticulous closure of the myometrial bed following myomectomy can be difficult via laparoscopy and could therefore interfere with the integrity of the scar [3]. Uterine rupture during pregnancy seems to occur more frequently as a consequence of laparoscopic than laparotomic myomectomy [2–16], although this finding is extremely limited because it depends on few reported cases (such as our submitted cases) and has provoked debate in the recent literature. After abdominal myomectomies the scars are of similar thickness to normal myometrium, whereas after laparoscopic procedures they are strained, more contracted, and thinner than normal myometrium. These differences are likely due to the use of sutures to achieve hemostasis during abdominal myomectomy, versus bipolar coagulation during laparoscopic myomectomy. In the latter, the resulting thermal damage to the myometrium induces a proliferation of connective tissue, which cannot undergo remodeling during pregnancy [6]. Malvasi et al. evaluated the presence of neuropeptide substance P and vasoactive intestinal peptide in the pseudocapsule of uterine myomas. Because these neuropeptides may affect wound healing and myometrial function in a subsequent pregnancy, the pseudocapsule neurovascular bundle should be carefully treated, avoiding damaging practices such as an extensive use of coagulation [1]. A study of uterine wound healing using magnetic resonance imaging demonstrated completion of the uterine healing process at 12 weeks after abdominal myomectomy in the absence of hematoma or oedema formation in the myometrium [6]. A study of laparoscopic myomectomy scars identified hematomas in 74% of women one day after surgery, probably due to closure of the uterine defect with only a single layer of sutures. Expert opinion recommends that intraoperative strategies to reduce uterine rupture in subsequent pregnancies include multilayer uterine closure, avoidance of entry into the endometrial cavity, avoidance of excessive electrosurgery to reduce devascularization, and the prevention of haematoma formation, which may affect wound strength [17, 18]. In our experience of two cases there were no surgical laparoscopic factors related to the risk of uterine rupture.

The size and number of the myomas removed, whether entering the endometrial cavity or not, have also been identified as potential factors affecting the risk of uterine rupture in subsequent pregnancies. In the seven uterine ruptures described by Pistofidis et al., the maximum myoma diameter was 4.4 cm, while in 5 patients it was ≤5 cm. Six patients had a single myoma. Only one patient had an intramural myoma, while all the others had subserosal and/or pedunculated myomas. In the research carried out by Parker et al. who described nineteen cases of uterine rupture, the greatest diameter of dissected myomas ranged from 1 to 11 cm (mean, 4.5 cm) [6]. Two small myomas (both 1.2 cm) were removed in 1 woman and 1 myoma in all the others. Pedunculated subserous myomas were removed in 4 women, subserosal myomas in 5, and intramural myomas in 10 [6]. In both our reported cases, the size (>4 cm), isthmic localization, and level of involvement of the myometrial wall (>50%, IM myoma-G5) [9] seem to be risk factors for uterine rupture. The MUSA classification [8] can be considered to better classify myomas before adenomyomectomy and to better predict the risk of uterine rupture in subsequent pregnancies, regarding site and size of myoma. However, due to limited evidence in this field, these factors remain a topic for debate [17].

In conclusion, despite evidence that laparoscopic myomectomy is associated with remarkable benefits, there is one concern that has still to be resolved: is this procedure associated with a higher risk of subsequent uterine rupture compared with open (via laparotomy) myomectomy? Excessive use of diathermy for hemostasis should be avoided and multiple layer suturing should always be done to repair the myometrial defect in cases of deep intramural and subserosal myomas. Our cases of uterine rupture despite observance of all the recent technical surgical recommendations during the previous laparoscopic multiple myomectomy underline the point. Larger studies are needed to better understand whether uterine rupture after laparoscopic myomectomy is a "real" complication of the procedure or a possible "malpractice."

Acknowledgments

The authors would like to thank the study investigators and surgeons that performed laparoscopic adenomyomectomy and emergency laparotomy in the described cases, including O. Ceci, S. Santamato, S. Bettocchi, and F. Caradonna.

References

[1] G. Pistofidis, E. Makrakis, P. Balinakos, E. Dimitriou, N. Bardis, and V. Anaf, "Report of 7 Uterine Rupture Cases After Laparoscopic Myomectomy: Update of the Literature," *Journal of Minimally Invasive Gynecology*, vol. 19, no. 6, pp. 762–767, 2012.

[2] K. J. Carlson, B. A. Miller, and F. J. Fowler, "The Maine Women's Health Study," *Obstetrics & Gynecology*, vol. 83, no. 4, pp. 556–565, 1994.

[3] D. C. Nkemayim, M. E. Hammadeh, M. Hippach, D. Mink, and W. Schmidt, "Uterine rupture in pregnancy subsequent to previous laparoscopic electromyolysis. Case report and review of the literature," *Archives of Gynecology and Obstetrics*, vol. 264, no. 3, pp. 154–156, 2000.

[4] C. Jin, Y. Hu, X.-C. Chen et al., "Laparoscopic versus open myomectomy—a meta-analysis of randomized controlled trials," *European Journal of Obstetrics & Gynecology and Reproductive Biology*, vol. 145, no. 1, pp. 14–21, 2009.

[5] C. Nezhat, F. Nezhat, S. L. Silfen, N. Schaffer, and D. Evans, "Laparoscopic myomectomy," *International Journal of Fertility & Sterility*, vol. 36, no. 5, pp. 275–280, 1991.

[6] W. H. Parker, J. Einarsson, O. Istre, and J.-B. Dubuisson, "Risk factors for uterine rupture after laparoscopic myomectomy," *Journal of Minimally Invasive Gynecology*, vol. 17, no. 5, pp. 551–554, 2010.

[7] J. Y. Woo, L. Tate, S. Roth, and A. C. Eke, "Silent Spontaneous Uterine Rupture at 36 Weeks of Gestation," *Case Reports in Obstetrics and Gynecology*, vol. 2015, Article ID 596826, 3 pages, 2015.

[8] T. Van Den Bosch, M. Dueholm, F. P. G. Leone et al., "Terms, definitions and measurements to describe sonographic features of myometrium and uterine masses: A consensus opinion from the Morphological Uterus Sonographic Assessment (MUSA) group," *Ultrasound in Obstetrics & Gynecology*, vol. 46, no. 3, pp. 284–298, 2015.

[9] F. D. Fascilla, P. Cramarossa, R. Cannone, C. Olivieri, A. Vimercati, and C. Exacoustos, "Ultrasound diagnosis of uterine myomas," *Minerva Ginecologica*, vol. 68, no. 3, pp. 297–312, 2016.

[10] V. Del Vecchio, A. Chincoli, F. Caradonna, and A. Vimercati, "US-color Doppler early diagnosis of uterine rupture with protrusion of umbilical cord," *Journal of Prenatal Medicine*, vol. 10, no. 1/2, p. 1, 2016.

[11] G. I. Ogbole, O. A. Ogunseyinde, and A. L. Akinwuntan, "Intrapartum rupture of the uterus diagnosed by ultrasound," *African Health Sciences*, vol. 8, no. 1, pp. 57–59, 2008.

[12] C. S. Claydon and M. L. Pernoll, "Third-trimester vaginal bleeding," in *Current Obstetric and Gynaecologic Diagnosis and Treatment*, A. H. DeCherney and L. Nathan, Eds., pp. 354–368, Lange/McGraw Hill, New York, NY, USA, 9th edition, 2003.

[13] Y. S. Jo, M. J. Kim, G. S. R. Lee, and S. J. Kim, "A large amniocele with protruded umbilical cord diagnosed by 3D ultra-sound," *International Journal of Medical Sciences*, vol. 9, no. 5, pp. 387–390, 2012.

[14] A. Golan, O. Sandbank, and A. Rubin, "Rupture of the pregnant uterus," *Obstetrics & Gynecology*, vol. 56, pp. 594–654, 1980.

[15] M. A. Pelosi III and M. A. Pelosi, "Spontaneous uterine rupture at thirty-three weeks subsequent to previous superficial laparoscopic myomectomy," *American Journal of Obstetrics & Gynecology*, vol. 177, no. 6, pp. 1547–1549, 1997.

[16] Y. Nagao, K. Osato, M. Kubo, T. Kawamura, T. Ikeda, and T. Yamawaki, "Spontaneous uterine rupture in the 35th week of gestation after laparoscopic adenomyomectomy," *International Medical Case Reports Journal*, vol. 9, pp. 1–4, 2015.

[17] C. Sutton, P. Standen, J. Acton, and C. Griffin, "Spontaneous Uterine Rupture in a Preterm Pregnancy following Myomectomy," *Case Reports in Obstetrics and Gynecology*, vol. 2016, Article ID 6195621, 4 pages, 2016.

[18] C. Koh and G. Janik, "Laparoscopic myomectomy: The current status," *Current Opinion in Obstetrics and Gynecology*, vol. 15, no. 4, pp. 295–301, 2003.

12

Profound Hypokalaemia Resulting in Maternal Cardiac Arrest: A Catastrophic Complication of Hyperemesis Gravidarum?

Anna Walch ⓘ,[1,2,3] Madeline Duke,[4,5,6] Travis Auty,[2,7,8] and Audris Wong[9,10,11,12]

[1] Doctor of Medicine (MD), Griffith University, Australia
[2] Lecturer, School of Medicine, Griffith University, Australia
[3] Obstetrics and Gynaecology Principal House Officer, Gold Coast University Hospital, Australia
[4] Bachelor of Medicine and Bachelor of Surgery (MBBS), Bond University, Australia
[5] Obstetric Medicine Fellow, Royal Brisbane and Women's Hospital, Australia
[6] Endocrine Advanced Trainee, Royal Brisbane and Women's Hospital, Australia
[7] Bachelor of Medicine and Bachelor of Surgery (MBBS), Griffith University, Australia
[8] Intensive Care Unit Registrar, Gold Coast University Hospital, Australia
[9] Obstetrics and Gynaecology Staff Specialist, Gold Coast University Hospital, Australia
[10] FRANZCOG (Fellowship of the Royal Australian and New Zealand College of Obstetricians and Gynaecologists), Australia
[11] MRCOG (Membership of the Royal college of Obstetricians and Gynaecologist), UK
[12] MRCPI (Membership of the Royal College of Physicians in Ireland (Obstetrics and Gynaecology and General Medicine)), Ireland

Correspondence should be addressed to Anna Walch; anna.walch@griffithuni.edu.au

Academic Editor: Kyousuke Takeuchi

We present a case of a 39-year-old G8P6 Pacific Islander woman who at 15+5 weeks' gestation had an out-of-hospital cardiac arrest secondary to profound hypokalaemia which was associated with severe hyperemesis gravidarum (HG). Her clinical course after arrest was complicated by a second 5-minute cardiac arrest in the Intensive Care Unit (ICU) (pre-arrest potassium 1.8), anuric renal failure requiring dialysis, ischaemic hepatitis, and encephalopathy and unfortunately fetal demise and a spontaneous miscarriage on day 2 of admission. Despite these complications, she was discharged home 4 weeks later with a full recovery. Following a plethora of inpatient and outpatient investigations, the cause of her cardiac arrest was determined to be profound hypokalaemia. The hypokalaemia was presumed second to a perfect storm of HG with subsequent nutritional deficiencies causing electrolyte wasting, extracellular fluid (ECF) volume reduction, and activation of the renin-angiotensin-aldosterone axis (RAAS). This combined with the physiological changes that promote potassium wasting in pregnancy including volume expansion, increased renal blood flow, increased glomerular filtration rate, and increase in cortisol contributed to the patient having a profoundly low total body potassium level. This diagnosis is further strengthened by the fact that her pre- and post-pregnancy potassium levels were within normal limits in the absence of supplementary potassium. This case highlights the potentially life-threatening electrolyte imbalances that can occur with HG and the importance of recognising the disease, comprehensive electrolyte monitoring, and aggressive management in pregnancy.

1. Background

Hyperemesis gravidarum (HG) is a severe form of nausea and vomiting that affects 0.3–3% of pregnancies [1]. It is characterised by severe, protracted nausea and vomiting associated with weight loss of more than 5% of pre-pregnancy weight, dehydration, and electrolyte imbalances [2, 3]. HG can be associated with significant morbidity including pneumomediastinum, renal failure, liver dysfunction, Boerhaave's syndrome, and Wernicke's encephalopathy [1]. In the fetus, it is also associated with an increased risk of adverse pregnancy outcomes including low birth weight, neurodevelopmental disorders, intrauterine growth restriction, preterm delivery, and fetal and neonatal death [4]. Although maternal death

TABLE 1: Serum electrolytes.

	Pre-pregnancy	On Admission	On discharge from hospital
Potassium K^+ (mmol/L) range 3.5-5.2	3.8	2.1	3.9
Magnesium Mg^{2+} (mmol/L) range 0.75-1.1	0.89	1.25	0.82
Phosphate PO^4_{3-} (mmol/L) range 0.75-1.50	1.32	4.95	1.27

TABLE 2: Venous blood gas (VBG) on arrival to the emergency department.

pH range 7.35-7.45	6.71	Haemoglobin (g/L) range 110-140	108
pC02 (mmHg) range 35-45	102	Sodium Na^+ (mmol/L) range 135-145	135
Bicarbonate HCO_3^- (mmol/L) range 22-28	12	Potassium K^+ (mmol/L) range 3.5-5.2	2.1
Anion gap (mmol/L) range 4-12	34	Chloride Cl^- (mmol/L) range 98-106	91
Lactate (mmol/L) range 0.5-2	26.0	Glucose (mmol/L) range 3.9-7.5	22.0

is a rare complication of HG, there are still reported cases of it annually in first-world countries [4]. This is the first case report detailing a case of cardiac arrest from hypokalaemia second to HG and presents the critical importance of proactively managing nutritional and metabolic imbalances associated with HG.

2. Case

We present a case of a 39-year-old G8P6M1 Pacific Islander woman who at 15+5 weeks gestation was brought in by ambulance following an out-of-hospital cardiac arrest. The arrest was witnessed by her family at home who contacted the ambulance service and commenced cardiopulmonary resuscitation (CPR). She was resuscitated at the scene involving CPR with approximately 40 minutes downtime, cold intubation, and multiple direct current cardioversions for stabilisation. On arrival to the emergency department she had fixed dilated pupils and was found to be significantly acidotic (pH 6.7, lactate 26mmol/L) with associated hypokalaemia of 2.1mmol/L (range 3.5-5.2mmol/L) (see Tables 1 and 2). Her initial resuscitation and stabilisation involved a potassium infusion up to 40 mmol/hr and an adrenaline and nora-drenaline infusion, 4 units of packed red blood cells, and 4 units of albumin. Following stabilisation and electrolyte repletion, she had a second 5-minute ventricular fibrillation (VF) arrest 4 hours later in the ICU, where her potassium on her preceding venous blood gas was 1.8mmol/L. She was commenced on 300mg of IV Thiamine daily from day one of her ICU admission. On day one of admission, the pregnancy was still viable with a FHR of 150beats per minute detected. Unfortunately, on day two of her admission, there was fetal demise and she spontaneously miscarried in the ICU and required a dilatation and curettage for retained products of conception. Her inpatient stay was complicated by multiorgan dysfunction including ischaemic hepatitis, mild encephalopathy requiring rehabilitation, and anuric renal failure requiring short-term dialysis.

The patient's pregnancy history was unremarkable preceding the out-of-hospital cardiac arrest except for an early positive oral glucose tolerance test (OGTT) (in the absence of evidence of type 2 diabetes mellitus with a normal HbA1C)

TABLE 3: Oral glucose tolerance test.

Fasting plasma glucose	5.4 mmol/L (range <5.1)
1-hour glucose	7.5 mmol/L (range <10.0)
2-hour glucose	7.6 mmol/L (range <8.5)

TABLE 4: Urinary electrolytes/cortisol (24hr collection).

Potassium K+	49 mmol/24hr (range 25-125)
Creatinine	12.5 mmol/24hr (range 6.0 – 14.0)
Cortisol (free)	26 nmol/24hr (range 10 - 120)

performed at 13 weeks' gestation (see Table 3). On the day of her arrest her husband did not notice any additional symptoms and her nausea and vomiting did not particularly worsen, but she did manage to tolerate a small lunch meal prior to arresting. She had a background history of 5 previous pregnancies to the same partner, complicated by some nausea and vomiting in those pregnancies, with no definitive evidence of HG. In this pregnancy, from an early gestation, the patient confirmed the presence of significant nausea and vomiting, with emesis occurring after every meal on most days. She had limited oral intake as a result and ensuing weight loss occured with approximately 10kg's lost in total (9% of total body weight).

The patient's background medical history was otherwise unremarkable with no symptoms or biochemical evidence of a disorder of potassium homeostasis preceding the pregnancy. Specifically, she denied symptoms to suggest hypokalaemic periodic paralysis and serial serum electrolyte testing revealed normal potassium levels before and after pregnancy (see Table 1). Urine electrolyte testing was also unremarkable postpartum, with no evidence of renal potassium wasting (see Table 4). Furthermore, she had no history to suggest an arrhythmogenic disorder with no palpitations, presyncope, or syncope reported. She had no significant family history of cardiomyopathy or sudden cardiac death and no personal history of valvular heart disease or rheumatic fever. She denied symptoms to suggest thyroid disease and pre-pregnancy had normal Thyroid Stimulating Hormone

(TSH) levels on serial testing, including a normal TSH level at 7-weeks gestation. She was not hypertensive, and there was no evidence of primary hyperaldosteronism on testing. There was no clinical evidence of cortisol excess, and screening 24-hour urinary free cortisol was normal. She was not on any regular medications and had no known drug allergies.

The patient was thoroughly investigated for causes and contributors to her cardiac arrest. Results of cardiac investigations included a normal coronary angiogram, normal left ventricle ventriculogram, and a transoesophageal echocardiogram which demonstrated preserved biventricular systolic function and structurally normal valves with moderate mitral regurgitation. She had a normal computed tomography pulmonary angiogram (CTPA) with no evidence of pulmonary embolism. She had a largely normal CT head with a 10mm filling defect in her left transverse sinus but nil other acute pathology. She had a normal baseline electrocardiogram (ECG) post-arrest with no evidence of long QT syndrome.

Following stabilisation and correction of her potassium (see Table 1) and acute renal failure, she was discharged home after a total 33-day admission. She transitioned well to home where she is continuing to care for her children, the youngest of which is 3 years old. She is independent with her activities of daily living and mobility and only suffered from mild short-term memory impairment and mild impairment in her concrete problem solving. Importantly, her serum potassium level remains normal.

3. Discussion

A case of maternal cardiac arrest second to profound hypokalaemia in a patient with HG presents a unique opportunity to discuss the potential implications of this common disorder. A patient with HG frequently vomits gastric juice and, thus, the loss of hydrogen ions, sodium, chloride, and water in gastric contents leads to chloride-sensitive metabolic alkalosis, dehydration, and extracellular fluid (ECF) volume reduction [5]. Our patient had lost approximately 9% in body weight and likely was volume deplete, causing elevated activity of the renin-angiotensin-aldosterone system (RAAS) [5]. This activated RAAS, in turn, increases the urinary excretion of potassium, compounding the hypokalaemia [6]. This severe hypokalaemia eventually led to her sudden cardiac arrest. On presentation, her potassium was low at 2.1mmol/L. This was an unexpected finding in a patient post-cardiac arrest. It is more common after arrest to see hyperkalaemia due to the exchange of potassium ions with hydrogen ions and the movement of intracellular potassium to the extracellular space in an attempt to correct the acidosis [6]. It was presumed that her hypokalaemia was much more severe prior to her arresting.

Many of the reported serious morbidity and even mortality second to HG in the literature have presented with Wernicke's encephalopathy (WE) or associated thyrotoxicosis. There are increasing reports of maternal mortality secondary to WE from HG which is caused by thiamine (vitamin B1) deficiency [7, 8]. WE typically manifests with nonspecific symptoms of headache, confusion, and irritability but then progresses to spastic paresis, ataxia, oculomotor dysfunction, myoclonus, and nuchal rigidity [7, 8]. Rarely, thiamine deficiency can cause cardiovascular compromise which is termed "wet beriberi" which could eventually lead to cardiac arrest [9]. Wet beriberi presents with clinical signs of congestive cardiac failure including tachycardia, dyspnoea, peripheral oedema, and cardiomegaly with normal sinus rhythm [9]. Our patient and her family denied any presence of these signs and symptoms as well as no preceding symptoms of WE including weakness, confusion, or ataxia. After arrest, our patient had no significant abnormalities on echocardiogram suggesting no involvement of thiamine deficiency as a cause for her cardiovascular compromise. Macgibbon reports a mortality of a pregnant patient who had respiratory failure second to HG, hypokalaemia, and Wernicke's encephalopathy [8]. That patient, however, presented with symptoms of slurred speech, confusion, and weakness and subsequently later died from rapid correction of hyponatremia causing osmotic demyelination syndrome and respiratory arrest [8]. However, given her history of HG, our patient was treated with 300mg of IV thiamine daily from admission which is the gold standard treatment for thiamine deficiency and WE.

There is a case report by Iwashita [10] that attributes hypokalaemia second to HG as a cause of arrest and maternal death. The authors report on an obese pregnant woman who suffered a respiratory arrest at 12+4 weeks' gestation that was attributed to severe HG causing profound hypokalaemia. They attributed the respiratory arrest to severe potassium deficiency causing respiratory muscle paralysis and this was compounded by obesity [10].

There have been several case reports of refeeding syndrome causing severe hypokalaemia in pregnancy. Refeeding syndrome is usually seen in the context of increased caloric intake after prolonged periods of malnutrition. For example, Majumdar reports a case of refeeding syndrome after treatment of severe HG with NJ feeds [11]. Refeeding syndrome manifests as severe hypophosphataemia, hypokalaemia, hypomagnesaemia, fluid retention, and altered glucose homeostasis [11]. Against this diagnosis, our patient presented with marked hyperphosphataemia (4.95mmol/L) and hypermagnesaemia (1.25mmol/L) which is inconsistent with the electrolyte derangement that are the hallmarks of refeeding syndrome [12, 13].

Fezjo et al. report that five out of six patients in their case series who died from complications secondary to HG, presented with hypokalaemia [4]. Therefore, patients who present with HG accompanied by hypokalaemia may represent a high-risk subgroup that should be closely monitored and treated until complete and prolonged stabilisation of potassium and other electrolyte levels is achieved. The importance of potassium homeostasis is highlighted by the finding that patients with potassium abnormalities have an increased rate of death from any cause [4].

First it must be highlighted that although the most likely cause of hypokalaemia in this case was hyperemesis; some rare differentials cannot be completely excluded. One is hypokalaemic periodic paralysis, which could be exacerbated by undiagnosed hyperthyroidism in pregnancy [14]. This cannot be completely disproved as there were no thyroid function tests (TFTs) performed at the time of the cardiac arrest. However, the fact that TFTs earlier in the pregnancy and subsequent TFTs shortly after the miscarriage were normal (*T4 9.8pmol/L ref 7.0-17, T3 5.4pmol/L ref 3.5-6.0 and TSH 1.1mU/L ref 0.3-4.5*) makes this diagnosis highly unlikely. Additionally, the patient reported no previous history to suggest periodic paralysis, even though this condition is more common in people of Pacific Islanders descent [15].

Other rare differential diagnoses include a tubulointerstitial disorder resulting in excessive renal potassium wasting. One example of such a disorder is Gitelman's syndrome [5]. This is extremely unlikely given that she had normal urinary electrolytes with no evidence of sodium or potassium wasting outside of pregnancy and no personal or family history to suggest this [16]. But it has been considered that the patient could excessively waste urinary potassium in pregnancy exclusively.

4. Conclusion

This is a unique case of profound hypokalaemia in pregnancy resulting in maternal cardiac arrest. The most likely aetiology was gestational emesis and gestational diabetes mellitus which aggravated the normal potassium wasting of pregnancy; however, it is impossible to exclude all potential contributors to the development of hypokalaemia in a patient with no preceding or post-event electrolyte derangements. This case highlights the fact that HG can cause profound metabolic and electrolyte disturbances in patients with the potential for resultant catastrophic consequences. Clinicians should consider performing a serum screening of electrolytes in all patients who report persistent severe nausea and vomiting in pregnancy with associated weight loss and appropriately correct the imbalances.

References

[1] P. C. Tan, R. Jacob, K. F. Quek, and S. Z. Omar, "Pregnancy outcome in hyperemesis gravidarum and the effect of laboratory clinical indicators of hyperemesis severity," *Journal of Obstetrics and Gynaecology Research*, vol. 33, no. 4, pp. 457–464, 2007.

[2] M. N. Niemeijer, I. J. Grooten, N. Vos et al., "Diagnostic markers for hyperemesis gravidarum: a systematic review and metaanalysis," *American Journal of Obstetrics & Gynecology*, vol. 211, no. 2, pp. 150.e1–150.e15, 2014.

[3] M. Bustos, R. Venkataramanan, and S. Caritis, "Nausea and vomiting of pregnancy - What's new?" *Autonomic Neuroscience: Basic and Clinical*, vol. 202, pp. 62–72, 2017.

[4] M. S. Fejzo and K. MacGibbon, "Why are women still dying from nausea and vomiting of pregnancy?" *Gynecology & Obstetrics Case Report*, vol. 2, article 2, 2016.

[5] M. C. Acelajado, R. M. Culpepper, and W. D. Bolton III, "Hyperemesis gravidarum in undiagnosed Gitelman's syndrome," *Case Reports in Medicine*, vol. 2016, Article ID 2407607, 4 pages, 2016.

[6] P. S. Aronson and G. Giebisch, "Effects of pH on potassium: New explanations for old observations," *Journal of the American Society of Nephrology*, vol. 22, no. 11, pp. 1981–1989, 2011.

[7] S. J. Scalzo, S. C. Bowden, M. L. Ambrose, G. Whelan, and M. J. Cook, "Wernicke-Korsakoff syndrome not related to alcohol use: a systematic review," *Journal of Neurology, Neurosurgery & Psychiatry*, vol. 86, no. 12, pp. 1362–1368, 2015.

[8] K. W. MacGibbon, M. S. Fejzo, and P. M. Mullin, "Mortality secondary to hyperemesis gravidarum: a case report," *Women's Health & Gynecology*, vol. 6, no. 2, 2015.

[9] N. Huertas-González, V. Hernando-Requejo, Z. Luciano-García, and J. L. Cervera-Rodilla, "Wernicke's encephalopathy, wet beriberi, and polyneuropathy in a patient with folate and thiamine deficiency related to gastric phytobezoar," *Case Reports in Neurological Medicine*, vol. 2015, Article ID 624807, 5 pages, 2015.

[10] A. Iwashita, Y. Baba, R. Usui, A. Ohkuchi, S. Muto, and S. Matsubara, "Respiratory arrest in an obese pregnant woman with hyperemesis gravidarum," *Case Reports in Obstetrics and Gynecology*, vol. 2015, Article ID 278391, 4 pages, 2015.

[11] S. Majumdar and B. Dada, "Refeeding syndrome: a serious and potentially life-threatening complication of severe hyperemesis gravidarum," *Journal of Obstetrics & Gynaecology*, vol. 30, no. 4, pp. 416-417, 2010.

[12] L. Chiarenza, A. Pignataro, and V. Lanza, "Refeeding syndrome in early pregnancy. Case report," *Minerva Anestesiologica*, vol. 71, no. 12, pp. 803–808, 2005.

[13] M. A. Marinella, "Refeeding syndrome and hypophosphatemia," *Journal of Intensive Care Medicine*, vol. 20, no. 3, pp. 155–159, 2005.

[14] A. W. C. Kung, "Clinical Review: thyrotoxic periodic paralysis: a diagnostic challenge," *The Journal of Clinical Endocrinology & Metabolism*, vol. 91, no. 7, pp. 2490–2495, 2006.

[15] M. S. Elston, B. J. Orr-Walker, A. M. Dissanayake, and J. V. Conaglen, "Thyrotoxic, hypokalaemic periodic paralysis: polynesians, an ethnic group at risk," *Internal Medicine Journal*, vol. 37, no. 5, pp. 303–307, 2007.

[16] I. Kurtz, "Molecular pathogenesis of Bartter's and Gitelman's syndromes," *Kidney International*, vol. 54, no. 4, pp. 1396–1410, 1998.

13

Interstitial Pregnancy: From Medical to Surgical Approach—Report of Three Cases

L. Di Tizio,[1] **M. R. Spina ⓘ,**[1,2] **S. Gustapane,**[3] **F. D'Antonio,**[4,5] **and M. Liberati**[1,2,6]

[1]*Department of Obstetrics and Gynecology, SS Annunziata Hospital, Chieti, Italy*
[2]*Department of Medicine and Aging Sciences University "G. d'Annunzio" of Chieti-Pescara, Italy*
[3]*Department of Obstetrics and Gynecology, Casa di Cura Salus srl, Brindisi, Italy*
[4]*Women's Health and Perinatology Research Group, Department of Clinical Medicine,*
Faculty of Health Sciences, UiT-The Arctic University of Norway, Tromsø, Norway
[5]*Department of Obstetrics and Gynaecology, University Hospital of Northern Norway, Tromsø, Norway*
[6]*"G. d'Annunzio" University, Chieti, Italy*

Correspondence should be addressed to M. R. Spina; mariarobertaspina@gmail.com

Academic Editor: Maria Grazia Porpora

Background. Interstitial pregnancy is a rare form of ectopic pregnancy that usually leads to uterine rupture resulting in sudden life-threatening haemorrhage, need for blood transfusion, and admission to intensive care unit. Mortality rate is 6–7 times higher than that in classical ectopic pregnancy. Uterine rupture has been typically reported to occur at more advanced gestational ages compared to tubal pregnancy although several recent reports have shown a high risk of rupture before 12 weeks of gestation. *Cases Presentation.* We report three cases of women affected by interstitial pregnancy, with different clinical symptoms, and managed to be treated with surgery or medical therapy. An emergency laparotomy was performed in the first case by the general surgeon, while in the second case laparoscopy was made by a gynecologist; last case shows the success of systemic administration of methotrexate. *Conclusion.* Interstitial pregnancy is still a challenging condition to diagnose and treat; early diagnosis may help to choose the proper management.

1. Background

The interstitial part of the fallopian tube is the proximal portion located into the muscular wall of the uterus. Pregnancies implanting in this site are defined as interstitial or cornual [1].

The interstitial part of the tube has a significantly greater capacity to expand before rupture because of its thickness; rupture can result in catastrophic haemorrhage with massive blood loss from the vascular anastomoses between the uterine and the ovarian arteries (Sampson's artery) [2].

Risk factors include assisted reproductive techniques, previous tubal pregnancies, tubal surgeries, a history of pelvic inflammatory disease, and sexually transmitted diseases [3].

Therefore, early detection is crucial to reduce morbidity and mortality.

Surgical approach consists of both laparotomy and laparoscopy techniques; conservative treatment is the administration of systemic methotrexate, checking the serum ß-hCG level on the 0th, the 4th, and the 7th day after, according to the Stovall protocol [4].

2. Cases Presentation

Three women were diagnosed with ectopic interstitial pregnancy from 2013 to 2016.

2.1. CASE no. 1. A 26-year-old woman (one previous Caesarean section and two previous voluntary terminations), with a history of irregular menstrual cycles, was admitted to the emergency unit with acute abdominal symptoms

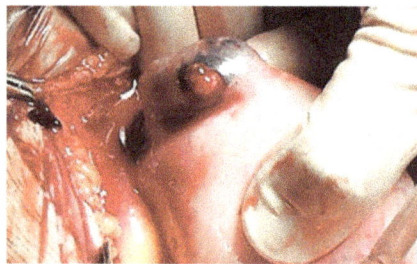

FIGURE 1

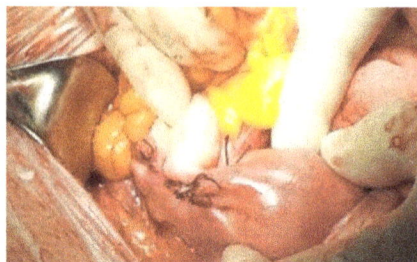

FIGURE 2

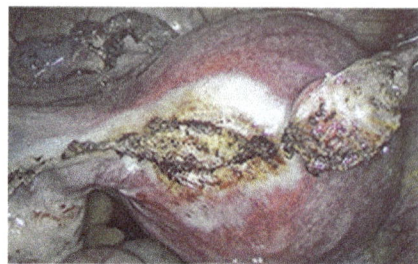

FIGURE 3

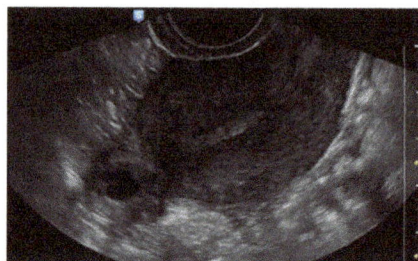

FIGURE 4

and vaginal bleeding. She was initially assessed by a general surgeon.

At first assessment, she presented with blood pressure of 70/40 mmHg and severe pallor; abdominal examination revealed guarding and tenderness in both iliac fossae and hypogastrium, while rectal examination revealed pain at the pressure of the pouch of Douglas. At ultrasound scan, corpusculated free fluid was detected. Laboratory test showed haemoglobin level of 10,1 g/dl. At vaginal examination, there was cervical tenderness with fullness in posterior fornix. Transvaginal ultrasound was not performed, since the patient conditions were worsening, and the general surgeon pushed to take the patient to the operating room, even though HCG test and the result of the CT were not ready.

Due to her unstable clinical conditions, the general surgeon decided on emergency laparotomy: subumbilical incision was performed, showing massive hemoperitoneum with blood loss from the uterine angle, due to a ruptured ectopic interstitial pregnancy (Figure 1).

Resection of the cornual area combined with an ipsilateral salpingectomy was performed and a tobacco pouch suture (Figure 2) made to provide an effective haemostasis.

In the operating theatre, multiple arterial blood samples were taken, and a decreasing haemoglobin trend was noticed, with the minimum value of 6,3 g/dl. Plasma expanders, crystalloids, and two blood units were administered. Pregnancy test proved to be positive and CT scan showed massive hemoperitoneum, without detecting any masses in the uterus or adnexal regions.

The following days, serum ß-hCG level showed a decreasing trend (1212,3 UI/L-514,6 UI/L-228,3 UI/L). A week after the discharge, serum ß-hCG level was 8,8 UI/L.

2.2. *CASE no. 2.* The second woman, thirty years old, (one previous voluntary termination) was referred to the emergency obstetrics department with pelvic pain and vaginal bleeding in the past three days.

A blood sample for haemoglobin and ß-hCG levels was taken at admission, while a transvaginal scan revealed the presence of a round mass containing an embryo with positive heart beat located in the isthmic portion of left tube. Furthermore, a small amount of free fluid in the pouch of Douglas was noticed; ß-hCG level at the access was 482,80 UI/L. The patient was haemodynamically stable, without any signs or symptoms of acute abdomen.

After extensive counselling, elective laparoscopic left salpingectomy was performed (Figure 3) and serum ß-hCG after surgery progressively decreased.

2.3. *CASE no. 3.* A third woman, thirty eight years old, (tertigravida, nullipara, one previous Caesarean section, and one previous voluntary termination) was admitted to the obstetrics and gynaecologic unit for vaginal blood loss and worsening pelvic pain. Laboratory tests and transvaginal ultrasound scan were immediately performed. The scan revealed the presence of a cornual anechoic mass with a hyperechoic border, compatible with tubal ring in the interstitial portion of the right tube, with maximum diameter of 0,87 cm, (Figure 4) and no free fluid in the pouch of Douglas. At admission, serum ß-hCG level was 3212 UI/L.

In view of the stable clinical conditions and the woman's wish to preserve the tube, intramuscular methotrexate was administered according to Stovall protocol [4]; serum ß–hCG levels were assessed on days 0, 4, and 7. Since the values did not decrease at least 15% between day 4 and day 7, a second dose of methotrexate was administered. ß-hCG levels showed a decreasing trend and became negative after 5 weeks.

3. Discussion

Interstitial pregnancy is a rare form of ectopic pregnancy, located in the proximal part of the fallopian tube, which usually leads to uterine rupture with resultant life-threatening hemorrhage [1]. It can be easily misdiagnosed with angular pregnancy; however, the latter is located within the endometrial cavity, in the corner where the tube connects with the fundal part of the uterus [5]. Most ruptures are reported later than in other tubal pregnancies because the myometrium is more distensible than the fallopian tube [1], but this common belief has been dispelled by more recent case series, reporting them at less than 12 weeks [6].

Major risk factors for interstitial pregnancies include assisted reproductive techniques, previous tubal pregnancy, tubal surgery, history of pelvic inflammatory disease, and sexually transmitted diseases [7].

Common symptoms of interstitial pregnancy are abdominal pain and vaginal bleeding, while signs of acute abdomen may occur in case of rupture and hemoperitoneum.

Haemorrhagic shock, due to interstitial pregnancy rupture, occurs in almost a quarter of the cases, thus explaining the relatively high mortality rate of interstitial pregnancies [3]; some authors have reported rupture of the interstitial pregnancy and formation of a hematoma of the broad ligament [8].

Early diagnosis is fundamental to manage this condition safely and it is accomplished using antenatal ultrasound and quantitative HCG assay.

Main diagnostic criteria using transvaginal ultrasound are as follows [9]: an empty uterine cavity, a separate chorionic sac at least 1 cm from the lateral edge of the uterine cavity, and a thin (5 mm) myometrial layer surrounding the gestational sac.

Ackerman et al. [10] described the interstitial line sign, which refers to the visualization of an echogenic line that runs from the endometrial cavity to the interstitial region, abutting the interstitial mass or gestational sac.

The paucity of the myometrium around the gestational sac is diagnostic of interstitial pregnancy, while an angular pregnancy has at least 5 mm of myometrium on all its sides [3]; in the first case the embryo is implanted lateral to the round ligament and in the second one embryo is implanted in the lateral angle of the uterine cavity, medial to the uterotubal junction and round ligament [6].

Sonographic findings in two dimensions can be further confirmed using three-dimensional ultrasound, where available, to avoid misdiagnosis with early intrauterine or angular (implantation in the lateral angles of the uterine cavity) pregnancy [11].

Early diagnosis with transvaginal ultrasound allows conservative treatment with methotrexate; if it is made later in gestation, surgical treatment can be required [12].

Traditionally, the treatment of interstitial pregnancy involves hysterectomy or cornual resection, although more conservative approaches have been recently introduced.

Systemic methotrexate is safe and effective, but early recognition is essential. Local injection of methotrexate, either transvaginal or laparoscopic, provides highly effective methods [6].

Recent studies have reported that a pharmacological approach using methotrexate is usually effective, although there is insufficient evidence to recommend local or systemic approach.

Major institution recommends that methotrexate should be the first-line management for hemodynamically stable women with no pain, those with an unruptured ectopic pregnancy, a mass smaller than 35 mm with no visible heartbeat, and a serum b-hCG between 1500 and 5000 IU/l [11].

Other authors have reported an alternative approach by performing a transvaginal ultrasound guided aspiration of the extracelomic fluid from the gestational sac, followed by intrasaccular injection of 25 mg of methotrexate with/without 0.2–0.4 mEq of potassium chloride [11].

The main advantages of local injection of methotrexate include smaller drug dosage, fewer systemic side effects, and higher tissue concentration [6].

Surgical treatment consists of conservative techniques, such as laparoscopic cornual resection, laparoscopic or laparotomic cornuostomy or hysteroscopic removal of interstitial ectopic tissue, and radical operations such as salpingectomy [6, 13] or hysterectomy [6].

Radical surgery is necessary in cases where haemorrhage is life threatening [14].

Due to the abundant blood supply in the cornual region from both uterine and ovarian vessels, rupture occurring after 12 weeks of gestation often leads to severe haemorrhage and eventually maternal death [5].

Laparotomy used to be the preferred surgical approach to the treatment of ruptured cornual pregnancy, especially when it occurs in advanced gestation [6].

Ipsilateral uterine artery ligation should be performed before attempting to repair a ruptured uterine cornu [6] or temporary clipping of the main structures (uterine and ovarian arteries) before the excision [15]; both techniques will help to achieve haemostasis and allow time to repair the cornu [16].

Even in women with ectopic pregnancy with significant hemoperitoneum, laparoscopic surgery has been reported to be safe in experienced hands [14, 17].

Both Tulandi (1995) [18] and Reich (1998) [19] used laparoscopic cornual excision to manage cornual pregnancies. Trends toward less extensive laparoscopic procedures are evident in further case reports using cornuostomy [6].

Most authors agree that the size of cornual gestation determines the best laparoscopic approach; Tulandi [18] reported that salpingostomy is appropriate for gestations of <3.5cm, whereas cornual excision was recommended by Grobman et al. [20] for gestations of >4 cm.

Various endoscopic approaches have been reported, such as electrocauterization, endoloop application, or the encircling suture before evacuation of the conceptus [21].

In a retrospective study, Moon et al. [21] reported that "the endoloop and the encircling suture methods are simple, safe, effective, and nearly bloodless." He also described a technique which uses highly diluted vasopressin for hemostasis during laparoscopic surgery (1 ampoule [20 U] of vasopressin diluted in 1000 ml of normal saline [1000-fold] and 150–250 ml [0.02 U/ml] of diluted vasopressin injected in the uterus below the interstitial pregnancy [22]. There were no uterine ruptures in the pregnancies following these methods of endoscopic management.

Other authors described other techniques such as the "purse-string" technique, a haemostatic suture passed at the base of the mass before removing it [13], or a sort of square knot at the border of the cornuostomy [23].

Hysteroscopic management can be particularly suitable for women who are reluctant to undergo medical treatment with methotrexate or in whom this treatment fails or is unavailable. Minelli et al. stated that, in expert hands, resection of the corneal endometrium, including the tubal ostium, can be successfully performed without perforation of the uterus [6].

Surgical treatment involving resection of the cornual region is associated with decreased fertility and increased uterine rupture rates in future pregnancies [24].

It is also described for uterine rupture in a pregnant woman with previous surgery of cornuostomy [25].

One of the concerns of future pregnancy is rupture of the interstitial portion of the tube (uterine rupture). The postulated mechanism is through a defective area of uterine wall [26].

Some authorities suggest suturing the uterine wall after surgical management to reinforce the defective area in the uterine wall. Term deliveries have, however, been reported following laparoscopic treatment of corneal pregnancy without reinforcing sutures [27, 28].

Most authors agreed that Caesarean section should be the optimum mode of delivery for all pregnancies following cornual pregnancy [14].

The second concern after conservative management of cornual pregnancy is recurrence of ectopic pregnancy, particularly cornual pregnancy on the same side [6].

Thus, conservative treatment should be the first treatment option if the patient is stable and there is the aim to preserve fertility; otherwise interstitial pregnancy should be removed via laparoscopy or laparotomy.

However, more cases and studies should be reported; limitations of our case report study are based on the paucity of the patients.

4. Conclusion

Cornual pregnancy poses a significant diagnostic and therapeutic challenge; early diagnosis may help to choose the proper management and treatment; according to the clinical presentation and the haemodynamic stability, it should be based on laboratory exams (serum ß-hCG level) and transvaginal ultrasound.

Abbreviations

ß-hCG: The β-subunit of human chorionic gonadotropin
CRL: Crown-rump length
3D scan: Three-dimensional scan
hCG: Human chorionic gonadotropin.

Consent

We got an authorization from the hospital to collect and publish data for research activity; we obtained consent for publication of data from the patients.

Authors' Contributions

Dr. Spina Maria Roberta collected data and wrote the manuscript; Dr. Di Tizio Luciano contributed by collecting data and performing the two surgical interventions; Dr. Gustapane Sarah helped in collecting data; and Prof. D'Antonio Francesco and Prof. Liberati Marco supervised the manuscript.

References

[1] S. Shiragur, V. R, M. J, R. Doshi, and S. Kori, "Ruptured cornual ectopic pregnancy at 8 weeks gestation- successful conservative approach: a case report," *International Journal of Reproduction, Contraception, Obstetrics and Gynecology*, vol. 2, no. 4, p. 671, 2013.

[2] K. E. Buch, M. Reiner, and C. M. Divino, "Hemoperitoneum following inguinal hernia repair: a case report," *Hernia*, vol. 11, no. 5, pp. 459–461, 2007.

[3] T. Tulandi and D. Al-Jaroudi, "Interstitial pregnancy: Results generated from the society of reproductive surgeons registry," *Obstetrics & Gynecology*, vol. 103, no. 1, pp. 47–50, 2004.

[4] T. G. Stovall and F. W. Ling, "Single-dose methotrexate: an expanded clinical trial," *American Journal of Obstetrics & Gynecology*, vol. 168, no. 6, pp. 1759–1765, 1993.

[5] S. M. Surekha, T. Chamaraja, N. Nabakishore Singh, L. Bimolchandra Singh, and T. S. Neeraja, "A ruptured left cornual pregnancy: A case report," *Journal of Clinical and Diagnostic Research*, vol. 7, no. 7, pp. 1455-1456, 2013.

[6] R. Faraj and M. Steel, "Management of cornual (interstitial) pregnancy," *The Obstetrician & Gynaecologist*, vol. 9, no. 4, pp. 249–255, 2007.

[7] D. Soriano, D. Vicus, R. Mashiach, E. Schiff, D. Seidman, and M. Goldenberg, "Laparoscopic treatment of cornual pregnancy: a series of 20 consecutive cases," *Fertility and Sterility*, vol. 90, no. 3, pp. 839–843, 2008.

[8] A. M. Abbas, A. M. Sheha, S. S. Ali, A. M. Maghraby, and E. Talaat, "A rare presentation of ruptured interstitial ectopic pregnancy with broad ligament hematoma: A case report," *Middle East Fertility Society Journal*, vol. 22, no. 1, pp. 80–83, 2017.

[9] I. E. Timor-Tritsch, A. Monteagudo, C. Matera, and C. R. Veit, "Sonographic evolution of cornual pregnancies treated without surgery," *Obstetrics & Gynecology*, vol. 79, no. 6, pp. 1044–1049, 1992.

[10] T. E. Ackerman, C. S. Levi, S. M. Dashefsky, S. C. Holt, and D. J. Lindsay, "Interstitial line: Sonographic finding in interstitial (cornual) ectopic pregnancy," *Radiology*, vol. 189, no. 1, pp. 83–87, 1993.

[11] C. J. Elson, R. Salim, N. Potdar, M. Chetty, J. A. Ross, and E. J. Kirk, "Diagnosis and management of ectopic pregnancy," *BJOG: An International Journal of Obstetrics & Gynaecology*, vol. 123, no. 13, pp. e15–e55, 2016.

[12] K. Jermy, J. Thomas, A. Doo, and T. Bourne, "The conservative management of interstitial pregnancy," *BJOG: An International Journal of Obstetrics & Gynaecology*, vol. 111, no. 11, pp. 1283–1288, 2004.

[13] G. Cucinella, S. Rotolo, G. Calagna, R. Granese, A. Agrusa, and A. Perino, "Laparoscopic management of interstitial pregnancy: The 'purse- string' technique," *Acta Obstetricia et Gynecologica Scandinavica*, vol. 91, no. 8, pp. 996–999, 2012.

[14] G. F. Grimbizis, T. Tsalikis, T. Mikos et al., "Case report: Laparoscopic treatment of a ruptured interstitial pregnancy," *Reproductive BioMedicine Online*, vol. 9, no. 4, pp. 447–451, 2004.

[15] S. Guven and E. S. Guven, "Laparoscopic temporary clipping of uterine and ovarian arteries for the treatment of interstitialectopic pregnancy," *Clinical and Experimental Obstetrics and Gynecology*, vol. 43, no. 1, pp. 128–130, 2016.

[16] N. Khawaja, T. Walsh, and B. Gill, "Uterine artery ligation for the management of ruptured cornual ectopic pregnancy," *European Journal of Obstetrics & Gynecology and Reproductive Biology*, vol. 118, no. 2, p. 269, 2005.

[17] G. A. Hill, J. H. Segars, and C. M. Herbert, "Laparoscopic Management of Interstitial Pregnancy," *Journal of Gynecologic Surgery*, vol. 5, no. 2, pp. 209–212, 1989.

[18] T. Tulandi, G. Vilos, and V. Gomel, "Laparoscopic treatment of interstitial pregnancy," *Obstetrics & Gynecology*, vol. 85, no. 3, pp. 465–467, 1995.

[19] H. Reich, D. A. Johns, J. DeCaprio, F. McGlynn, and E. Reich, "Laparoscopic treatment of 109 consecutive ectopic pregnancies," *Obstetrics, Gynaecology and Reproductive Medicine*, vol. 33, no. 11, pp. 885–890, 1988.

[20] W. A. Grobman and M. P. Milad, "Conservative laparoscopic management of a large cornual ectopic pregnancy," *Human Reproduction*, vol. 13, no. 7, pp. 2002–2004, 1998.

[21] H. S. Moon, Y. J. Choi, Y. H. Park, and S. G. Kim, "New simple endoscopic operations for interstitial pregnancies," *American Journal of Obstetrics & Gynecology*, vol. 182, no. 1, Article ID 102710, pp. 114–121, 2000.

[22] H. S. Moon, S. G. Kim, G. S. Park, J. K. Choi, J. S. Koo, and B. S. Joo, "Efficacy of bleeding control using a large amount of highly diluted vasopressin in laparoscopic treatment for interstitial pregnancy," *American Journal of Obstetrics & Gynecology*, vol. 203, no. 1, pp. 30–e6, 2010.

[23] M. Huang, T. Su, and M. Lee, "Laparoscopic management of interstitial pregnancy," *International Journal of Gynecology & Obstetrics*, vol. 88, no. 1, pp. 51-52, 2005.

[24] R. Ross, S. R. Lindheim, D. L. Olive, and E. A. Pritts, "Cornual gestation: A systematic literature review and two case reports of a novel treatment regimen," *Journal of Minimally Invasive Gynecology*, vol. 13, no. 1, pp. 74–78, 2006.

[25] A. M. Abbas, F. M. Fawzy, M. N. Ali, and M. K. Ali, "An unusual case of uterine rupture at 39 weeks of gestation after laparoscopic cornual resection: A case report," *Middle East Fertility Society Journal*, vol. 21, no. 3, pp. 196–198, 2016.

[26] S. Lau and T. Tulandi, "Conservative medical and surgical management of interstitial ectopic pregnancy," *Fertility and Sterility*, vol. 72, no. 2, pp. 207–215, 1999.

[27] N. Gleicher, V. Karande, D. Rabin, and D. Pratt, "Laparoscopic removal of twin cornual pregnancy after in vitro fertilization," *Fertility and Sterility*, vol. 61, no. 6, pp. 1161-1162, 1994.

[28] H. S. Moon, Y. J. Choi, Y. H. Park, and S. G. Kim, "New simple endoscopic operations for interstitial pregnancies," *American Journal of Obstetrics & Gynecology*, vol. 182, no. 1, pp. 114–121, 2000.

14

Retroperitoneal Endometriotic Cyst Infiltrated in the Iliopsoas Incidentally Found in a Patient with Acute Back Pain

Nanami Tsukasaki, Takuro Yamamoto, Akihisa Katayama, Nozomi Ogiso, and Tomoharu Okubo

Department of Obstetrics and Gynecology, Japanese Red Cross Society Kyoto Daiichi Hospital, 15-749 Honmachi, Higashiyama-ku, Kyoto 605-0981, Japan

Correspondence should be addressed to Nanami Tsukasaki; n-tksk@koto.kpu-m.ac.jp

Academic Editor: Seung-Yup Ku

We describe a rare case of retroperitoneal endometriotic cyst infiltrated in the iliopsoas incidentally found in a patient with acute back pain. Endometriosis at the pelvic peritoneum, including the Douglas pouch, has been reported often; there are few reports of cystic endometriosis in the retroperitoneal cavity. Today there are various theories regarding how endometriosis occurs. By pathological findings and lesion sites of the present case, we concluded that the endometrial tissues in the menstrual blood might metastasize lymphatically and implant and form the retroperitoneal cyst.

1. Introduction

An endometriotic lesion occurs frequently in the ovary, pelvic peritoneum, and Douglas pouch but rarely at other sites. In recent years, an endometriotic lesion that occurs at an atypical site has been defined as scarcity endometriosis in Japan. We describe a case of a retroperitoneal endometriotic cyst that infiltrated the iliopsoas and was incidentally found in a patient with acute back pain. Here, we describe the patient's clinical course and pathological findings and discuss the pathogenic mechanisms.

2. Case Presentation

The patient was a 43-year-old, gravida 0, para 0, woman with a history of leiomyomectomy at the age of 28 years. She felt sudden pain between the left lower abdomen and lower back 3 days before her first visit, and she took analgesic drugs; however, the pain persisted. Originally, she did not have additional menstrual disorders and the lumbar backache was not related to menstruation cycle. The computed tomography (CT) scan showed enlargement of the uterus, which led us to suspect uterine sarcoma and para-aortic lymph node metastasis that infiltrated the iliopsoas. She was referred

to our hospital for a detailed examination. Her abdomen was enlarged 5 cm above the umbilicus, and we recognized the left costovertebral angle knock pain. The transvaginal ultrasonogram showed a great mass with echo-free space in the uterus, and we suspected uterine fibroma. The serum levels of CA-125 and CA-19-9 were increased to 514.3 U/mL and 299.2 U/mL, respectively. However, the levels of CEA and lactate dehydrogenase were within normal ranges. The pelvic magnetic resonance imaging scan showed adenomyosis of the uterus and a mass lesion measuring $19 \times 15 \times 7$ cm on the left side of the uterus with many cystic and hemorrhagic cavities. The mass had low-intensity enhancement on T1-weighted and T2-weighted images, and it did not have decreased diffusion. The bilocular cystic mass with hemorrhaging was found in the retroperitoneal cavity. The retroperitoneal cyst was $5.3 \times 2.7 \times 4.0$ cm and did not have solid parts, and it had high-intensity enhancement on T1-weighted and T2-weighted images with shading. Therefore, we diagnosed the patient as having endometriotic cysts. Using contrast-enhanced CT, we found that this bilocular cystic mass was located caudally from the left renal hilus. The cranial cystic wall was relatively thick; however, it did not have solid parts (Figures 1(a) and 1(b)). The cyst was close to the left renal artery cranially, left ureter caudally, left kidney laterally, and

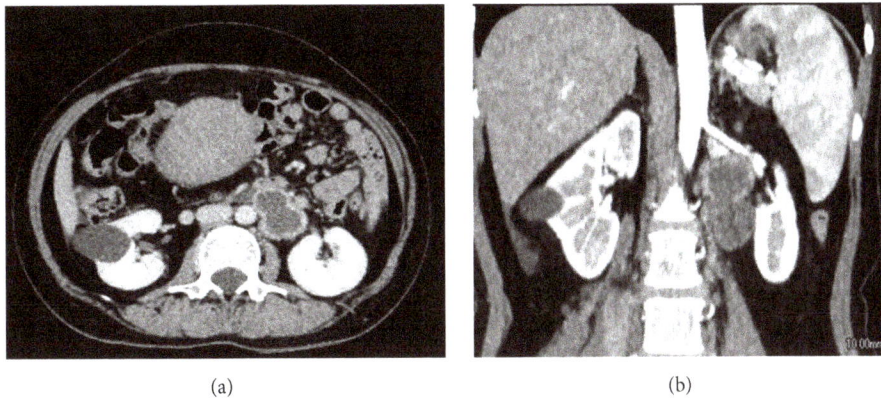

(a)

(b)

FIGURE 1: Computed tomography scan showing that the bilocular cystic mass is located caudally from the left renal hilus without solid parts.

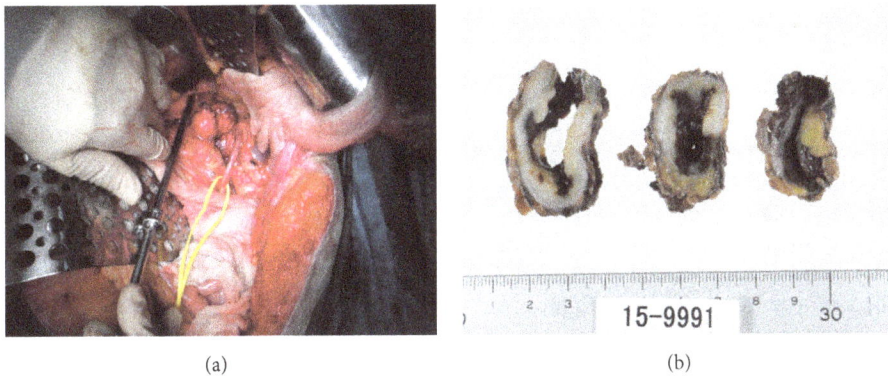

(a)

(b)

FIGURE 2: (a) Intraoperative findings showing that the peritoneal cyst in the left inferior kidney is bilocular, and it is firmly adhered to the left iliopsoas and ureter. (b) Photographs of the resected retroperitoneal cyst showing that it is bilocular with cystic space with old and new bleeding.

left psoas major muscle medially. Therefore, we suspected that the cyst had adhered to peripheral tissues and infiltrated the left psoas major muscle, which resulted in transformation. There was no metastasis to the lung, bone, or lymph nodes (mediastinal, axillary, subclavian, and so on). All these findings led us to suspect degenerated uterine fibroma and hemorrhagic cyst growth in the retroperitoneum; thus, we performed total abdominal hysterectomy and bilateral salpingo-oophorectomy and retroperitoneal cystectomy. The surface of the uterus was smooth, and there were no malignant findings macroscopically. Both adnexa had no abnormal findings. The result of cytology of ascites was negative, and the intraoperative rapid pathological diagnosis was leiomyoma. The peritoneal cyst in the left inferior kidney was bilocular, and it adhered firmly to the left iliopsoas and ureter (Figure 2(a)). We exfoliated the cyst from the peripheral tissues being careful not to disrupt the stream of the left renal artery and ureter, and we removed the cyst by resecting a part of the iliopsoas that was infiltrated. During this process, a part of the cyst perforated, and chocolate-like fluid leaked out. There were no disseminated lesions or lymph node swelling. Therefore, we concluded that the lesions were uterine fibroma and an endometriotic cyst had formed in the left inferior renal hilus. Her postoperative course was uneventful, and

she was discharged on postoperative day 7. The serum levels of CA-125 and CA19-9 were normalized to 5.7 U/mL and 8.2 U/mL and lumbar backache was improved. Pathologically, the final diagnosis was leiomyomas and endometriotic cysts in the retroperitoneal space. So far, we have not seen recurrent findings.

3. Pathologic Findings

3.1. Gross Findings.
Gross findings showed a 22-cm mass at the uterine corpus. Poorly marginated adenomyosis existed in the left side of the uterus (Figure 2(b)). The retroperitoneal cyst was bilocular, and it had cystic space with old and new bleeding (Figure 3(a)).

3.2. Light Microscopy Findings.
The mass of the uterine corpus was associated with bleeding, and hyalinizing and eosinophilic spindle cells grew with a fascicle-like structure. Adenomyotic tissues existed in the surrounding area. The retroperitoneal cyst had exfoliated epithelia, and most cystic walls were fibrous tissues with bleeding and hemosiderosis. However, we recognized the endometrium-like tissues and endometrial stromata with CD10 expression (Figure 3(b)).

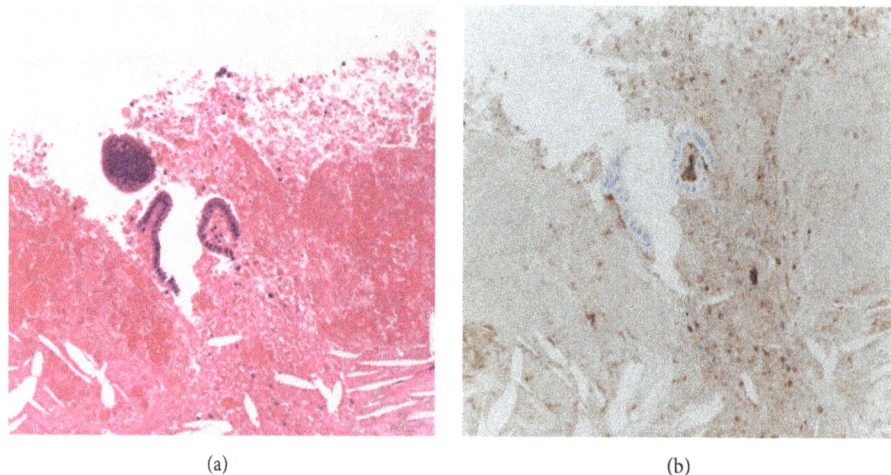

(a)

(b)

FIGURE 3: Microscopic findings using hematoxylin and eosin (HE) staining (a) and CD10 (b). We identified the endometrial gland tissues using HE staining and CD10-positive stromal cells using immunohistochemical staining.

4. Discussion

Atypical endometriosis that occurs at sites other than female genitals has been defined as scarcity endometriosis, which develops at various sites, such as the intestine, bladder, urinary duct, diaphragm, chest cavity, and abdominal wall. Various symptoms occur depending on the original site and invasion depth. Intestinal endometriosis occurs most frequently among those with scarcity endometriosis, and the common sites are the rectum and sigmoid colon [1]. Although endometriosis at the pelvic peritoneum, including the Douglas pouch, has been reported often, there are few reports of cystic endometriosis in the retroperitoneal cavity. Since endometrial stromal cells express CD10 during proliferation, secretion, and the atrophic stage of endometrium and endometriotic lesions, CD10 is a useful marker for diagnosing endometriosis, including ectopic endometriosis [2–4]. This case pathologically showed that the epithelium was exfoliated remarkably, and most of the cystic wall was covered with fibrous tissues with bleeding and hemosiderosis. We made a diagnosis of cyst endometriosis based on the identification of endometrial gland tissues with hematoxylin and eosin staining and CD10-positive stromal cells.

There are various theories regarding how endometriosis occurs, such as the implantation theory, coelomic metaplasia theory, embryonic residual theory, hematogenous dissemination theory, and lymphatic dissemination theory [5, 6]. These hypotheses are not compatible, and it is thought that some of the mechanisms contribute to the generation of endometriosis. The coelomic metaplasia theory states that mesothelial cells and stromata on the peritoneum and ovarian surface metamorphose into endometrium-like tissues where the endometriotic tissues occur. The embryonic residual theory states that endometriotic tissues occur from the residual tissue of Müllerian and Wolffian ducts. The backflow of menstrual blood occurs in approximately 90% of reproductive females; therefore, the implantation theory makes sense in that menstrual blood moves back into the fallopian tubes and reaches the peritoneal cavity, and the endometrial

tissues in the menstrual blood become implanted in the peritoneum [7]. However, in our patient, endometriosis occurred in the retroperitoneal cavity, which contradicts the implantation theory. Corpus uterine cancer frequently metastasizes lymphatically. Our patient's metastasis occurred at a very rare site of the left inferior renal hilus, which corresponds with the 325 type b lymph nodes that were the metastatic site of uterine corpus cancer. There were some lymph nodes around the retroperitoneal cystic mass pathologically. All these findings led us to conclude that the endometrial tissues in the menstrual blood metastasized lymphatically in the left inferior renal hilus and implanted and formed the retroperitoneal cyst. Similar to the present case, when physicians recognize hemorrhagic cysts in the retroperitoneal cavity in patients with lumbar backache, it is necessary to suspect an endometriotic cyst in the retroperitoneal cavity as a differential diagnosis even if there are no other findings of endometriosis. To definitively diagnose endometriosis, it is necessary to perform a pathological examination with immunostaining and to not overlook few endometrial epithelia and stromata.

References

[1] I. K. Orbuch, H. Reich, M. Orbuch, and L. Orbuch, "Laparoscopic treatment of recurrent small bowel obstruction secondary to ileal endometriosis," *Journal of Minimally Invasive Gynecology*, vol. 14, no. 1, pp. 113–115, 2007.

[2] W. G. McCluggage, V. P. Sumathi, and P. Maxwell, "CD10 is a sensitive and diagnostically useful immunohistochemical marker of normal endometrial stroma and of endometrial stromal neoplasms," *Histopathology*, vol. 39, no. 3, pp. 273–278, 2001.

[3] V. P. Sumathi and W. G. McCluggage, "CD10 is useful in demonstrating endometrial stroma at ectopic sites and in

confirming a diagnosis of endometriosis," *Journal of Clinical Pathology*, vol. 55, no. 5, pp. 391-392, 2002.

[4] G. Capobianco, J. M. Wenger, V. Marras et al., "Immuno-histochemical evaluation of epithelial antigen Ber-Ep4 and CD10: new markers for endometriosis?" *European Journal of Gynaecological Oncology*, vol. 34, no. 3, pp. 254–256, 2013.

[5] E. Seli, M. Berkkanoglu, and A. Arici, "Pathogenesis of endo-metriosis," *Obstetrics and Gynecology Clinics of North America*, vol. 30, no. 1, pp. 41–61, 2003.

[6] C. A. Witz, "Pathogenesis of endometriosis," *Gynecologic and Obstetric Investigation*, vol. 53, no. 1, pp. 52–62, 2002.

[7] J. A. Sampson, "The development of the implantation theory for the origin of peritoneal endometriosis," *American Journal of Obstetrics & Gynecology*, vol. 40, no. 4, pp. 549–557, 1940.

15

Abruptio Placentae Caused by Hypertriglyceridemia-Induced Acute Pancreatitis during Pregnancy: Case Report and Literature Review

Pınar Yalcin Bahat ⓘD, Gokce Turan ⓘD, and Berna Aslan Cetin

*Department of Obstetrics and Gynecology, Kanuni Sultan Suleyman Training and Research Hospital,
Istanbul Health Sciences University, Istanbul, Turkey*

Correspondence should be addressed to Pınar Yalcin Bahat; dr_pinaryalcin@hotmail.com

Academic Editor: Erich Cosmi

Background. Hormonal effects during pregnancy can compromise otherwise controlled lipid levels in women with hypertriglyceridemia and predispose to pancreatitis leading to increased morbidity for mother and fetus. Elevation of triglyceride levels is a risk factor for development of pancreatitis if it exceeds 1000 mg/dL. Pancreatitis should be considered in emergency cases of abdominal pain and uterine contractions in Emergency Department at any stage of pregnancy. We report a case of abruptio placentae caused by hypertriglyceridemia-induced acute pancreatitis. Also, literature review of cases of acute pancreatitis induced by hypertriglycaemia in pregnancy has been made. *Case.* A 22-year-old woman presented to our Emergency Department, at 35 weeks of gestation, for acute onset of abdominal pain and uterine contractions. Blood tests showed a high rate of triglyceride. The patient was diagnosed with abruptio placentae caused by hypertriglyceridemia-induced acute pancreatitis. Immediate cesarean section was performed and it was observed that blood sample revealed a milky turbid serum. Insulin, heparin, and supportive treatment were started. She was discharged on the 10th day. *Conclusion.* Consequently, patients with known hypertriglyceridemia or family history should be followed up more closely because any delay can cause disastrous conclusions for mother and fetus. Acute pancreatitis should be considered in pregnant women who have sudden onset, severe, persistent epigastric pain and who have a risk factor for acute pancreatitis.

1. Introduction

Acute pancreatitis (AP) is a rare complication in pregnancy, occurring in approximately three in 10000 pregnancies [1, 2]. Hypertriglyceridemia is recognized as the third most common cause of gestational acute pancreatitis after gallstones and alcohol and occurs in about 4% of all cases [2]. An increase in plasma lipid level during pregnancy has been well documented. It is thought to represent a physiologic response to the hormonal changes; however, it is not sufficient to cause acute pancreatitis. Gestational pancreatitis due to hypertriglyceridemia usually occurs in pregnant women with preexisting abnormalities of the lipid metabolism. There are effective treatment choices during pregnancy such as dietary restriction of fat, intravenous heparin, and insulin and plasmapheresis. We report a case of abruptio placentae caused by hypertriglyceridemia-induced acute pancreatitis.

2. Case Report

A 22-year-old patient, Para 1, Gravida 2, presented to our Emergency Department of Gynecology and Obstetrics, at 35 weeks of gestation for acute onset of abdominal pain and uterine contraction. It was learned that the patient's history had no follow-up hypertriglyceridemia. On physical exam, her heart rate was at 100 pulses per minute, and her blood pressure was at 110/70 mm-Hg, respiratory rate 18 /min. Her abdomen was defensive. Her cervical os was dilated to 1-2 cm and minimal bleeding. The patient had mild epigastric tenderness. Decelerations were seen in pregnant cardiotocography follow-ups with abnormal abdominal pain and uterine contractions continued and simultaneous wide bleeding area (like abruptio placenta) was seen on the posterior part of placenta in ultrasound. Immediate cesarean section was performed under general anesthesia because of contraction of the tetanic type in the manual contraception. She gave birth to a healthy infant of 2980 g. Amylase, lipase, triglyceride, HDL, and LDL were studied in the patient's blood after emulsion of chylous fluid from abdomen during the cesarean section. Liver enzymes were high: ast: 241, sub. 147. It was observed that blood sample revealed a milky turbid serum. Laboratory finding included a triglyceride at 3297 mg/dl and amylase 827 U/L, lipase 1576 U/L. Abdominal ultrasound showed thickened pancreas without necrosis; acute pancreatitis compatible with diffuse edema was observed on pancreas. Biliary tract was naturally observed. Other causes of cholestasis of pregnancy, such as cholangitis, acute hepatitis, and hemophagocytic syndrome, were ruled out. Oral intake of the patient was stopped; intravenous fluid replacement therapy, antibiotherapy, proton pump inhibitor, insulin, and heparin therapy were started. She was discharged on the 10th day of treatment. Even though the patient did not have previous history of diabetes or gestational diabetes, the baby was born 4 to 3 weeks earlier. It was thought that this condition might be related to maternal hyperlipidemia for newborn's doctors.

3. Discussion

Acute pancreatitis (AP) is a rare complication in pregnancy. Diagnosis becomes difficult because it can interfere with the physiological findings in pregnancy. Acute pancreatitis should be considered in pregnancies with nausea, vomiting, and epigastric pain. Gallstones, hypertriglyceridemia, and alcohol especially play a role in the etiology of acute pancreatitis.

Hypertriglyceridemia is the second most common cause of acute pancreatitis in pregnancy. Diagnosis is made when the serum triglyceride is > 1000 mg/dl. Hypertriglyceridemia in pregnant patients can occur with preexisting dyslipidemia, associated with others diseases (hypertension, diabetes mellitus, and alcoholism), or without any predisposing factor. Triglycerides concentration rises gradually, 2.5-fold over prepregnancy levels, reaching a peak during the third trimester to almost twice as high value of nonpregnant value. This is thought to be due to estrogen-induced increases in triglyceride synthesis and very low-density lipoprotein secretion [29]. Therefore, AP is more common in the third trimester of pregnancy. Lipids decrease gradually postpartum to reach prepregnancy level in 6 weeks [30, 31]. Epigastric pain, spreading pain, nausea, vomiting, and distension can be seen at the beginning of the symptoms in acute pancreatitis cases. Findings of peritoneal irritation are not seen in general, especially when there is epigastric pain in mild cases as indicated by physical examination findings. In severe cases, epigastric tenderness and peritoneal irritation findings may be accompanied by ileus, fever, and tachycardia. The increase in serum amylase reaches peak values 6-12 hours after the onset of the event. The exact diagnosis of pancreatitis is based on the amylase/creatinine clearance rate. Serum lipase values also increase. Imaging methods can be used in the diagnosis of acute pancreatitis from ultrasonography, computed tomography, and magnetic resonance imaging. Ultrasound is the most appropriate method for pregnancy.

Acute pancreatitis treatment in pregnancy is similar to nonpregnant treatment of hyperlipidemia. Pregnancy pancreatitis treatment is primarily medicinal and approximately 90% of patients respond to medical treatment. Medical treatment of AP is mostly supportive. These treatments include low fat diet [32, 33], antihyperlipidemic therapy [32, 33], insulin [32, 34] (to increase lipoprotein lipase activity), heparin [33, 35] (to increase lipoprotein lipase activity), and even plasmapheresis [32, 35].

Our patient was admitted with acute onset of abdominal pain and uterine contraction to our clinics in the 35th week of gestation. She had lipid abnormality in her history, but her history had no follow-up hypertriglyceridemia. Pregnancy had induced aggravation of hypertriglyceridemia and associated pancreatitis. In addition, acute pancreatitis induced by the pregnancy was accompanied by abruptio placenta and delivery was performed with an emergency cesarean section. It was observed that blood sample revealed a milky turbid serum. We managed our patient conservatively in postoperative period. Oral intake of the patient was stopped; intravenous fluid replacement therapy, antibiotherapy, proton pump inhibitor, insulin, and heparin therapy were started. The patient's clinical condition subsequently improved.

Cases of acute pancreatitis induced by hypertrigliceridemia during pregnancy published in the literature are listed in Table 1. In the majority of published case, medical treatment was first tired. Oral intake was closed, supportive treatment started. However, pregnancy-induced pancreatitis has been mortal in some cases and has gone as far as maternal death.

Ihuang et al. performed a retrospective study on 21 pregnant women diagnosed with acute pancreatitis (AP). Patients were divided into acute biliary pancreatitis (A BP), hypertriglyceridemia-induced acute pancreatitis (HTG P), and idiopathic groups according to etiology. 95% of the patients were in the third trimester of gestation. The percentage of patients with HTGP was higher than that of ABP (48% versus 14%). The percentage of severe acute pancreatitis (SAP) in the HTGP group was higher than that in the ABP group (40.0% versus 0%). In the HTGP group, five patients given were plasma exchange therapy and five were not. According to the results of this study it was found that plasma exchange may be safe and effectively administered for HTGP patients during pregnancy with SIRS or multiple organ dysfunction syndrome (MODS) [36].

In a study by Lingyu Luo et al., they retrospectively reviewed 121 acute pancreatitis in pregnancy (APIP) cases. The correlation between APIP types, severity, biochemical parameters, and mortality was analyzed. The most common causes of APIP were gallstone and hypertriglyceridemia. Lower level of serum calcium could be used as an indicator for the severity of the APIP. According to the result s of this study it was found that the severity of APIP was associated with higher risk for neonate asphyxia and maternal and fetal death [37].

In a prospective study performed by Athyros VG et al., 17 cases of acute pancreatitis induced by hypertriglyceridemia were included in the study. These patients were followed for 42 months. In the content of the study causative conditions

TABLE 1: Case literatures of acute pancreatitis induced by hypertriglyceridemia during pregnancy.

First Author	Year	Age	G/P	Birth	Medication	Other	Mode BW	Indication	Laboratory *	After Treatment **
Billion JM [3]	1991	32		35	TPN					
Achard JM [4]	1991				Two Lipaphereses					
Perrone G [5]	1996	37		35	Diet, Gemfibrozil					
ibrahim Bildirici [6]	2002	26	G2P2	24	Insulin, Plasmapheresis		C/S	Fetal Distress (750 g)	Serum Amylase: 487 Panc. Amylase:184 Panc Lipase:786 TG: 2316	
Chee-Chuen Loo [7]	2002	37	G3P2	37	Ranitidine, Heparin, Insulin		SVD		Serum Amylase: 956 TG: 2066	Serum Amylase: 39 TG: 492
J.C. Sleth [8]	2004	28	G2P1	37	Heparin		C/S	Unstable Condition of the Mother	TG: 2316 Cholesterol: 1000 Panc. Amylase: 574 Panc. Lipase: 1310	TG: 100
A. Abu Musa [9]	2006	39	G2P1	28	Plasmapheresis		C/S	A Repeat C/S Delivery	TG: 3810 Panc. Amylase: 525 Panc. Lipase: 3524	TG: 591 Panc. Amylase: 79 Panc. Lipase: 396
Shih-Chang Chuang [10]	2006	28	G1P0	34	Antibiotics, TPN	Pancreatic Necrosectomy, Right Hemicolectomy Ileostomy, Cholecys-tostomy, Gastrostomy, Feeding Jejunostomy		Unstable Condition of the Mother	TG: 2184 Panc. Amylase: 1365 Panc. Lipase: 533	TG: 319

TABLE 1: Continued.

First Author	Year	Age	G/P	Birth	Medication	Other	Mode BW	Indication	Laboratory *	After Treatment **
Alptekin Gürsoy [11]	2006	24	G1P0	37			C/S (3230 g)	Fetal Distress	TG: 10092 Cholesterol: 1159 Panc. Amylase: 367 Panc. Lipase: 797	TG: 143 Cholesterol: 274 Panc Amylase: 23 Panc Lipase: 41
V. Exbrayat [12]	2007	31		33	Plasmapheresis, Heparin		C/S	Fetal Distress	TG: 11300 Cholesterol: 2500 Panc Amylase: 334 Panc Lipase: 168	TG: 1000
Luminita S. Crisan [13] - 1	2008	27	G2P0	35	TPN, Analgesics, Bowel Rest	ARDS	C/S (2653 g)	Fetal Distress		
Luminita S. Crisan [13] - 2	2008	29	G3P1	30	TPN, Analgesics, Bowel Rest	Acute Myocardial Infarction	Forceps–Assisted Vaginal Delivery (1854 g)			
Luminita S. Crisan [13] - 3	2008	34	G3P0	33	TPN, Analgesics, Bowel Rest	ARDS	SVD (2147 g)			
Luminita S. Crisan [13] - 4	2008	23	G1P0	35	TPN, Analgesics, Bowel Rest		C/S (2498 g)	Low BPP		
L. Vandenbroucke [14]	2009	34		37	Heparin, A Low-Fat Diet		C/S (3940 g)	Fetal Distress	TG: 8447	TG: 240
Dilek Altun [15] -1	2012	27	G1P0	5	Plasmapheresis, Heparin			Termination	TG: 2225 Cholesterol: 470 Panc. Amylase: 959	TG: 278 Cholesterol: 181
Dilek Altun [15] - 2	2012	24	G1P0	34	Plasmapheresis, A Low-Fat Diet		C/S (3100 g)		TG: 2699 Cholesterol: 230 Panc. Amylase: 956 Panc. Lipase: 2580	TG: 570 Cholesterol: 2500 Panc. Amylase: 208 Panc. Lipase: 208
Mindaugas Serpytis [16]	2012	31	G2P0	33	Heparin, Insulin, Plasmapheresis				TG: 1576	TG:183

TABLE 1: Continued.

First Author	Year	Age	G/P	Birth	Medication	Other	Mode BW	Indication	Laboratory *	After Treatment **
Kumar Thulasidass [17] - 1	2013	37	G3P0	14	Insulin, Metformin, Fish Oil Therapy	Termination			TG: 1421 Cholesterol: 481 Serum Amylase: 1464	TG: 111 Cholesterol: 93
Kumar Thulasidass [17] - 2	2013	24	G1P0	8		ARDS	Spontaneous Abortion		TG: 839 Cholesterol: 300 Serum Amylase: 8962	TG: 57 Cholesterol: 77
Rafet Basar [18] - 1	2013	32	G3P0	37	Heparin, Fatty Acids, DF		C/S	Elective	TG: 1400	TG: 380
Rafet Basar [18] - 2		30	G2P1	36	Heparin, Fatty Acids, DF, Plasmapheresis		C/S	Elective	TG: 12000	TG: 758
Ying Hang [19]	2013	31	G2P0	27		Noninvasive Positive Pressure Ventilation (NPPV), Drainage of Chylous Ascites, Peritoneal Lavage, ARDS	C/S (1180 g)	Fetal Distress	TG: 523 Cholesterol: 325 Panc. Amylase: 178	TG: Normal Cholesterol: Normal
Bahiyah Abdullah [20]	2014	25	G4P3	8		Diagnostic Laparoscopy, Acute Hemorrhagic Pancreatitis	Spontaneous Abortion		Serum Amylase: 1273	Serum Amylase: 147
Tejal Amin [21]	2014	40	G5P4	18	Insulin	IUMF			TG: 836 Cholesterol: 300	TG: 90
Natasha Gupta [22]	2014	32	G5P4	38	Plasmapheresis	Preeclampsia, Pleural Effusion, Chronic Pericarditis, Retinal Detachment	C/S	Unstable Condition of the Mother	TG: 12.570 Cholesterol: 1067 Panc. Amylase: 1617 Panc. Lipase: 1330	TG: 295 Cholesterol: 179
Fadi Safi [23]	2014	24	G9P8	35	Plasmapheresis		C/S (1720 gr)	Unresponsiveness to Treatment	TG: 2661 Cholesterol: 683 Serum Amylase: 802	TG: 425

TABLE 1: Continued.

First Author	Year	Age	G/P	Birth	Medication	Other	Mode BW	Indication	Laboratory *	After Treatment **
Rachel Lim [24]	2015	27	G1P0	33	Insulin, Plasmapheresis	Placental Abruption	SVD		TG: 720 Cholesterol: 90 Panc. Lipase: 504	TG: 41
Ying Liu [24]	2015	30	G1P0	32	Plasmapheresis	Compound Heterozygosity (Glu242Lys and Leu252VaL)	C/S	Fetal Distress	TG: 2160 Cholesterol: 670 Panc. Amylase: 132	TG: 420
Funda Gok [25]	2015	37	G1P0	31	Insulin, DF	IUMF	SVD		TG: 9742 Cholesterol: 705 Panc. Amylase: 570 Panc. Lipase: 319	TG: 556 Panc. Amylase: 107 Panc. Lipase: 77
Hae Rin Jeon [26]	2016	28	G1P0	23		IUMF, Pancreatic Cells Necrotized, Diabetic Ketoacidosis, Metabolic Acidosis, Cardiac Arrest, EX			TG: 10392 Cholesterol: 1006 Panc. Amylase: 1833 Panc. Lipase: 1863	
Ioanna Poly-pathelli [27]	2017	38	G2P1	30	Heparin, Fatty Acids, Antibiotics		C/S	Resistant Exaggerated Thrombocytosis	TG: 14440 Cholesterol: 1600 Serum Amylase: 540	TG: 521
Tamanna Chibber [28]	2017	38		11		Cardiac Arrest, EX			TG: >1254 Cholesterol: 648 Panc. Lipase: 1079	

BW: birth weight, G: gravida, P: parity, SVD: spontaneous vaginal delivery, BPP: biophysical profile, TPN: total parenteral nutrition, DF: double filtration apheresis, C/S: cesarean section, TG: triglyceride, ARDS: Adult Respiratory Distress Syndrome, and IUMF: Intra-Uterine Mort Fetus.
Triglyceride and total cholesterol units are calculated in mg/dL. Other units are converted to mg/dL.
Serum Amylase: normal range is between 30 and 110 (U/L) [11].
Pancreatic Amylase: normal range is between 17 and 115 (U/L) [11].
Pancreatic Lipase: normal range is between 13 and 60 U/L (U/L) [11].
TG: normal range is between 50 and 160 mg/dL (mg/dL) [11].
Cholesterol: normal range is between 130 and 230 (mg/dL) [11].
* Highest values.
** Lowest values.

of HTG-induced A P were familial HTG in eight patients, HTG caused by uncontrolled diabetes mellitus in five, HTG aggravated by drugs in two (one by tamoxifen and one by fluvastatin), familial hyperchylomicronemia (HCM) in one, and lipemia of pregnancy in one. During the acute phase of pancreatitis, patients underwent standard treatment. After that, HTG was efficiently controlled with high dosages of fibrates or a fibrate plus acipimox, except for the patient with H CM, who was on a specific diet (the only source of fat was a special oil consisting of medium chain triglyceride) and taking a high dosage of acipimox. One of the patients died during the acute phase of pancreatitis with acute respiratory distress syndrome. According to the results of the study it was found that appropriate diet and drug treatment, including dose titration, of severe HTG are very effective in preventing relapses of HTG-induced AP [38].

As a result, pancreatitis can be seen in pregnancy in cases with uncontrolled hypertriglyceridemia. Patients with known hypertriglyceridemia or family history should be followed up more closely. Acute pancreatitis should be considered in pregnant women who have sudden onset, severe, persistent epigastric pain and who have a risk factor for acute pancreatitis.

References

[1] J. J. Eddy, M. D. Gideonsen, J. Y. Song, W. A. Grobman, and P. O'Halloran, "Pancreatitis in pregnancy," *Obstetrics & Gynecology*, vol. 112, no. 5, pp. 1075–1081, 2008.

[2] K. D. Ramin, S. M. Ramin, S. D. Richey, and F. G. Cunningham, "Acute pancreatitis in pregnancy," *American Journal of Obstetrics & Gynecology*, vol. 173, no. 1, pp. 187–191, 1995.

[3] K. Ohmoto, Y. Neishi, I. Miyake, and S. Yamamoto, "Severe acute pancreatitis associated with hyperlipidemia: Report of two cases and review of the literature in Japan," *Hepato-Gastroenterology*, vol. 46, no. 29, pp. 2986–2990, 1999.

[4] J. M. Achard, P. F. Westeel, P. Moriniere, J. D. Lalau, B. de Cagny, and A. Fournier, "Pancreatitis related to severe acute hypertriglyceridemia during pregnancy: Treatment with lipoprotein apheresis," *Intensive Care Medicine*, vol. 17, no. 4, pp. 236-237, 1991.

[5] G. Perrone and C. Critelli, "Severe hypertriglyceridemia during pregnancy. A case report," *Minerva Ginecologica*, vol. 48, no. 12, pp. 573–576, 1996.

[6] I. Bildirici, I. Esinler, O. Deren, T. Durukan, B. Kabay, and L. Onderoglu, "Hyperlipidemic pancreatitis during pregnancy," *Acta Obstetricia et Gynecologica Scandinavica*, vol. 81, no. 5, pp. 468–470, 2002.

[7] C.-C. Loo and J. Y. L. Tan, "Decreasing the plasma triglyceride level in hypertriglyceridemia-induced pancreatitis in pregnancy: A case report," *American Journal of Obstetrics & Gynecology*, vol. 187, no. 1, pp. 241-242, 2002.

[8] J. C. Sleth, E. Lafforgue, R. Servais et al., "A case of hypertriglycideremia-induced pancreatitis in pregnancy: Value of heparin," *Annales Françaises d'Anesthésie et de Réanimation*, vol. 23, no. 8, pp. 835–837, 2004.

[9] A. A. Abu Musa, I. M. Usta, J. B. Rechdan, and A. H. Nassar, "Recurrent hypertriglyceridemia-induced pancreatitis in pregnancy: A management dilemma [5]," *Pancreas*, vol. 32, no. 2, pp. 227-228, 2006.

[10] S.-C. Chuang, K.-T. Lee, S.-N. Wang, K.-K. Kuo, and J.-S. Chen, "Hypertriglyceridemia-associated acute pancreatitis with chylous ascites in pregnancy," *Journal of the Formosan Medical Association*, vol. 105, no. 7, pp. 583–587, 2006.

[11] A. Gürsoy, M. Kulaksizoglu, M. Sahin et al., "Severe hypertriglyceridemia-induced pancreatitis during pregnancy," *Journal of the National Medical Association*, vol. 98, no. 4, pp. 655–657, 2006.

[12] V. Exbrayat, J. Morel, J. P. De Filippis, G. Tourne, R. Jospe, and C. Auboyer, "Pancréatite aiguë secondaire à une hypertriglycéridémie majeure dorigine gestationnelle. À propos dun cas," in *In Annales françaises danesthésie et de réanimation*, vol. 26, pp. 677–679, Elsevier Masson, 2007.

[13] L. S. Crisan, E. T. Steidl, and M. E. Rivera-Alsina, "Acute hyperlipidemic pancreatitis in pregnancy," *American Journal of Obstetrics & Gynecology*, vol. 198, no. 5, pp. e57–e59, 2008.

[14] L. Vandenbroucke, S. Seconda, L. Lassel, G. Le Bouar, and P. Poulain, "Pancréatite aiguë secondaire à une hypertriglycéridémie majeure au cours de la grossesse. À propos dun cas," *Journal de Gynécologie Obstétrique et Biologie de la Reproduction*, vol. 38, no. 5, pp. 436–439, 2009.

[15] D. Altun, G. Eren, Z. Cukurova, O. Hergünsel, and L. Yasar, "An alternative treatment in hypertriglyceridemia-induced acute pancreatitis in pregnancy: plasmapheresis," *Journal of Anaesthesiology Clinical Pharmacology*, vol. 28, no. 2, pp. 252–254, 2012.

[16] M. Serpytis, V. Karosas, R. Tamosauskas et al., "Hypertriglyceridemia-induced acute pancreatitis in pregnancy," *Journal of the Pancreas*, vol. 13, no. 6, pp. 677–680, 2012.

[17] K. Thulasidass and T. A. Chowdhury, "Hypertriglyceridemic pancreatitis in pregnancy: case reports and review of the literature," *JRSM Short Reports*, vol. 4, no. 8, pp. 1–3, 2013.

[18] R. Basar, A. K. Uzum, B. Canbaz et al., "Therapeutic apheresis for severe hypertriglyceridemia in pregnancy," *Archives of Gynecology and Obstetrics*, vol. 287, no. 5, pp. 839–843, 2013.

[19] S. Gupta, M. Jayant, and R. Kaushik, "Acute hyperlipidemic pancreatitis in a pregnant woman," *World Journal of Emergency Medicine*, vol. 4, no. 3, p. 311, 2013.

[20] B. Abdullah, T. K. Pillai, L. H. Cheen, and R. J. Ryan, "Severe acute pancreatitis in pregnancy," *Case reports in obstetrics and gynecology*, 2015.

[21] T. Amin, L. C. Y. Poon, T. G. Teoh et al., "Management of hypertriglyceridaemia-induced acute pancreatitis in pregnancy," *The Journal of Maternal-Fetal and Neonatal Medicine*, vol. 28, no. 8, pp. 954–958, 2015.

[22] N. Gupta, S. Ahmed, L. Shaffer, P. Cavens, and J. Blankstein, "Severe hypertriglyceridemia induced pancreatitis in pregnancy," *Case Reports in Obstetrics and Gynecology*, 2014.

[23] F. Safi, A. Toumeh, M. A. A. Qadan, R. Karaz, B. AlAkdar, and R. Assaly, "Management of familial hypertriglyceridemia-induced pancreatitis during pregnancy with therapeutic plasma exchange: A case report and review of literature," *American Journal of Therapeutics*, vol. 21, no. 5, pp. e134–e136, 2014.

[24] Y. Liu, Y. Lun, Y. Lv, X. Hou, and Y. Wang, "A Chinese patient with recurrent pancreatitis during pregnancy induced by hypertriglyceridemia associated with compound heterozygosity (Glu242Lys and Leu252VaL) in the lipoprotein lipase gene," *Journal of Clinical Lipidology*, vol. 10, no. 1, pp. 199–203e1, 2016.

[25] F. Gök, S. Köker, A. Kılıçaslan, G. Sarkılar, A. Yosunkaya, and Ş. Otelcioğlu, "Acute pancreatitis due to hypertriglyceridaemia in pregnancy," *Turk Anesteziyoloji ve Reanimasyon Dernegi Dergisi*, vol. 43, no. 2, pp. 116–118, 2015.

[26] H. R. Jeon, S. Y. Kim, Y. J. Cho, and S. J. Chon, "Hypertriglyceridemia-induced acute pancreatitis in pregnancy causing maternal death," *Obstetrics gynecology science*, vol. 59, no. 2, pp. 148–151, 2016.

[27] I. Polypathelli, C. Demosthenous, M. Gavra, E. Matsaridou, and G. Tzatzagou, "Hypertriglyceridemia-induced acute pancreatitis in third trimester of pregnancy: A case report," *Atherosclerosis*, vol. 263, pp. e203–e204, 2017.

[28] T. Chibber and P. S. Gibson, "Fatal Abdominal Compartment Syndrome Due to Severe Triglyceride-Induced Pancreatitis in Early Pregnancy," *Journal of Obstetrics and Gynaecology Canada*, 2017.

[29] G. Lippi, A. Albiero, M. Montagnana et al., "Lipid and lipoprotein profile in physiological pregnancy," *Clinical Laboratory*, vol. 53, no. 3-4, pp. 173–177, 2007.

[30] R. Klingel, B. Göhlen, A. Schwarting, F. Himmelsbach, and R. Straube, "Differential indication of lipoprotein apheresis during pregnancy," *Therapeutic Apheresis*, vol. 7, no. 3, pp. 359–364, 2003.

[31] R. H. Knopp, M. R. Warth, D. Charles et al., "Lipoprotein metabolism in pregnancy, fat transport to the fetus, and the effects of diabetes," *Biology of the Neonate*, vol. 50, no. 6, pp. 297–317, 1986.

[32] J. H. Bae, S. H. Baek, and H. S. Choi, "Acute pancreatitis due to hypertriglyceridemia: report of 2 cases," *The Korean Journal of Gastroenterology*, vol. 46, no. 6, pp. 475–480, 2005.

[33] E.-Q. Mao, Y.-Q. Tang, and S.-D. Zhang, "Formalized therapeutic guideline for hyperlipidemic severe acute pancreatitis," *World Journal of Gastroenterology*, vol. 9, no. 11, pp. 2622–2626, 2003.

[34] A. Monga, A. Arora, R. P. S. Makkar, and A. K. Gupta, "Hypertriglyceridemia-induced acute pancreatitis—treatment with heparin and insulin," *Indian Journal of Gastroenterology*, vol. 22, no. 3, pp. 102-103, 2003.

[35] S. B. Iskandar and K. E. Olive, "Plasmapheresis as an adjuvant therapy for hypertriglyceridemia-induced pancreatitis," *The American Journal of the Medical Sciences*, vol. 328, no. 5, pp. 290–294, 2004.

[36] C. Huang, J. Liu, Y. Lu et al., "Clinical features and treatment of hypertriglyceridemia-induced acute pancreatitis during pregnancy: A retrospective study," *Journal of Clinical Apheresis*, vol. 31, no. 6, pp. 571–578, 2016.

[37] L. Luo, H. Zen, H. Xu et al., "Clinical characteristics of acute pancreatitis in pregnancy: experience based on 121 cases," *Archives of gynecology and obstetrics*, pp. 1–7, 2017.

[38] V. G. Athyros, O. I. Giouleme, N. L. Nikolaidis et al., "Long-term follow-up of patients with acute hypertriglyceridemia-induced pancreatitis," *Journal of Clinical Gastroenterology*, vol. 34, no. 4, pp. 472–475, 2002.

16

A Case of Haematometra Secondary to Cervical Stenosis after Vesicle Vaginal Fistula Surgical Repair

Athanase Lilungulu,[1] Willy Mwibea,[2] Mzee Nassoro,[3] and Balthazar Gumodoka[4]

[1]Department of Obstetrics and Gynaecology, Dodoma University, College of Health Sciences, P.O. Box 395, Dodoma, Tanzania
[2]Department of Obstetrics and Gynaecology, Kibaha Clinical Officer Training College, P.O. Box 30282, Coast Regional, Tanzania
[3]Department of Obstetrics and Gynaecology, Dodoma Regional Referral Hospital, P.O. Box 43, Dodoma, Tanzania
[4]Department of Obstetrics & Gynaecology, Catholic University of Health and Allied Sciences, Bugando Medical Centre, P.O. Box 1370, Mwanza, Tanzania

Correspondence should be addressed to Athanase Lilungulu; athalilungulu@yahoo.com

Academic Editor: Giampiero Capobianco

Background. Haematometra is a rare postobstetrics fistula surgical repair outcome complication; however the condition can be misinterpreted especially in limited resource areas that lack routine ultrasound guidance and with a slowly progressed increase in size of abdomen accompanied with a history of amenorrhoea together with a history of having unprotective sexual intercourse which may increase the possibility of being controversial to full-term gravid uterus. The causes of haematometra might be either due to congenital abnormality of the vaginal canal or acquired iatrogenically. However, any other cause that involved vaginal canal can be a predisposing factor of haematometra. We present a case of a 32-year-old female patient, who had obstetric fistula which was successfully repaired over the past two years. She presented with one-year-and-two-month history of an amenorrhoea that was progressive accompanied with distended abdomen to the extent of looking typically as the gravid uterus. Explorative laparotomy was performed successfully and surgical incision managed by hysterotomy and salpingotomy, whereby approximately ten liters of serosanguinous blood fluid mixed with blood clots was completely suctioned. Despite being a rare condition after vesicle vaginal fistula repair complication outcome, haematometra remains to be relatively common gynaecological condition among female adolescence during postpubertal period.

1. Introduction

Haematometra, also known as haematocolpos, is a common gynaecological condition among postpubertal female adolescence caused by congenital abnormality of vaginal canal [1]; however, any other cause involved vaginal canal regardless of the specific age can be a predisposing factor [2]. The causes of haematometra might be due to either congenital abnormality of the vaginal canal or acquired factor [3, 4]. The most lifetime risk factor of haematometra is congenital abnormality of the vaginal canal. It is reported that postpubertal female adolescence having normal secondary sexual characteristics but presented with primary amenorrhoea must be ruled out with the risk of developed haematometra [5].

Haematometra secondary to any gynaecological surgical procedure involving approach through vaginal canal is extremely rare and usually characterized by clinical feature of secondary amenorrhoea [6]. It usually occurs to female of reproductive age group with the specific history of known gynaecological condition involving specific gynaecological surgical procedure [7]. The management of haematometra regardless of the cause is still remaining to be surgical approach through either abdominal or vaginal technique [8]. We report a case of 32-year-old female patient, who presented with one-year-and-two-month history of an amenorrhoea that was progressive accompanied with distended abdomen to the extent of looking typically as the gravid uterus. Explorative laparotomy was performed successfully and surgical incision managed by hysterotomy and salpingotomy, whereby approximately ten liters of serosanguinous blood fluid mixed with blood clots was completely suctioned.

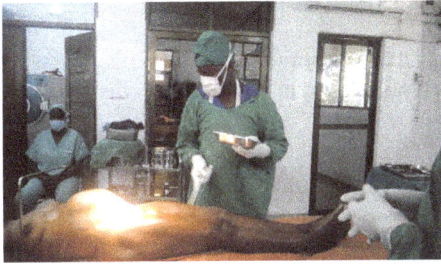

FIGURE 1: Distended abdomen due to haematometra appears likely to be a full-term pregnancy woman.

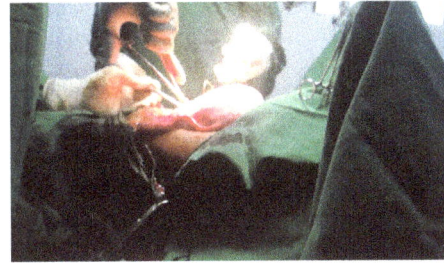

FIGURE 2: Intraoperative finding of giant haematometra and huge distended bilateral haemosalpinx.

2. Case Presentation

A 32-year-old woman, prime para, came at the obstetric department at Kibaha Tumbi Referral Hospital, after an onset of progressive abdomen distention with a history of amenorrhea of one year and two months. Her medical history was unremarkable. However, her past obstetric history was prime para with previous history of prolonged obstructed labor which took three days to be in labor and she had difficult attempted vaginal deliveries of fresh stillbirth male baby at term. On the 14 days after removing the catheter, she started to experience a continuous uncontrolled urine leakage. Before being seen at our obstetric clinic, she had been already having three consecutive obstetric fistula surgical repairs, whereby the third one was done one year and two months prior to this admission. The third fistula surgical repair went successful whereby she could not notice urine leakage and resume her normal sexual life without using any unprotected gear but she could not get a normal menstrual flow throughout the all period, when later she started to notice a progressive abdomen distended and amenorrhea contradict herself as if she had a full-term pregnancy (Figure 1).

Due to the distended abdomen she was thought to have pregnancy despite the fact that she had never seen her normal menstruated blood. Therefore, she was decided to return to the hospital seeking for further evaluation and obstetrics care at our clinic.

Physically she looked healthy with significant normal body weight. Afebrile with her blood pressure measured 120/70 mmHg and pulse rate measured 78 beats/min. Her abdomen was distended with approximated fundal height corresponding to the gestational age of 39 weeks, tense abdomen and tympanic sound, no palpable fetal part, no fluid thrill, and no shifted dullness with the marked tenderness of the lower abdomen.

On speculum examination, a normal cervix could be clearly visualized, and adhesive scared tissue was visualized filling the lateral fornix and the upper part of the vaginal vault. The bimanual examination was performed which revealed that the mass was originated from the uterus with bilateral adnexal difficult to be appreciated.

Haematology laboratory findings revealed a hemoglobin level of 9.6 g/dl, the haematocrit value was 35.7%, and complete blood count was 4.5 billion cells/L with a platelet

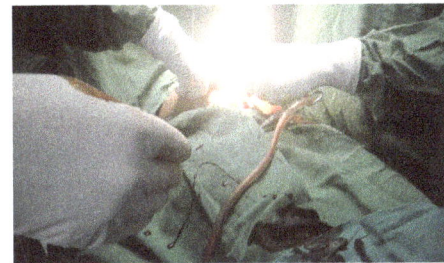

FIGURE 3: Haematometra blood debris amount measured approximately 10 liters.

count of 125 billion/L. Other hematological findings include serum creatinine, BUN, electrolytes, prothrombin time, and partial thromboplastin time appearing in the normal range and biochemistry panel: ALAT-26.71 IU/L ASAT-24.48 IU/L.

Transabdominal ultrasound revealed echogenic opacification with free fluids filled in the uterus, endometrial thickening which measured 10 mm, and markedly thinned elongated closed cervix with free fluid.

The ultrasonography conclusion was a presence of lower genital tract occlusion with haematometra and bilateral haemosalpinx secondarily to acquire obstruction of the lower female genital tract. Detailed examination and planned dilation of the endocervical canal to allow egress of the depicted fluid and subsequent menstruation were attempted under general anesthesia, yet no dimple indicating the external cervical os could be visualized or palpated.

The patient was informed to have explorative laparotomy and the possibility of undergoing abdominal hysterotomy.

Peritoneal cavity was exposed and found a huge haematometra with distended bilateral haemosalpinx and blood debris leaking at the end of ampulla (Figure 2).

The urinary bladder was identified and the lower uterine segment was not obviously formed, hysterotomy was done, and menstruated blood debris was suction which was approximately 10 liters (Figure 3). Using Hegar dilator numbers 6 and 9 repeated alternatively to dilated uterine cervix through abdominally were performed until successful cervical dilatation has been observed and Hegar pass was allowed through the internal os of cervix to the vaginal canal, respectively. Finally, hemostasis was achieved and hysterotomy incision repaired in layers using Vicryl number 2 and abdomen wall closed successfully.

Pathologic assessment of the surgical menstrual blood debris specimen showed the recently evacuated blood clots and endometrial tissues, respectively. The approximate blood loss was one liter and intraoperatively she was transfused one unit of blood. Postoperative period was unremarkable and she was discharged on the seventh day in good condition and advised to continue with cervical dilatation using Hegar at GOPD whereby she was lost to follow-up.

3. Discussion

The complications of vaginal occlusion, vaginal stenosis, and vaginal shortening following obstetric fistula surgical repair are almost rare. The risk of complications depends on fistula hole if it has been extended to such an extent that it involved the nearest pelvic organs and presence of postsurgery inflammatory scared band formation [9].

Haematometra defined as the present retention of menstruation cycle blood in the uterine cavity which can be due to congenital or acquired causes. Congenital causes may be due to cervical agenesis, transverse vaginal septum, and imperforate hymen and acquired cause may be iatrogenically as a result of healing by secondary intention with the scared formation [10].

Haematometra has also been described in elderly women secondary to radiotherapy. Cone biopsy can also rarely lead to cervical stenosis followed by haematometra formation.

Cases of haematometra formation after Cesarean section have been reported in various reviewed articles [11].

Haematometra has been reported not only during postabortion evacuation [12], but also during postpartum cervical tear repair, dilatation, and curettage and cervical ablation therapy. Again during caesarian section procedure when attempting to arrest acute uterine blood loss by applying multiple hemostatic sutures material at the placental bed in a case of placenta previa section can lead to synechiae formation, cervical stenosis, and haematometra [13]. Inappropriate closure of anterior and posterior wall of the uterus during lower segment Cesarean scar can create a uterine pouch and lead to haematometra [14].

We report this unusual case of haematometra and bilateral hydrosalpinx due to cervical stenosis after a successful vesicle vaginal fistula surgical repair. In this case, the archived cervical canal obtained successfully by canalizing the cervical internal os by going through the abdominal approach and attempting to do hysterotomy incision whereby an intrauterine cavity dilatation was achieved using different size of Hegar's dilator to allow easy passage and communication between cervical internal os and upper part of the vaginal canal. Later, after cervical os recanalized repair she was stayed in a ward for the fourteen days and then she was discharged based on seeing her in routinely two-week interval for recanalized cervical os by using Hegar dilator. She was again seen at the GOPD clinic in a period of one month after the first surgical repair and found to have being on dilatation schedule which was shown to be successful cervical os canalization. However, she was lost to follow-up to the clinic.

4. Conclusion

After surgical fistula repair, cervical stenosis causing haematometra is an uncommon complication diagnosis that can be made in a case of prior cervical surgeries.

Consent

A written informed consent was obtained from the patient for publication of this case report.

Acknowledgments

The authors acknowledge the help of the gynaecological ward staff team and theatre operating room staffs.

References

[1] T. Gasim and F. E. Al Jama, "Massive Hematometra due to Congenital Cervicovaginal Agenesis in an Adolescent Girl Treated by Hysterectomy: A Case Report," *Case Reports in Obstetrics and Gynecology*, vol. 2013, pp. 1–3, 2013.

[2] P. S. Vishwekar and G. Sawant, "Cervical Stenosis and Hematometra: a Rare Complication of Cesarean Section and Vvf Repair," *Journal of Evolution of Medical and Dental Sciences*, vol. 4, no. 81, pp. 14245–14247, 2015.

[3] O. I. Odugu BU, U. I. Oko DS, and E. P. Onyekpa IJ, "Imperforate Hymen Presenting with Massive Hematometra and Hematocolpos: A Case Report," *Gynecology & Obstetrics*, vol. 5, no. 10, 2015.

[4] G. Samuel et al., "Hematometra – An unusual cause of suprapubic pain in an adult," *Israeli Journal of Emergency Medicine*, vol. 5, no. 3, pp. 13–17, 2005.

[5] N. Atci, K. S. Dolapcioglu, A. G. Okyay, A. Karateke, I. Kartal, and H. Bayarogullari, "Case Report A case of imperforated hymen in a regularly menstruating girl," vol. 2, no. 3, pp. 56–58, 2015.

[6] M. Subhadra, R. Chitra, and B. Sunanda, "Postabortal hematometra," *The Journal of Obstetrics and Gynecology of India*, vol. 57, no. 3, pp. 257-258, 2007.

[7] V. K. Dalton, N. A. Saunders, L. H. Harris, J. A. Williams, and D. I. Lebovic, "Intrauterine adhesions after manual vacuum aspiration for early pregnancy failure," *Elsevier J Fertil Steril*, vol. 85, no. 6, pp. 2005–2007, 2006.

[8] A. M. Awara, "Abdominal surgical management of partial cervical agenesis in a virgin," *Medical Practice and Reviews*, vol. 3, pp. 5–8, 2012.

[9] A. Di Spiezio Sardo, R. Campo, S. Gordts et al., "The comprehensiveness of the ESHRE/ESGE classification of female genital tract congenital anomalies: A systematic review of cases not classified by the AFS system," *Human Reproduction*, vol. 30, no. 5, pp. 1046–1058, 2015.

[10] M. Bakacak, "Management of hematometrocolpos due to dysfunctional uterine bleeding following progestin use: a case report," *Northern Clinics of Istanbul*, vol. 1, no. 1, pp. 45–48, 2014.

[11] S. Thomas, P. Roy, B. Biswas, and R. Jose, "Complete Cervical Stenosis Following Cesarean Section & VVF Repair," *The*

Journal of Obstetrics and Gynecology of India, vol. 62, no. S1, pp. 49–51, 2012.

[12] M. Subhadra and R. Chitra, "Postabortal hematometra," *Blood*, vol. 57, no. 3, pp. 257-258, 2007.

[13] G. Kaur, S. Jain, A. Sharma, and N. B. Vaid, "Hematometra formation- A rare complication of cesarean delivery," *Journal of Clinical and Diagnostic Research*, vol. 8, no. 8, pp. OD03–OD04, 2014.

[14] A. Kharat and S. Kumari, "Cervical Stenosis: A Rare Complication of Cesarean Section," vol. 24, no. 11, 2014.

17

Advanced Stage Breast Sarcoma Treatment in a Third World Country Public Hospital

Amanda Lino de Faria ⓘ,[1] **Cinthia Moreno Garcia,**[1] **Gabriela de Andrade Rodrigues,**[1] **Lais Helena Dumbra Toloni dos Santos,**[2] **Gabriela B. K. Uyeda,**[2] **Simone Elias,**[2] **Marair G. F. Sartori,**[2] **Afonso Celso Pinto Nazário,**[2] **and Gil Facina**[2]

[1]*Federal University of São Paulo (UNIFESP), São Paulo, Brazil*
[2]*Department of Gynecology, Federal University of São Paulo (UNIFESP), São Paulo, Brazil*

Correspondence should be addressed to Amanda Lino de Faria; amanda.lino@unifesp.br

Academic Editor: Seung-Yup Ku

The case reports a 49-year-old patient, drug-addicted, undernourished, and homeless, who was referred to our service presenting a diagnostic of breast sarcoma and ulcerating tumor which extended from the right breast to the right flank. She underwent hygienic mastectomy and, as it developed, she presented a range of complications, culminating in the recurrence of the tumor and pulmonary metastasis few months after her initial treatment. There is relevance in our study not only because it reports the development of the breast sarcoma, rare neoplasm, and its aggressiveness with fast recurrence, but also because it exposes the impact of biopsychosocial behavior of this patient in her clinical outcome.

1. Introduction

Nowadays, breast cancer is the most common malignant cancer in Brazilian women, excluding nonmelanoma skin cancer, while soft tissue sarcomas are rare tumors derived from mesenchymal cells, comprising 1% of the malignant neoplasms in the adult population [1].

The highest incidence of soft tissue sarcomas is after the fifth decade of the life. Tumors appear as a firm and high volume painless mass, with a rapid growth that reaches around 5 to 6 cm. In circumstances in which there is a tardy diagnosis, these tumors can outgrow to the skin and ulcerate, causing bleeding and infection. The best prognostic predictor is the tumor size since masses smaller than 5 cm have a better prognostic [2].

Considering it a rare neoplasm, the diagnosis of sarcoma is not always easy and it is made by histopathology after removing the lesion [3]. The treatment is guided by the histological grade and adequacy of the surgical margins. Surgery with clear surgical margins is the initial treatment recommended for most patients, and the adjuvant chemotherapy and radiotherapy are individualized according to each patient.

2. Case Report

The case reports patient CAGF, female, 49 years old, homeless in São Paulo, crack addict for ten years, and smoker 70 years/pack of cigarettes, G10P10, without breast cancer in her family history. She mentioned that three years ago she noticed a progressive increase of her right breast and the appearing of bleeding ulcers. She noted a not measured ponderal loss and progressive weakness. She sought primary healthcare service for the first time three months before where a biopsy of the lesion was performed. The anatomopathological examination evidenced an atypical fusiform proliferation, ulcerated and necrotic. The patient was referred to the São Paulo Hospital with a bulk tumor mass, which extended from the right breast to the right flank, friable, bleeding, and sore with a malodorous (Figure 1). She was undernourished (BMI $15,57/m^2$), in a regular, state feverish and pale +/4+. Her physical examination performed by medical equipment did

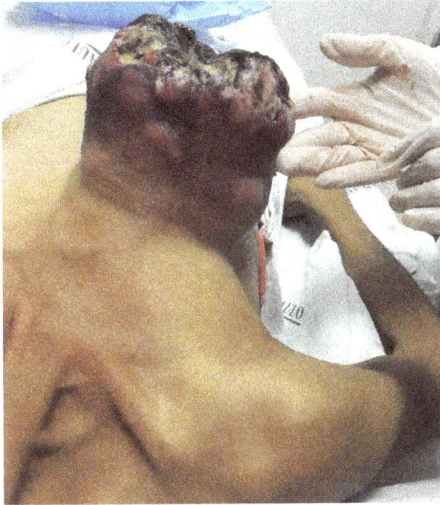

FIGURE 1: Aspect of the lesion in the admission of the patient.

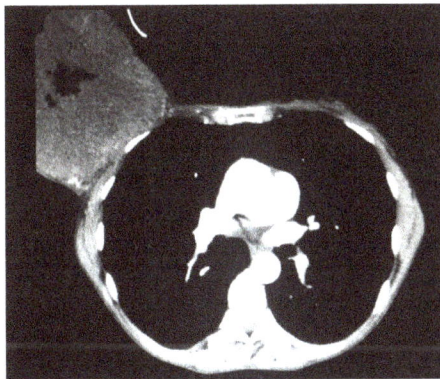

FIGURE 2: Chest tomography at the admission.

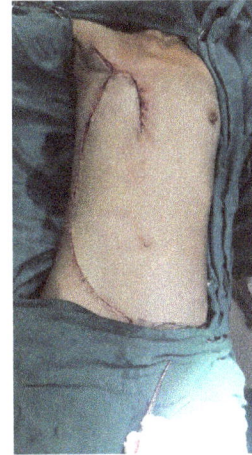

FIGURE 3: Immediate postoperative.

not show alterations. The chest tomography showed the cystic injury and lungs without signs of metastasis (Figure 2).

Initially, due to the infectious character of the wound, antibiotic therapy was performed with intravenous clindamycin. After a discussion of the medical board, a hygienic mastectomy, and reconstruction unilateral thoracoabdominal, the surgical specimen performed had the following dimensions: 14,5x12x9 cm and 1.375g (Figure 3).

The anatomopathological exam resulted in a malignant mesenchymal tumor of a high histological grade. The immunohistochemistry showed pleomorphic undifferentiated sarcoma of high grade (Ki-67 positive in 70% of the sample, negative CD34, negative S-100, and negative vimentin).

Two weeks after the surgical procedure (14° PO), the patient evolved with necrosis in part of the thoracoabdominal flap; it was necessary to perform the debridement of the necrotic area (Figures 4(a) and 4(b)). On the 26° PO, a new debridement of the surgical wound was performed applying skin graft from the right thigh.

During the hospital stay, the patient presented symptoms and laboratory aspects of anemia, being necessary transfusion with red blood cells. The antibiotic therapy with

ceftriaxone and metronidazole was staged for clindamycin (POI) and cephalothin (12° PO) and, later, for piperacillin and tazobactam (17th PO) due to remaining infectious signs in the surgical wound.

After 21 days of antibiotic therapy with piperacillin and tazobactam (39° PO), the patient developed fever (40,3°C), tachycardia, and sweating progressing to a decreased level of consciousness. The patient was transferred to the ICU, where she remained for 48 hours, due to a sepsis of unknown origin and neutropenia of 146 U/L, secondary to sepsis. She initiated meropenem and vancomycin remaining stable, without the use of vasoactive drugs, but maintaining the fever. Infectious screening was performed without the identification of origin.

After 48 hours of admission in the UCI, the patient had an improvement in its fever and neutropenia status, being transferred back to the Gynecology Ward where she presented diffuse maculopapular rash over all integument and face worsening after the contrasted CT on the following day. Vancomycin was suspended due to a suspicion of the pharmacodermy, which was confirmed in skin biopsy.

The patient evolved with a rapid and significant recovery of her skin rash without the need of continued corticotherapy after suspending the vancomycin. Then, the linezolid was initiated to cover the Gram + germs.

After 14 days of meropenem and 7 days of linezolid, the patient presented a satisfactory progression, remaining afebrile and asymptomatic for 12 days.

Despite the clinical improvement and stability, on the 38° PO clinical staff noted the appearance of ulcerated nodule of around 1 cm of diameter in in the right parasternal region, suggestive of local recurrence, which increased progressively, presenting a measure of around 3 cm at the moment of the patient discharge (Figure 5). Besides, during the hospitalization, small pulmonary lesions were identified on computed tomography, absent at the moment of the diagnosis, suggestive of tumor metastasis (Figure 6).

The case was followed and discussed with the Clinical Oncology, which opted to perform outpatient chemotherapy, with Doxorubicin, due to the impossibility of another surgical intervention at the moment. Resources such as transport and

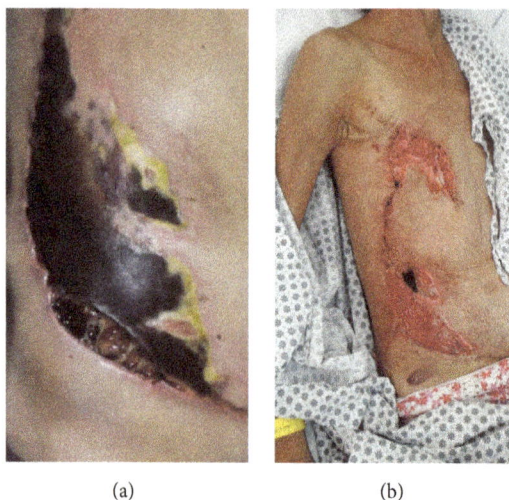

(a)   (b)

FIGURE 4: Necrosis of the surgical flap (a) and final aspect after debridement (b).

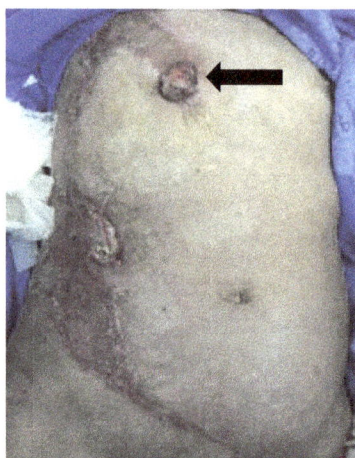

FIGURE 5: Local recurrence (arrow).

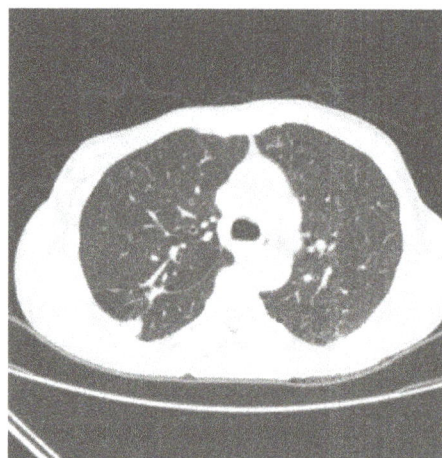

FIGURE 6: Chest tomography at the hospital discharge.

psychological follow-up with CAPS (Psychosocial Attention Center) were provided for the adherence and maintenance of the treatment, besides management by the infectious and plastic surgery staff.

During the outpatient follow-up, 4 chemotherapy cycles were performed, but the recurrence progression was maintained, returning 4 months after the hospital discharge, with an extensive lesion, fever, and local refractory pain, with diagnostic hypothesis of sepsis of cutaneous origin (Figure 7).

The antibiotic therapy was initiated, and the patient was hospitalized for stabilization. A new tomography was performed, presenting pulmonary extensive metastatic lesions, bilateral, besides the massive lesion (Figure 8). The patient remained hospitalized for six days, without complications, and introduced to the palliative care after the hospital discharge.

3. Discussion

Breast sarcoma, as the primary site, is extremely rare, being found in very few cases like this one of our patient. Along with being rare, it is an aggressive tumor, considering that the overall survival in five years ranges between 50% and 66% and the disease-free survival between 33% and 52%. The best prognostic predictor is the tumoral size, considering lesions smaller than 5 cm as the ones with a more favorable prognostic. The bigger the lesions, the worse the disease prognostic that metastasizes hematogenously [4]. Therefore, it is crucial that its detection happens in the early stages, allowing the initial institution of the treatment, with high chances of cure [5]. As most of the disease recurrence is local, the surgery is the recommended first treatment, whether conservative, respecting the margins, or radical.

In the case of our patient, the social condition and the difficulty to access some health care end up in a late diagnosis which shows extensive and infected lesions. Concomitant to the unfavorable external factors, the anatomopathological and immunohistochemical characteristics confirm the aggressiveness of the tumor and the reserved prognostic. Due to the size and the condition of the lesion, the therapeutic surgery could not be performed; then it is recommended to

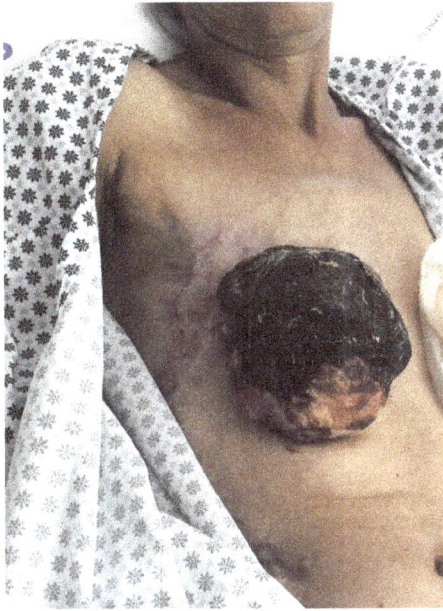

FIGURE 7: An aspect of the lesion in the readmission of the patient.

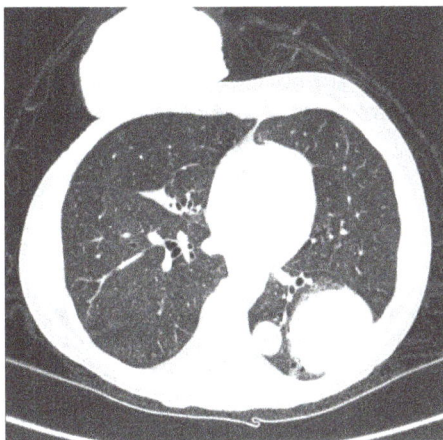

FIGURE 8: Chest tomography in the rehospitalization.

perform a hygienic mastectomy to reduce the morbidity of the lesion and enable a posttreatment.

The evolution on the postsurgical, with necrosis of the flap and neutropenia, precludes the use of adjuvant therapy. The use of chemotherapy is controversial, having few comparative studies to prove its efficiency in increasing the survival expectation [2, 6], while the radiotherapy may be performed in the sarcoma of high grade, being associated with the decrease of the probability of recurrence and dissemination, being the lung the most affected place [5, 7, 8]. However, although the adjuvant therapy is of extreme importance, the clinic conditions of the patient limited the use of those treatments as well as its prognostic and made recurrence progression easier.

In conclusion, we had an uncommon experience, mentioning not only the rare neoplasm but also facing a differentiated clinic course ahead of limitations that are inherent to the social and clinic condition of the patient. Both culminated in a series of nonideal events, creating clinical evolution permeated by complications which took to an unfavorable outcome, showing quick recidivism of the tumor and few therapeutic possibilities. However, even in this situation, it was possible to make a wide approach, with improvement of the clinical condition of the patient, enabling the outpatient follow-up in the attempt of evaluating the best therapeutic possibilities. Nevertheless, considering the complications, recurrence and metastatic lesions, today the patient presents a reserved prognosis being in palliative care.

Conflicts of Interest

The authors declare that there are no conflicts of interest regarding the publication of this paper.

References

[1] M. Yin, H. B. MacKley, J. J. Drabick, and H. A. Harvey, "Primary female breast sarcoma: Clinicopathological features, treatment and prognosis," *Scientific Reports*, vol. 6, 2016.

[2] S. Al-Benna, K. Poggemann, H.-U. Steinau, and L. Steinstraesser, "Diagnosis and management of primary breast sarcoma," *Breast Cancer Research and Treatment*, vol. 122, no. 3, pp. 619–626, 2010.

[3] T. D. Pencavel and A. Hayes, "Breast sarcoma - a review of diagnosis and management," *International Journal of Surgery*, vol. 7, no. 1, pp. 20–23, 2009.

[4] N. Li, M. T. Cusidó, B. Navarro et al., "Breast sarcoma. A case report and review of literature," *International Journal of Surgery Case Reports*, vol. 24, pp. 203–205, 2016.

[5] L. Zelek, A. Llombart-Cussac, P. Terrier et al., "Prognostic factors in primary breast sarcomas: a series of patients with long-term follow-up," *Journal of Clinical Oncology*, vol. 21, no. 13, pp. 2583–2588, 2003.

[6] E. Nizri, O. Merimsky, and G. Lahat, "Optimal management of sarcomas of the breast: An update," *Expert Review of Anticancer Therapy*, vol. 14, no. 6, pp. 705–710, 2014.

[7] R. C. Fields, R. L. Aft, W. E. Gillanders, T. J. Eberlein, and J. A. Margenthaler, "Treatment and outcomes of patients with primary breast sarcoma," *The American Journal of Surgery*, vol. 196, no. 4, pp. 559–561, 2008.

[8] C. Adem, C. Reynolds, J. N. Ingle, and A. G. Nascimento, "Primary breast sarcoma: clinicopathologic series from the Mayo Clinic and review of the literature," *British Journal of Cancer*, vol. 91, no. 2, pp. 237–241, 2004.

18

Malignant Transformation of an Ovarian Endometrioma during Endometriosis Treatment: A Case Report

Hiroaki Takagi ⓘ, Emi Takata, Jinichi Sakamoto, Satoko Fujita, Masahiro Takakura, and Toshiyuki Sasagawa

Department of Obstetrics and Gynecology, Kanazawa Medical University, School of Medicine, Japan

Correspondence should be addressed to Hiroaki Takagi; terry-1@kanazawa-med.ac.jp

Academic Editor: Kyousuke Takeuchi

Dienogest (DNG) is considered to be effective against ovarian endometrioma (OMA). We report a rare case of OMA transformation to ovarian cancer during long-term endometriosis treatment with a periodic administration of a gonadotropin-releasing hormone agonist (Gn-RH agonist) and DNG. The patient was a 41-year-old Japanese woman. OMA and adenomyosis of the uterus were revealed via computed tomography. Consequently, she underwent conservative treatment without undergoing surgery because her overall status was poor. She received cyclic therapy (Gn-RH agonist and DNG) for approximately eight years. However, she reported lumbago and underwent close medical examination at our hospital after about eight years of treatment. Under the suspicion of malignant transformation, she underwent surgery. The pathological diagnosis was clear cell carcinoma of the right ovary (stage 2B). After surgery, she received six courses of chemotherapy (conventional TC). No evidence of disease was observed after chemotherapy. Our findings suggest that malignant transformation of OMA can occur during DNG treatment. Since the delayed detection of ovarian cancer greatly affects the prognosis, women older than 40 with OMA are encouraged to undergo regular check-ups every few months.

1. Introduction

Currently, Japanese women are marrying later in life, which greatly increases the number of menstruations and the risk of endometriosis [1]. Treatment with dienogest (DNG) has helped reduce pelvic pain and improved quality of life in patients with endometriosis [2]. In addition, DNG is expected to reduce the size of an ovarian endometrioma (OMA) [3], and the treatment of endometriosis has been expanded. Herein, we report a rare case of OMA transformation to ovarian cancer during long-term endometriosis treatment with the periodic administration of a gonadotropin-releasing hormone agonist (Gn-RH agonist) and DNG.

2. Case Presentation

A 41-year-old Japanese woman (gravid: 0; para: 0; height: 154 cm; weight: 52.2 kg; body mass index: 22.0 kg/m^2) visited our department due to severe vomiting. Although hyperglycemia and hypertension had been identified upon screening at her workplace, she neglected these findings. She underwent medical examination for the vomiting at a local clinic; however, because her condition did not improve, she was referred to our emergency medical center. She had a history of appendicitis at 20 years of age, and she had undergone bilateral ovarian cystectomy for OMA at 28 years of age. She did not have any additional relevant medical or family history.

Her physical examination findings were as follows: blood pressure, 208/94 mmHg; heart rate, 96 beats/min; respiratory rate, 20 breaths/min; temperature, 36.6°C; and arterial oxygen saturation, 98%. In addition, her blood examination findings were hemoglobin level: 6.3 g/dL; hematocrit: 20.1%; white blood cell count: $17.35 \times 10^3/\mu L$; neutrophil percentage: 91.5%; platelet count: $637 \times 10^3/\mu L$; C-reactive protein level: 14.04 mg/dL; albumin level: 1.8 g/dL; blood sugar level: 450 mg/dL; HbA1c (NGSP): 13.7%; and brain natriuretic peptide level: 922.8 pg/mL. Moreover, her tumor marker findings included cancer antigen (CA) 125 level of 636.0 U/mL and CA19-9 level of 610.0 U/mL. Furthermore, her blood gas

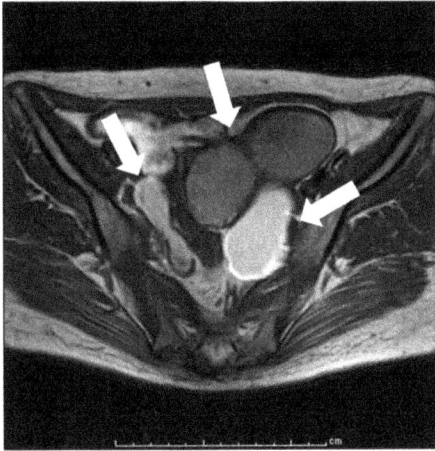

FIGURE 1: Pretreatment magnetic resonance imaging of our patient with endometriosis. Axial T1-weighted imaging at the first consultation. Two ovarian tumors (tumor size: right < left) show high-intensity signals (arrows), and the internal structure shows a blood-resistant component.

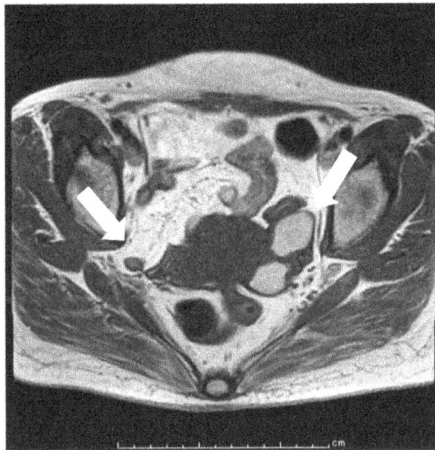

FIGURE 2: Posttreatment magnetic resonance imaging of our patient with endometriosis. Axial T1-weighted imaging after seven years of treatment. The two tumors show high-intensity signals with a diameter of 35 mm or less (arrow), and the tumor size was a partial response.

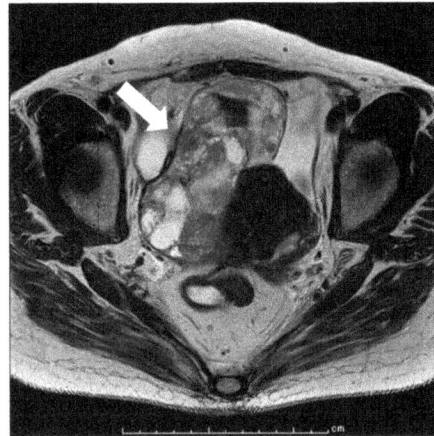

FIGURE 3: Posttreatment magnetic resonance imaging of our patient with endometriosis. MRI after eight years of treatment. The right ovary shows a mass with a maximum diameter of 114 mm (arrow). The solid part of the mass exhibits a low-intensity signal.

analysis findings were pH, 7.490; pCO_2, 34.0 mmHg; and pO_2, 64.9 mmHg. Chest radiography indicated a cardiothoracic ratio of ≤ 50% and a small pleural effusion. T1- and T2-weighted magnetic resonance images (MRI) revealed high-intensity signals in two ovarian tumors (tumor size: right < left) and masses with a maximum diameter of 59 mm in the left ovary (Figure 1). Notably, positron emission tomography-computed tomography (PTT/CT) did not show abnormal uptake. No clear malignant lesions were observed with MRI and PET/CT findings.

She was diagnosed with heart failure, type 2 diabetes mellitus, hypertension, hypoalbuminemia, and iron deficiency anemia at the initial assessment. In addition, OMA and adenomyosis of the uterus were indicated on CT. Consequently,

she underwent conservative treatment without undergoing surgery since her overall status was poor.

Cyclic therapy (Gn-RH agonist, leuprolide acetate 1.88 mg, or goserelin acetate 1.8 mg via subcutaneous injection six times every 4 weeks for 24 weeks; DNG, 2 mg/day, oral administration 24 - 108 weeks) was continued alternately for approximately eight years as endometriosis treatment. Moreover, regular medical examination for tumor markers and ultrasonography was performed every three months.

After approximately seven years of treatment, MRI findings revealed high-intensity signals in two ovarian tumors with a diameter of 35 mm or less, and the tumor size indicated a partial response (Figure 2). Moreover, the level of tumor marker had decreased.

However, she reported lumbago and underwent careful medical examination at our hospital after approximately eight years of treatment. Malignant transformation of the right ovarian tumor was suspected on ultrasonography (tumor enlargement and a solid mass). MRI findings revealed a mass with a maximum diameter of 114 mm in the right ovary. The solid part of the mass exhibited a low-intensity signal (Figure 3). PET/CT findings showed increased focal fludeoxyglucose accumulation (SUV max = 10.00) in the solid elements of the right ovary (Figure 4). Tumor marker findings were as follows: 125 levels, 455.2 U/mL; and CA19-9 levels, 1429.0 U/mL and surgery was performed. She underwent multiple debulking surgeries, including an abdominal total hysterectomy, bilateral salpingooophorectomy, and omentectomy. The pathological diagnosis was clear cell carcinoma of the right ovary (stage 2B [FIGO], T2b), endometriosis of the right ovary, left ovarian metastasis from right ovarian cancer, uterine infiltration from right ovarian cancer, and infiltration of clear cell carcinoma to the tissue in front of the rectum. H&E staining displayed ovarian endometriosis and clear cell carcinoma of the right ovary (Figures 5 and 6). Immunohistochemical staining results showed that the cancer cells were positive for paired box gene 8, tumor protein p53, and epithelial membrane antigen (partial positivity).

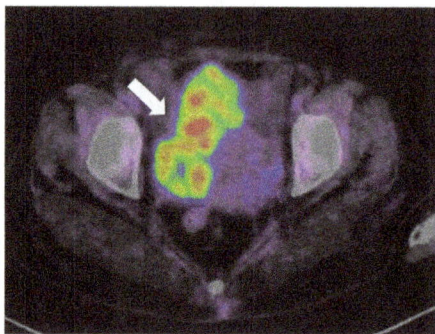

FIGURE 4: Posttreatment magnetic resonance imaging of our patient with endometriosis. PET/CT after eight years of treatment. Increased focal fludeoxyglucose accumulation (SUV max = 10.00) is observed in the solid elements of the right ovary (arrow).

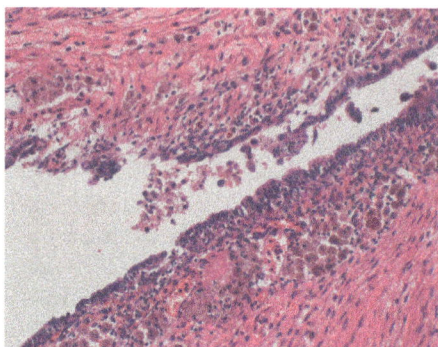

FIGURE 6: Pathological findings of the right ovary: clear cell carcinoma of the right ovary (H-E ×20) and proliferation infiltration of hobnail-like cells with pale eosinophilic cytoplasm.

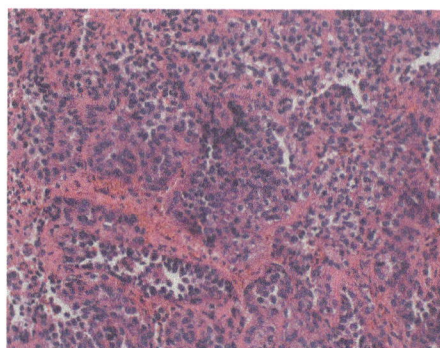

FIGURE 5: Pathological findings of the right ovary. Ovarian endometriosis of the right ovary. (H-E ×20). Ectopic endometrial tissues exist in the cyst wall, and macrophages with hemosiderin are observed.

Additionally, the cells were negative for the estrogen receptor, progesterone receptor, Ki-1, and Wilms' tumor suppressor gene 1.

Following surgery, she received six courses of conventional TC (paclitaxel, 175 mg/m^2; carboplatin, AUC 5). After chemotherapy, PET/CT did not show abnormal uptake. Currently, she exhibits no evidence of disease after chemotherapy.

Her clinical course is presented in Figure 7.

3. Discussion

OMA has a 0.5% – 1.0% probability of undergoing malignant transformation [4]. The inhibitory effect of an oral contraceptive (OC) on ovarian cancer development is remarkable in the long-term as the inhibition rates have been reported to be approximately 30%, 40%, and 50% for 5-, 10-, and 15-year OC treatments, respectively [5]. It has been demonstrated that an OC can epidemiologically prevent ovarian cancer, and the risk and reduction effects are known to correlate with the administration period [5]. An OC inhibits ovulation and appears to protect against the development of ovarian cancer by preventing major stress in the ovary [6]. DNG has both progestin effects and the ability to suppress endometriotic tissue growth, angiogenesis, and inflammation and promote

apoptosis [7]. Since these mechanisms could also reduce ovarian cancer growth, we speculate that DNG may help to reduce malignant transformation of OMA [8]. The Pharmaceuticals and Medical Devices Agency (PMDA) is the government organization in Japan responsible for reviewing drugs and medical devices, overseeing post-market safety, and providing relief for adverse health effects. The PMDA reported that adverse events resulted in ovarian cancer during DNG treatment in only three cases over 10 years. In Japan, the reported cases of malignant transformation from OMA during DNG treatment are negligible [9]. Thus, malignant transformation of OMA during DNG treatment is very rare.

It has been reported that patients with diabetes mellitus have an increased risk of cancer [10, 11]. Moreover, a previous report mentioned the occurrence of ovarian cancer in patients with diabetes mellitus (n = 74 [5 with diabetes mellitus]; hazard ratio, 2.42; 95% confidence interval, 0.96–6.09) [12]. Thus, patients with diabetes mellitus in the general Japanese population may be at an increased risk of developing ovarian cancer. Since the present patient had severe diabetes, her diabetic condition might have been strongly involved in the occurrence of ovarian cancer.

In a previous pathological study on the malignant transformation of endometrioma, Heaps et al. [13] reported that a transition from endometriosis to cancer was noted in 17% of endometrioid adenocarcinoma and 24% of clear cell carcinoma cases. Moreover, Sainz et al. [14] reported that, among the cases of stage 1 ovarian cancer, endometrial carcinoma was involved in 40% of the cases, with endometrioid adenocarcinoma accounting for 41% of these cases, clear cell adenocarcinoma accounting for 31%, and mixed carcinoma (endometrioid and/or clear cell types) accounting for 18%. The transition from endometriosis to cancer is often noted in endometrioid and clear cell adenocarcinomas, and it has been suggested that endometrioma is associated with the pathogenesis of these cancers.

According to the tissue type associated with ovarian epithelial adenocarcinoma (classified by the related genes) [15], type 1 ovarian cancer includes well-differentiated serous carcinoma, well-differentiated endometrioid adenocarcinoma, clear cell adenocarcinoma, mucinous adenocarcinoma, and carcinoma from a borderline malignant tumor

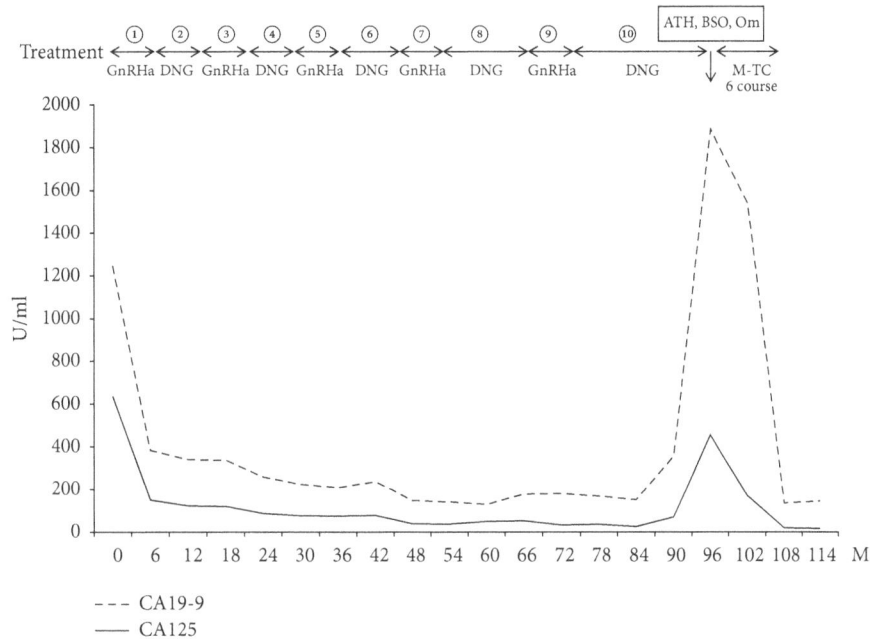

FIGURE 7: Clinical course of the patient. Increases in the level of the tumor markers, CA125 and CA19-9, are noted after six years of treatment. There was an observed decrease in the tumor markers following TC treatment.

or chocolate cyst. Type 1 cancer causes mutations in genes, including *PTEN*, *KRAS*, and *BRAF*, and shows progressively increasing malignancy from low-grade tumors to highly differentiated adenocarcinomas. Many categories show the gradual progression to cancer over several years. Type 2 ovarian cancer includes poorly differentiated serous adenocarcinoma, poorly differentiated endometrioid adenocarcinoma, undifferentiated carcinoma, and carcinosarcoma. It is considered that most serous adenocarcinomas are derived from the fallopian tube epithelium and that many serous adenocarcinomas are accompanied by a p53 mutation and tend to show peritoneal seeding from the initial stage. Furthermore, many categories show quick progression to cancer. In the present case, the tumor could be classified as type 1 ovarian cancer, and it is presumed that OMA underwent malignant transformation over several years. In clear cell adenocarcinoma, which is considered to have a poor prognosis, dense screening is important for the early detection of ovarian malignant transformation.

The factors associated with the differential diagnosis of OMA and ovarian cancer include age, size of the ovarian cyst, tumor marker levels, and diagnostic imaging findings (i.e., ultrasonography and MRI). The risk of malignant transformation of OMA increases with age over 40 years and a maximum tumor diameter of 6 cm [16]. Serum CA125 is a typical tumor marker for endometriosis-associated ovarian carcinoma. Among patients with non-serous ovarian carcinoma (mucinous, endometrioid, and clear cell types), approximately 50% showed bordering elevation of CA125 ($35 < CA125 < 65$ U/mL) within a period of 3.8 years [17]. Transvaginal ultrasonography is accurate for detecting abnormalities with regard to ovarian volume and morphology; however, it is less reliable for differentiating benign ovarian

tumors from malignant ovarian tumors [18]. MRI performed for clear cell adenocarcinoma typically shows a unilocular large cyst with solid protrusions, which are often round and few in number [19]. Recently, it has been shown that magnetic resonance spectroscopy might be an accurate approach for determining the total iron concentration in the cyst fluid and might represent a noninvasive method of predicting the malignant transformation of OMA [20]. This method might be clinically useful for differentiating endometriosis-associated ovarian cancer from OMA.

In conclusion, the malignant transformation of OMA is rare during DNG treatment. Since diabetes in women with endometriosis might be associated with ovarian malignant transformation, it should be carefully assessed and treated. Moreover, because a delay in the detection of ovarian cancer greatly affects prognosis, women older than 40 with OMA are encouraged undergo regular check-ups every few months.

Acknowledgments

The authors would like to thank Enago (www.enago.jp) for the English language review.

References

[1] T. Harada, "Dysmenorrhea and endometriosis in young women," *Yonago Acta Medica*, vol. 56, no. 4, pp. 81–84, 2013.

[2] S. A. Kim, M. J. Um, H. K. Kim, S. J. Kim, S. J. Moon, and H. Jung, "Study of dienogest for dysmenorrhea and pelvic

pain associated with endometriosis," *Obstetrics and Gynecology Science*, vol. 59, no. 6, pp. 506–511, 2016.

[3] A. E. Schindler, "Dienogest in long-term treatment of endometriosis," *International Journal of Women's Health*, vol. 3, no. 1, pp. 175–184, 2011.

[4] H. Kobayashi, "Epidemiological study for development of ovarian cancer among women with ovarian endometrioma," *Acta Obstet Gynaec*, vol. 59, no. 4, pp. 1051–1055, 2007.

[5] Collaborative Group on Epidemiological Studies of Ovarian Cancer, V. Beral, R. Doll, C. Hermon, R. Peto, and G. Reeves, "Ovarian cancer and oral contraceptives: collaborative reanalysis of data from 45 epidemiological studies including 23 257 women with ovarian cancer and 87 303 controls," *Lancet*, vol. 371, no. 9609, pp. 303–314, 2008.

[6] W. J. Murdoch and A. C. McDonnel, "Roles of the ovarian surface epithelium in ovulation and carcinogenesis," *Reproduction*, vol. 123, no. 6, pp. 743–750, 2002.

[7] M. D. P. Andres, L. A. Lopes, E. C. Baracat, and S. Podgaec, "Dienogest in the treatment of endometriosis: systematic review," *Archives of Gynecology and Obstetrics*, vol. 292, no. 3, pp. 523–529, 2015.

[8] D. L. Pup and M. Berretta, "As dienogest effectively suppresses endometriosis, could it also reduce endometriosis-associated ovarian cancers? A further motivation for long-term medical treatment," *WCRJ*, vol. 2, no. 2, p. e526, 2015.

[9] S. Kawai, R. Ichikawa, T. Ueda, M. Urano, M. Kuroda, and T. Fujii, "Ovarian clear cell adenocarcinoma revealed in a young patient during hormone therapy: a case report," *Fujita Medical Journal*, vol. 2, no. 4, pp. 77–79, 2016.

[10] P. Vigneri, F. Frasca, L. Sciacca, G. Pandini, and R. Vigneri, "Diabetes and cancer," *Endocrine-Related Cancer*, vol. 16, no. 4, pp. 1103–1123, 2009.

[11] E. Giovannucci, D. M. Harlan, M. C. Archer et al., "Diabetes and cancer: a consensus report," *Diabetes Care*, vol. 33, no. 7, pp. 1674–1685, 2010.

[12] M. Inoue, M. Iwasaki, T. Otani, S. Sasazuki, M. Noda, and S. Tsugane, "Diabetes mellitus and the risk of cancer: results from a large-scale population-based cohort study in Japan," *Archives of Internal Medicine*, vol. 166, no. 17, pp. 1871–1877, 2006.

[13] J. M. Heaps, R. K. Nieberg, and J. S. Berek, "Malignant neoplasms arising in endometriosis," *Obstetrics & Gynecology*, vol. 75, no. 6, pp. 1023–1028, 1990.

[14] R. Sainz De La Cuesta, J. H. Eichhorn, L. W. Rice, A. F. Fuller Jr., N. Nikrui, and B. A. Goff, "Histologic transformation of benign endometriosis to early epithelial ovarian cancer," *Gynecologic Oncology*, vol. 60, no. 2, pp. 238–244, 1996.

[15] R. J. Kurman and I.-M. Shih, "Pathogenesis of ovarian cancer: lessons from morphology and molecular biology and their clinical implications," *International Journal of Gynecological Pathology*, vol. 27, no. 2, pp. 151–160, 2008.

[16] H. Kobayashi, "Risk of ovarian cancer among women with ovarian endometrioma," *Acta Obstet Gynaec Jpn*, vol. 57, no. 9, pp. 351–355, 2005.

[17] J.-J. Wei, J. William, and S. Bulun, "Endometriosis and ovarian cancer: A review of clinical, pathologic, and molecular aspects," *International Journal of Gynecological Pathology*, vol. 30, no. 6, pp. 553–568, 2011.

[18] J. van Nagell and J. Hoff, "Transvaginal ultrasonography in ovarian cancer screening: current perspectives," *International Journal of Women's Health*, vol. 20, no. 6, pp. 25–33, 2013.

[19] Y. Matsuoka, K. Ohtomo, T. Araki, K. Kojima, W. Yoshikawa, and S. Fuwa, "MR imaging of clear cell carcinoma of the ovary," *European Radiology*, vol. 11, no. 6, pp. 946–951, 2001.

[20] C. Yoshimoto, J. Takahama, T. Iwabuchi, M. Uchikoshi, H. Shigetomi, and H. Kobayashi, "Transverse relaxation rate of cyst fluid can predict malignant transformation of ovarian endometriosis," *Magnetic Resonance in Medical Sciences*, vol. 16, no. 2, pp. 137–145, 2017.

19

A Case of Intrathoracic Gastric Duplication Cyst Detected on Prenatal Ultrasound Examination

Hisako Yagi,[1] Yoshino Kinjyo,[1] Yukiko Chinen,[1] Hayase Nitta,[1] Tadatsugu Kinjo,[1] Keiko Mekaru (iD),[1] Hitoshi Masamoto (iD),[1] Hideki Goya,[2] Tomohide Yoshida,[2] Naoya Sanabe,[3] and Yoichi Aoki (iD)[1]

[1]*Department of Obstetrics and Gynecology, Graduate School of Medicine, University of the Ryukyus, 207 Uehara, Nishihara, Okinawa 903-0215, Japan*
[2]*Department of Pediatrics, Graduate School of Medicine, University of the Ryukyus, 207 Uehara, Nishihara, Okinawa 903-0215, Japan*
[3]*Department of Digestive and General Surgery, Graduate School of Medicine, University of the Ryukyus, 207 Uehara, Nishihara, Okinawa 903-0215, Japan*

Correspondence should be addressed to Yoichi Aoki; yoichi@med.u-ryukyu.ac.jp

Academic Editor: Edi Vaisbuch

A 37-year-old (G4P3) woman was referred to our hospital at 32 weeks of gestation for the evaluation of a fetus with an intrathoracic cystic lesion. Ultrasonography and magnetic resonance imaging revealed that a fetal cystic lesion without a mucosal layer was located in the posterior mediastinum. These findings were consistent with a bronchogenic cyst. At 38 3/7 weeks of gestation, an elective cesarean section was performed because of her previous cesarean section. A female neonate without any external anomalies, weighing 2,442 g, with Apgar scores of 8 and 9, and requiring no resuscitation was born. Four weeks after delivery, the neonate was admitted because of respiratory distress due to mass effect. At right lateral thoracotomy, a 105 × 65 mm of solitary smooth-walled cyst containing serosanguineous fluid was found in the posterior mediastinum, which was excised completely. Histologic examination revealed the diagnosis of the mediastinal gastric duplication cyst. The neonate made an uneventful recovery. Accurate diagnosis is not necessary, but detection and continuous observation are logical. Although gastric duplication, particularly intrathoracic, is a rare pathology, it should be considered in the differential diagnosis of any intrathoracic cyst.

1. Introduction

Foregut duplication cysts are rare congenital anomalies of enteric origin; they constitute 10%–18% of all mediastinal lesions. They are further subdivided into bronchogenic, esophageal, gastric, enteric, and pancreatic cysts [1]. Gastric duplications account for less than 4% of all enteric duplications and most of them are located in the abdomen [2]. Although prenatal or early neonatal diagnosis is very important to avoid a complicated course, it is sometimes difficult. We report a case of an intrathoracic gastric duplication cyst detected on a prenatal ultrasound (US) examination.

2. Case Presentation

A 37-year-old (G4P3) woman was referred to the University of the Ryukyus Hospital at 32 weeks of gestation for the evaluation of a fetus with an intrathoracic cystic lesion. An US examination revealed a 39 × 30 × 44-mm sized monocystic lesion in the mediastinum, in which the aortic arch was displaced upward (Figure 1). Magnetic resonance imaging (MRI) revealed that a fetal cystic lesion was located in the posterior mediastinum without communication to surrounding organs (Figure 2). A mucosal layer in the cyst could not be depicted by US and MRI; these findings were consistent with a bronchogenic cyst. Thereafter, her pregnancy course was uneventful. At 38 3/7 weeks of gestation, an elective cesarean section was performed because of her previous cesarean section. A female neonate without any external anomalies, weighing 2,442 g, with Apgar scores of 8 and 9, and requiring no resuscitation was born. Computed tomography (CT) scan revealed a monocystic lesion in the posterior mediastinum consistent with a bronchogenic cyst.

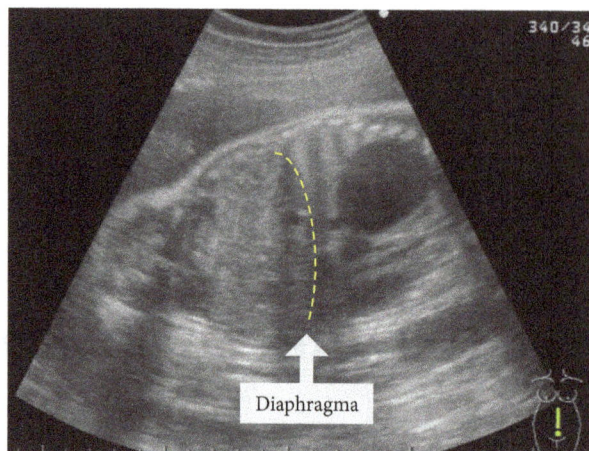

FIGURE 1: Ultrasound examination shows a 39 × 30 × 44-mm sized monocystic lesion in the mediastinum, in which the aortic arch was displaced upward.

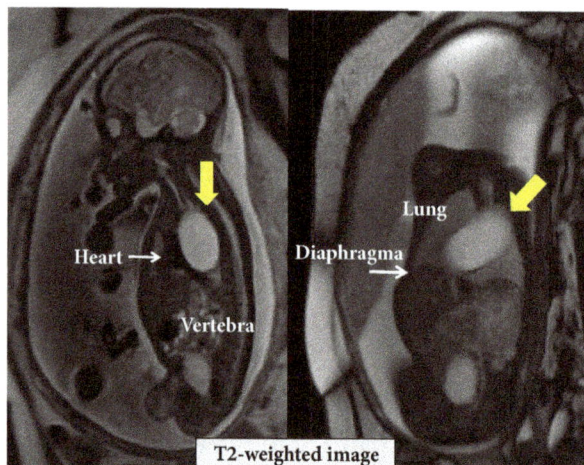

FIGURE 2: T2-weighted magnetic resonance imaging shows fetal cystic lesion located in the posterior mediastinum without communication to surrounding organs.

Four weeks after delivery, the neonate was admitted to the pediatric surgery ward because of respiratory distress due to mass effect. CT scan revealed enlargement of the mediastinal cystic lesion (Figure 3), and surgery was performed. At right lateral thoracotomy, a 105 × 65 mm of solitary smooth-walled cyst containing serosanguineous fluid was found in the posterior mediastinum, which was excised completely. Histologic examination revealed an inner lining of gastric mucosa and an outer smooth muscle coat (Figure 4), leading to the diagnosis of the mediastinal gastric duplication cyst. The neonate made an uneventful recovery and was discharged on the seventh postoperative day.

3. Discussion

The diagnosis of intrathoracic cysts is challenging because of several possible pathologic findings, including bronchogenic cysts, neurenteric cysts, and other foregut duplication cysts. Most intrathoracic alimentary tract duplications present

before the age of 2 years [3, 4]. Therefore, detecting the cyst prenatally is important, thereby leading to appropriate management at birth. Nakazawa et al. observed a mucosal layer in the cyst by postnatal CT scan, leading to the diagnosis of foregut duplication cyst [5]. In our patient, intrathoracic cyst was detected prenatally, and the cyst was monochamber and had smooth thin wall. We diagnosed it as bronchogenic cyst and not gastric duplication cyst. An accurate prenatal diagnosis seems difficult. Moreover, indications for antenatal intervention are limited, other than existence of hydrops fetalis [6]. Accurate diagnosis is not necessary, but detection and continuous observation are logical.

Duplication cysts can present various symptoms, such as dyspnea, stridor, or persistent cough, according to the location and type of the cysts. Asymptomatic patients later become symptomatic because of cyst enlargement, which was seen in our patient [1]. However, choosing between conservative treatment and resection for asymptomatic patients is controversial [7]. In our case, we were concerned about

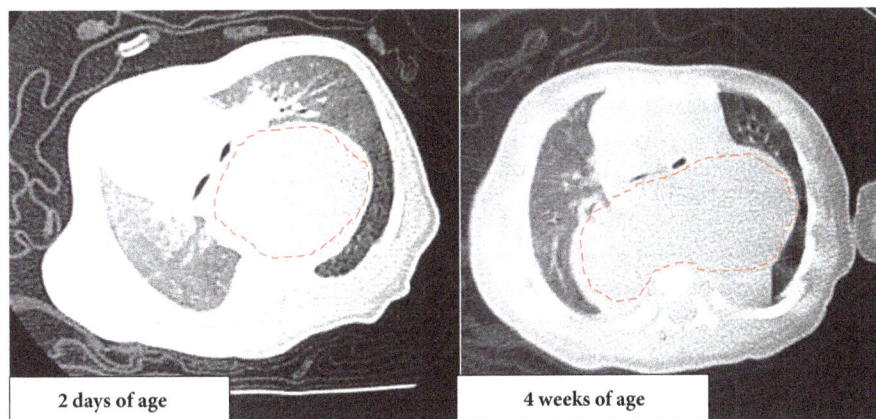

FIGURE 3: Four weeks after delivery, the neonate was admitted because of respiratory distress due to mass effect. Computed tomography scans (right panel: age 2 days, left panel: age 4 weeks) show enlargement of the mediastinal cystic lesion.

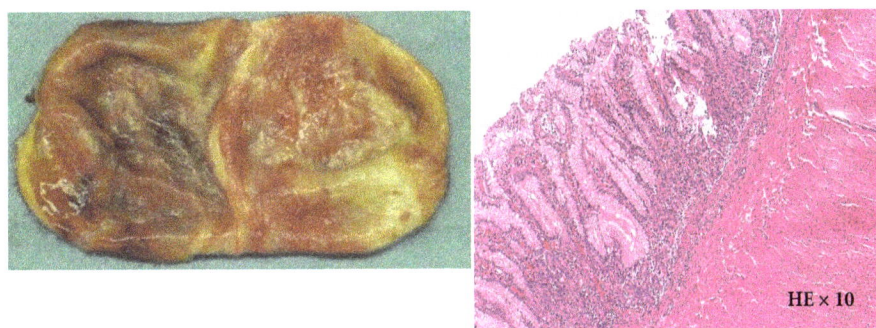

FIGURE 4: A 105 × 65 mm of solitary smooth-walled cyst containing serosanguineous fluid was excised completely (right panel). Histologic examination shows an inner lining of gastric mucosa and an outer smooth muscle coat (left panel), leading to the diagnosis of the mediastinal gastric duplication cyst.

the potential complications of cyst removal in early neonatal period. However, serious mediastinitis due to cyst infection, malignant transformation [8], life threatening hematemesis or hemoptysis, and risk of bleeding from mucosal erosion [9] were reported. Early cyst removal should also be considered.

The etiology of enteric duplication remains speculative. The most accepted theory "split notochord syndrome" postulated the abnormal separation of the notochord from the endoderm, leading to enteric duplications [10]. Although gastric duplication, particularly intrathoracic, is a rare pathology [11, 12], it should be considered in the differential diagnosis of any intrathoracic cyst.

Acknowledgments

The authors would like to thank Enago (https://www.enago.jp/) for the English language review.

References

[1] G. Azzie and S. Beasley, "Diagnosis and treatment of foregut duplications," *Seminars in Pediatric Surgery*, vol. 12, no. 1, pp. 46–54, 2003.

[2] A. Perek, S. Perek, M. Kapan, and E. Göksoy, "Gastric duplication cyst," *Digestive Surgery*, vol. 17, no. 6, pp. 634–636, 2000.

[3] S. T. Ildstad, D. J. Tollerud, R. G. Weiss, D. P. Ryan, M. A. McGowan, and L. W. Martin, "Duplications of the alimentary tract. Clinical characteristics, preferred treatment, and associated malformations," *Annals of Surgery*, vol. 208, no. 2, pp. 184–189, 1988.

[4] C. P. Iyer and G. H. Mahour, "Duplications of the alimentary tract in infants and children," *Journal of Pediatric Surgery*, vol. 30, no. 9, pp. 1267–1270, 1995.

[5] N. Nakazawa, T. Okazaki, and T. Miyano, "Prenatal detection of isolated gastric duplication cyst," *Pediatric Surgery International*, vol. 21, no. 10, pp. 831–834, 2005.

[6] D. J. Markert, K. Grumbach, and P. J. Haney, "Thoracoabdominal duplication cyst: Prenatal and postnatal imaging," *Journal of Ultrasound in Medicine*, vol. 15, no. 4, pp. 333–336, 1996.

[7] S. R. Patel, D. P. Meeker, C. V. Biscotti, T. J. Kirby, and T. W. Rice, "Presentation and management of bronchogenic cysts in the adult," *CHEST*, vol. 106, no. 1, pp. 79–85, 1994.

[8] M. T. Chuang, A. S. Teirstein, F. A. Barba, and M. Kaneko, "Adenocarcinoma arising in an intrathoracic duplication cyst of foregut origin: A case report with review of the literature," *Cancer*, vol. 47, no. 7, pp. 1887–1890, 1981.

[9] P. T. Foley, N. Sithasanan, R. McEwing, J. Lipsett, W. D. A. Ford, and M. Furness, "Enteric Duplications Presenting as Antenatally Detected Abdominal Cysts: Is Delayed Resection Appropriate?" *Journal of Pediatric Surgery*, vol. 38, no. 12, pp. 1810–1813, 2003.

[10] J. R. Bentley and Smith. J. R., "Developmental posterior enteric remnants and spinal malformations. Arch Dis Child," *Arch Dis Child*, vol. 35, pp. 527–530, 1960.

[11] P. Daher, L. Karam, and E. Riachy, "Prenatal diagnosis of an intrathoracic gastric duplication: a case report," *Journal of Pediatric Surgery*, vol. 43, no. 7, pp. 1401–1404, 2008.

[12] C. Turkyilmaz, E. Onal, Y. Atalay et al., "Two isolated giant gastric duplication cysts in thorax in a newborn," *Scottish Medical Journal*, vol. 58, no. 3, pp. e28–e30, 2013.

20

Nonsurgical Intervention in a Preeclamptic Patient with Spontaneous Spinal Epidural Hematoma

Michelle Nguyen ⓘ**,**[1] **Maria Raquel Kronen,**[1] **Alex Nhan** ⓘ**,**[2] **and Antonio Liu**[3]

[1]*Department of Obstetrics and Gynecology, White Memorial Medical Center, Los Angeles, CA 90033, USA*
[2]*University of Central Florida College of Medicine, Orlando, FL 32827, USA*
[3]*Department of Neurology, White Memorial Medical Center, Los Angeles, CA 90033, USA*

Correspondence should be addressed to Michelle Nguyen; nguyenmt02@ah.org

Academic Editor: Maria Grazia Porpora

Background. Spontaneous epidural hematoma (SEH) is a rare finding in pregnancy, especially since most pregnant women do not have risk factors for developing SEH. The presence of epidural anesthesia can delay the diagnosis of SEH in pregnant patients. Immediate surgical decompression is the current standard of care for treating SEH. *Case Presentation.* We present the case of a 37-year-old pregnant woman with preeclampsia with severe features who developed neurological deficits that were initially attributed to her epidural anesthesia. She was eventually found to have SEH with spinal stenosis at T5-T6 on MRI. Oral antihypertensives were used to keep the patient's blood pressures within normal limits, and she subsequently had complete resolution of her neurological symptoms and her SEH on imaging. *Conclusion.* Preeclampsia may contribute to the development of SEH in pregnancy, and strict blood pressure control may potentially provide a safe and effective alternative to neurosurgery for these patients.

1. Introduction

Spontaneous epidural hematoma (SEH) is a particularly rare and devastating complication in the peripartum period. SEH in pregnant patients may remain undetected for a significant amount of time as these patients are less likely to have predisposing factors for SEH, such as anticoagulation, arteriovenous (AV) malformations, hemophilia, or trauma [1]. Furthermore, the administration of epidural anesthesia can confound the clinical picture, posing another challenge in making the diagnosis. Prompt recognition of SEH in laboring patients is extremely important because urgent treatment is required to prevent long-term neurological damage and other associated complications, including seizure, placental abruption, hepatic rupture, and coagulopathy [2]. The standard treatment for SEH is immediate surgical decompression, as demonstrated in the rare cases of SEH in pregnancy that have been reported in the literature [3–7].

While SEH may present under a variety of conditions in the intrapartum period [8–14], SEH that is diagnosed postpartum in preeclamptic patients is especially challenging to treat. Maintaining the perfusion pressure of the spinal

cord is important because decreased blood pressure can lead to decreased spinal cord blood flow, which could further compromise the segment of spinal cord that has already been injured by the spontaneous hemorrhage [15, 16]. However, lowering blood pressure is important in order to reduce the preeclampsia-associated risks of seizures, stroke, hepatic rupture, and renal injury. The ACOG Task Force on Hypertension in Pregnancy recommends antihypertensive therapy in the postpartum period when blood pressure is persistently higher than 150 mm Hg systolic or 100 mm Hg diastolic [17]. This case study describes a preeclamptic patient with SEH who was conservatively managed with antihypertensive medication in the postpartum period to maintain blood pressures within a normal range (i.e., systolic <140, diastolic <90, below current literature recommendations) and made a full neurological recovery without invasive surgical intervention.

2. Case Report

A 37-year-old woman with a history of chronic back pain and sciatica presented to our teaching hospital at 36.5 weeks' gestation in early labor. At the time of presentation, she was noted to have acute onset of mild-range elevated blood pressures (140s-150s/90s) with a urine protein-to-creatinine ratio of 0.37, consistent with a diagnosis of preeclampsia. Six hours after admission, her blood pressures progressed to severe-range, with a maximum of 195/105. Per protocol, she was given IV labetalol and $MgSO_4$ for preeclampsia with severe features. Shortly thereafter, the patient retrospectively reported that she began to have mid-back pain along with numbness, tingling, and weakness in her right lower extremity, but she did not report these symptoms initially to her healthcare team, as she was more concerned about her pelvic pain with contractions. Approximately 3 hours after the onset of her neurological symptoms, a labor epidural was administered to help control her contraction pain and blood pressures. The epidural catheter was placed uneventfully at L3-L4 with the tip threaded to the maximum height of T11. As the epidural was being placed, the patient then reported to the anesthesiologist that she had been feeling weak. The patient was noted to appear lethargic on exam, but she was able to sit up with minimal assistance for her labor epidural. Therefore, her weakness was attributed to labor. She progressed to complete cervical dilation and had a vaginal delivery with vacuum assistance due to a 5-minute prolonged deceleration on FHT.

The patient continued to complain of leg weakness after delivery. At 14 hours postpartum, the nurse encouraged the patient to attempt ambulation. However, even with her best efforts, the patient was unable to move her body from a distinct line below her breasts down to her toes. She also noticed numbness, burning, and electrical sensations to light touch from that line down to her toes. At this time the resident team was notified, and a Foley catheter was inserted. There was low suspicion for magnesium toxicity as she had intact reflexes with no complaints of shortness of breath, and her magnesium level was 5.9. She still had mild-range elevated blood pressures at the time, and she remained on IV magnesium for 24 hours postpartum.

A stat CT scan of the head without contrast resulted in normal findings with no evidence of stroke. MRI of the spine showed a fluid sac suggestive of epidural blood, measuring 3.5 cm in the craniocaudal plane and 0.4 cm in the anteroposterior plane. There was also a mild-to-moderate degree of spinal stenosis at T5-T6 due to extrinsic mass effect of the epidural hemorrhage but no direct spinal cord compression (Figures 1(a) and 1(b)). The patient was immediately started on IV dexamethasone 4 mg q6h. Upon evaluation by neurosurgery, the patient was not considered to be a surgical candidate because the MRI showed no clear evidence of spinal cord hemorrhage or spinal cord compression.

On the morning of postpartum day #1, the patient remained with paresthesia in her lower extremities and flaccid paralysis from the waist down, but she was able to wiggle her toes. Her blood pressures were predominately normal (120-140/80-90) with a few mild-range elevated blood pressures. Per protocol, she was kept on IV magnesium for seizure prophylaxis until she was 24 hours postpartum. Diffusion-weighted imaging of the spine later that day showed an epidural lesion with a hemosiderin ring that had

decreased in size to 2-3 mm in maximal depth, suggestive of a resolving epidural hematoma when compared to the most recent MRI (Figure 2).

On postpartum day #2, the patient was started on PO nifedipine XL 30 mg daily to consistently maintain her blood pressures within normal range. Her mobility improved with demonstrated flexion and extension at the hips bilaterally, in addition to return of normal sensation in her lower extremities.

The patient's movements and sensation continued to improve day by day while she was kept on IV dexamethasone and PO nifedipine. By postpartum day #4, the patient was ambulating with a walker and had good bladder and bowel control. On postpartum day #6, the patient was ambulating without assistance and reported complete resolution of her pain in the back and lower extremities. She was discharged home in stable condition.

A follow-up MRI 6 weeks later showed complete resolution of the spinal epidural hematoma (Figure 3). At the time, she was still ambulating independently and had full control of her bladder and bowel function.

3. Discussion

The underlying pathogenesis of preeclampsia involves abnormalities in the placental vasculature, which lead to decreased circulating levels of VEGF (vascular endothelial growth factor) and other angiogenic growth factors. Decreased VEGF in turn causes endothelial cell dysfunction, which leads to vasoconstriction (i.e., spasms in the vascular smooth muscle) and elevated blood pressures [18]. Preeclampsia may have played a role in the development of SEH. Our patient first noticed back pain along with numbness, tingling, and weakness in her right lower extremity around the same time that her blood pressures progressed from mild-range (i.e., systolic 140-159 mm Hg, diastolic 90-109 mm Hg) to severe-range (i.e., systolic ≥160, diastolic ≥110). We suspect that the patient's increased blood pressures may have initiated her SEH at the T5-T6 region, which subsequently led to a transient extrinsic compression of the spinal cord and eventually cord edema. Epidural placement was likely a coincident rather than causative factor, given that the patient's neurological symptoms began prior to epidural anesthesia, and the lesion occurred above the level of epidural placement. Although epidural anesthesia made the diagnosis of SEH more difficult, the patient's cord edema was fortunately reversible with IV dexamethasone. Consistently maintaining her blood pressures within normal range (120-140/80-90) using PO antihypertensive medication likely also facilitated neurologic recovery.

Several challenges emerged in the diagnosis and treatment of this patient. First of all, our patient was a relatively healthy pregnant woman in her 30s with no preexisting medical conditions, prior surgeries, or trauma history. In contrast, SEH typically presents in the fourth or fifth decade of life, and it is more likely to occur in males [19]. The epidemiology of SEH is in part secondary to natural history of AV malformations, which are among the most

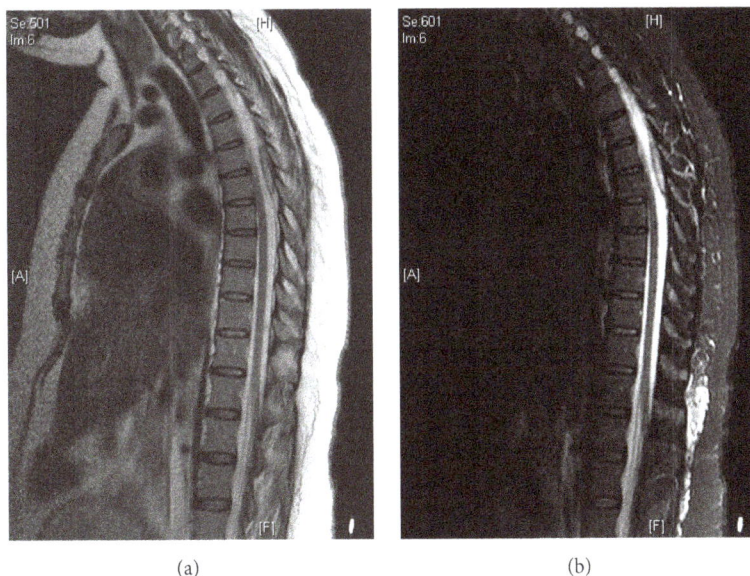

(a)

(b)

FIGURE 1: (a, b) MRI images at 14 hours postpartum showing a spinal epidural hematoma measuring 3.5 cm x 0.4 cm. There is also spinal stenosis at T5-T6 due to extrinsic mass effect of the epidural hemorrhage.

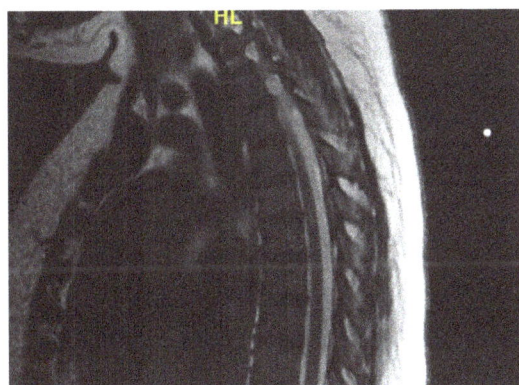

FIGURE 2: MRI T2 sagittal view of epidural blood collection which has decreased in size to 2-3 mm.

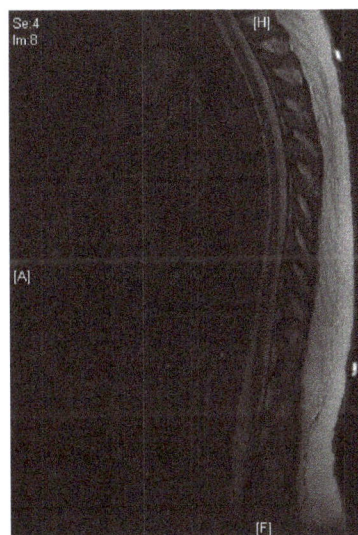

FIGURE 3: MRI at 6 weeks postpartum showing complete resolution of the spontaneous epidural hematoma.

significant predisposing factors. Spinal AV malformations, particularly dural AV fistulas, affect males more often than females, with the average age at diagnosis being 50s-60s [20]. This makes the presence of AV malformations in obstetric patients significantly less likely, and the diagnosis of ruptured SEH easy to miss. This is clinically significant because AV malformations have the potential to precipitate spontaneous hemorrhage and/or cord ischemia, and pregnancy increases the risk of hemorrhage from AV malformations [21].

may warrant revisiting in obstetric patients whose cases are complicated by preeclampsia, in light of this study.

Consent

The patient has signed an informed consent form stating that she agrees to give the authors full permission to use her protected health information, with all personal identifiers removed, for the purposes of clinical research, discussion, presentation, and publication. A copy of this signed informed consent form is available upon request.

4. Conclusion

Our patient achieved excellent outcomes from strict blood pressure control without undergoing invasive neurosurgery. The standard of care of neurosurgical treatment of SEH

References

[1] J. Figueroa and J. G. Devine, "Spontaneous spinal epidural hematoma: literature review," *Journal of Spine Surgery*, vol. 3, no. 1, pp. 58–63, 2017.

[2] D. D. Doblar and S. D. Schumacher, "Spontaneous acute thoracic epidural hematoma causing paraplegia in a patient with severe preeclampsia in early labor," *International Journal of Obstetric Anesthesia*, vol. 14, no. 3, pp. 256–260, 2005.

[3] C. W. Kong and W. W. K. To, "Spontaneous spinal epidural haematoma during pregnancy," *Journal of Obstetrics & Gynaecology*, vol. 38, no. 1, pp. 129–131, 2018.

[4] S. M. Hussenbocus, M. J. Wilby, C. Cain, and D. Hall, "Spontaneous spinal epidural hematoma: A case report and literature review," *The Journal of Emergency Medicine*, vol. 42, no. 2, pp. e31–e34, 2012.

[5] P. Wang, X.-T. Xin, H. Lan, C. Chen, and B. Liu, "Spontaneous cervical epidural hematoma during pregnancy: Case report and literature review," *European Spine Journal*, vol. 20, no. 2, pp. S176–S179, 2011.

[6] I. Haraga, Y. Sugi, K. Higa, S. Shono, K. Katori, and K. Nitahara, "Spontaneous spinal subdural and epidural haematoma in a pregnant patient," *The Japanese Journal of Anesthesiology*, vol. 59, no. 6, pp. 773–775, 2010.

[7] M. P. Steinmetz, I. H. Kalfas, B. Willis, A. Chalavi, and R. C. Harlan, "Successful surgical management of a case of spontaneous epidural hematoma of the spine during pregnancy," *The Spine Journal*, vol. 3, no. 6, pp. 539–542, 2003.

[8] M. Samali, A. Elkoundi, A. Tahri, M. Bensghir, and C. Haimeur, "Anesthetic management of spontaneous cervical epidural hematoma during pregnancy: A case report," *Journal of Medical Case Reports*, vol. 11, no. 1, 2017.

[9] P. Krishnan and R. Kartikueyan, "Spontaneous spinal epidural hematoma: A rare cause of paraplegia in pregnancy," *Neurology India*, vol. 62, no. 2, pp. 205–207, 2014.

[10] Z.-L. Wang, H. X. Bai, and L. Yang, "Spontaneous spinal epidural hematoma during pregnancy: Case report and literature review," *Neurology India*, vol. 61, no. 4, pp. 436-437, 2013.

[11] S. Tada, A. Yasue, H. Nishizawa, T. Sekiya, Y. Hirota, and Y. Udagawa, "Spontaneous spinal epidural hematoma during pregnancy: Three case reports," *Journal of Obstetrics and Gynaecology Research*, vol. 37, no. 11, pp. 1734–1738, 2011.

[12] F. Badar, S. Kirmani, M. Rashid, S. F. Azfar, S. Yasmeen, and E. Ullah, "Spontaneous spinal epidural hematoma during pregnancy: A rare obstetric emergency," *Emergency Radiology*, vol. 18, no. 5, pp. 433–436, 2011.

[13] A. Jea, K. Moza, A. D. Levi, and S. Vanni, "Spontaneous spinal epidural hematoma during pregnancy: Case report and literature review," *Neurosurgery*, vol. 56, no. 5, p. E1156, 2005.

[14] G. Masski, B. Housni, K. Ibahiouin, and M. Miguil, "Spontaneous cervical epidural haematoma during pregnancy," *International Journal of Obstetric Anesthesia*, vol. 13, no. 2, pp. 103–106, 2004.

[15] Y. Y. Jo, D. Lee, Y. J. Chang, and H. J. Kwak, "Anesthetic management of a spontaneous spinal-epidural hematoma during pregnancy," *International Journal of Obstetric Anesthesia*, vol. 21, no. 2, pp. 185–188, 2012.

[16] J. W. Squair, L. M. Bélanger, A. Tsang et al., "Spinal cord perfusion pressure predicts neurologic recovery in acute spinal cord injury," *Neurology*, vol. 89, no. 16, pp. 1660–1667, 2017.

[17] Hypertension in pregnancy, "Report of the American College of Obstetricians and Gynecologists' Task Force on Hypertension in Pregnancy," *Obstetrics & Gynecology*, vol. 122, no. 5, pp. 1122–1131, 2013.

[18] E. Funai, "Preeclampsia," in *High-Risk Obstetrics: The Requisites in Obstetrics and Gynecology*, E. Funai, M. Evans, and C. Lockwood, Eds., Mosby, Philadelphia, PA, USA, 2008.

[19] B. S. Baek, J. W. Hur, K. Y. Kwon, and H. K. Lee, "Spontaneous spinal epidural hematoma," *Journal of Korean Neurosurgical Society*, vol. 44, no. 1, pp. 40–42, 2008.

[20] J. E. Fugate, G. Lanzino, and A. A. Rabinstein, "Clinical presentation and prognostic factors of spinal dural arteriovenous fistulas: An overview," *Neurosurgical Focus*, vol. 32, no. 5, article no. E17, 2012.

[21] B. A. Gross and R. Du, "Hemorrhage from arteriovenous malformations during pregnancy," *Neurosurgery*, vol. 71, no. 2, pp. 349–355, 2012.

21

Placenta Percreta in First Trimester after Multiple Rounds of Failed Medical Management for a Missed Abortion

**Jaimin Shah,[1] Eduardo Matta,[2] Fernando Acosta,[3]
Natalia Golardi,[3] and Cristina Wallace-Huff[1]**

[1]*Department of Obstetrics, Gynecology and Reproductive Sciences, McGovern Medical School, The University of
Texas Health Science Center at Houston, Houston, TX, USA*
[2]*Department of Diagnostic and Interventional Imaging, McGovern Medical School, The University of
Texas Health Science Center at Houston, Houston, TX, USA*
[3]*Department of Pathology and Laboratory Medicine, McGovern Medical School, The University of
Texas Health Science Center at Houston, Houston, TX, USA*

Correspondence should be addressed to Jaimin Shah; jaimin.shah@uth.tmc.edu

Academic Editor: Giampiero Capobianco

Background. The detection of a morbidly adherent placenta (MAP) in the first trimester is rare. Risk factors such as multiparity, advanced maternal age, prior cesarean delivery, prior myomectomy, placenta previa, or previous uterine evacuation place patients at a higher risk for having abnormal placental implantation. If these patients have a first trimester missed abortion and fail medical management, it is important that providers have a heightened suspicion for a MAP. *Case.* A 24-year-old G4P3003 with 3 prior cesarean deliveries underwent multiple rounds of failed medical management for a missed abortion. She had a dilation and curettage that was complicated by a significant hemorrhage and ultimately required an urgent hysterectomy. *Conclusion.* When patients fail medical management for a missed abortion, providers need to assess the patient's risk factors for a MAP. If risk factors are present, a series of specific evaluations should be triggered to rule out a MAP and help further guide management. Early diagnosis of a MAP allows providers to coordinate a multidisciplinary treatment approach and thoroughly counsel patients. Ensuring adequate resources and personnel at a tertiary hospital is essential to provide the highest quality of care and improve outcomes.

1. Introduction

The detection of a morbidly adherent placenta (MAP) in early pregnancy is rare. Routine first trimester transvaginal ultrasounds (TVUS) usually do not focus on localization and implantation of the placenta [1]. Generally, a MAP is not clinically detected until later in pregnancy [2]. Risk factors such as multiparity, advanced maternal age, prior cesarean delivery, prior myomectomy, placenta previa, or previous uterine evacuation place patients at a higher risk for having abnormal placental implantation in future pregnancies [2, 3]. The incidence of MAPs in early gestation has been increasing likely due to the rising rates of cesarean deliveries and prior uterine surgery [1, 4–7]. In patients with risk factors for abnormal placental implantation and who fail medical management for a first trimester abortion, it is important

that providers have an increased suspicion for a MAP. We report a case of a patient with a 7-week missed abortion with three prior cesarean deliveries that failed multiple rounds of medical management. She subsequently had an attempted dilation and curettage that was complicated by a significant hemorrhage and she ultimately required an urgent hysterectomy.

2. Case

A 25-year-old G4P3003 at 7 weeks and 1 day by last menstrual period with a medical history of 3 previously documented low transverse cesarean deliveries and obesity (BMI: 34) presented for management at a county hospital for a missed abortion diagnosed at an outlying rural clinic. The patient reported that this was a planned pregnancy and desired future pregnancies; she denied any spotting, cramping, or passage of any tissue. The formal TVUS report at the outside clinic showed an intrauterine pregnancy with a 27.8 mm mean sac diameter consistent with 8 weeks and no fetal cardiac activity seen; no evidence of a MAP was noted in the report. A repeat bedside TVUS in clinic by a resident physician showed an irregular shaped gestational sac with a crown rump length of 1.5 cm.

After thoroughly counseling the patient on expectant, medical, and surgical management, she elected for medical management. The patient was uninsured and declined surgical management as she did not want to incur the expense of the procedure. The patient received 800 mcg of misoprostol per vagina (PV) in clinic and she was sent home with a prescription to take two additional doses of 800 mcg buccally every 24–48 hours if needed until she noted passage of clots or tissue. She was instructed to return to clinic in one week unless she developed heavy bleeding soaking greater than two pads an hour for two hours or fever greater than 100.4 degrees Fahrenheit [8]. She followed up one week later and denied spotting, cramping, or passage of tissue. A bedside TVUS by a resident physician showed no change from the week prior. Given that the patient's insurance eligibility status was still pending, the patient declined surgical management due to the potential financial burden and declined expectant management. The patient was counseled that no data supports multiple rounds of medical management but, given her insurance eligibility status and strong desire to not incur surgical fees, she received two more rounds of medical management without resolution of her missed abortion. The patient was then able to acquire insurance approval. She then opted for surgical management. She presented three days later to the ambulatory outpatient surgical center.

She was Rh positive with a hemoglobin of 12.7 g/dL. During her procedure, the cervix was dilated followed by insertion of the suction curette; some products of conception were evacuated but the canister filled quickly with bright red blood. Upon removing the curette, she continued to bleed heavily. Methergine was administered intramuscularly which helped decrease the amount of bleeding. The estimated blood loss (EBL) was 1200 cc; two units of packed red blood cells (PRBC) were given and the main operating room (OR) and hospital were notified for her immediate transfer since the ambulatory surgery center was not sufficiently equipped for this level of care. A foley balloon was placed into the uterus and inflated to 60 cc. This was able to tamponade and minimize the bleeding.

The patient was transferred to the main hospital by ambulance. A TVUS was performed which showed products of conception versus a 5 cm hematometra. Given that the patient had refractory abdominal pain unrelieved by intravenous morphine and a concern for an expanding hematometra, the patient was taken back to the OR for an exploratory laparotomy. The patient was consented for a possible total abdominal hysterectomy versus evacuation of hematometra. Upon entry into the abdomen, dense abdominal adhesions were noted; there was approximately 200 cc of hemoperitoneum in the rectouterine pouch. It was noted that there was a 7-8 cm portion of the lower uterine segment that displayed placental

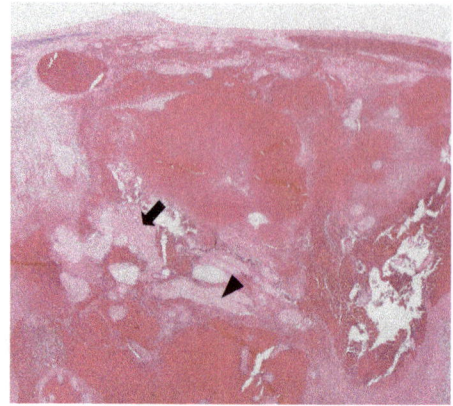

FIGURE 1: Necrotic myometrium (arrow) with degenerating chorionic villi (arrowhead) transecting through the entire myometrial thickness to the serosal surface with extensive hemorrhage (H&E stain, 20x magnification).

tissue overlying the uterine serosa by 1 mm. The decision was made to proceed with a hysterectomy. She received 1 unit each of fresh frozen plasma and PRBC intraoperatively. The EBL intraoperatively was 500 cc bringing the total blood loss to 1900 cc. A cystoscopy was performed and bladder involvement was ruled out. The patient met all postoperative milestones and recovered well.

Final pathology showed a placenta percreta. Sectioning through the patient's myometrium showed extensive hemorrhage dissecting through the entire myometrial thickness at the level of the lower uterine segment (Figure 1). Microscopic evaluation showed numerous chorionic villi penetrating through the entire thickness of the myometrial wall and through the uterine serosa which is diagnostic of a placenta percreta [9].

3. Discussion

Upon review of the literature, a MAP is a rare finding to detect in the first trimester. Of the MAPs, placenta accreta occurs 75%, placenta increta 18%, and placenta percreta 7% of the time [2, 5]. To our knowledge, there have been 26 prior MAPs diagnosed in the first trimester and treated before 15 weeks' gestation (Table 1). Most patients had a history of a prior cesarean delivery leaving possible scar tissue in the anterior uterine wall [1, 4]. Twenty-two patients required a hysterectomy while four had conservative management and retained their uterus. The majority of patients had a risk factor for a MAP but a few cases occurred in patients with a nonscarred uterus [1]. It is our understanding there were only two other cases that attempted one round of medical management in which both cases ended up with an hysterectomy [3, 10]. Per The American College of Obstetricians and Gynecologists (ACOG), they recommend one round of medical management for missed abortions and then consider alternate management options [8]. Our patient did not have insurance coverage so the option of surgery after her failed first round of medical management was not financially feasible. Given patient's socioeconomic constraints, offering

TABLE 1: Morbidly adherent placentas (MAPs) diagnosed in the first trimester and treated before 15 weeks' gestation [1, 3, 4].

Author and year	Type of MAP	Prior CS[§]	Prior D&C[†]	GA at Diagnosis[#]	Presenting symptoms	US diagnostic of MAP	Management & outcome
Helkjaer et al., 1982	n/a[^]	1	0	11 wks	VB[*]	n/a	Laparotomy, repair
Woolcott et al., 1987	Percreta	2	0	10 wks	VB	No; missed abortion	Laparotomy, hysterectomy + bladder repair
Haider, 1990	Percreta	1	0	10 wks	VB	No; missed abortion	Laparotomy, hysterectomy
Ecker et al., 1992	Increta	n/a	n/a	1st trimester	n/a	n/a	Laparotomy, hysterectomy
Arredondo et al., 1995	Accreta	0	3	1st trimester	None	No; missed abortion	Laparotomy, hysterectomy
Gherman et al., 1999	Increta	1	1	8 wks	VB/abd pain	Yes; suspected MAP	Laparoscopy/laparotomy, hysterectomy
Walter et al., 1999	Increta	1	0	11 wks	VB	n/a	D&C/laparotomy, hysterectomy
Marcus et al., 1999	Percreta	2	0	13 wks	VB	n/a	UAE**/D&C/laparotomy, hysterectomy
Chanrachakul et al., 2001	Increta	1	0	7 wks	VB	No; missed abortion	D&C/laparotomy, hysterectomy
Hopker et al., 2002	Percreta	1	1	10 wks	Abd pain	Yes; suspected MAP versus invasive mole	Laparotomy, hysterectomy
Shih et al., 2002	Accreta	0	0	8 wks	VB	Yes; suspected MAP	Elective laparotomy at 15 wks, hysterectomy
Buetow, 2002	Percreta	1	0	1st trimester	VB/pelvic pain	Yes; suspected MAP	Laparotomy, hysterectomy
Chen et al., 2002	Accreta	2	1	9 wks	VB	Yes; suspected MAP	Laparotomy, hysterectomy
Liang et al., 2003	Percreta	2	n/a	1st trimester	Abd pain/shock	n/a	Laparotomy, hysterectomy
Liu et al., 2003	Increta	1	0	1st trimester	n/a	n/a	UAE/laparotomy, hysterectomy
Coniglio and Dickinson, 2004	Accreta	2	0	8 wks	Abd pain/shock	Yes; suspected Cesarean scar pregnancy	Laparotomy, repair

TABLE 1: Continued.

Author and year	Type of MAP	Prior CS[§]	Prior D&C[†]	GA at Diagnosis[#]	Presenting symptoms	US diagnostic of MAP	Management & outcome
Dabulis and McGuirk, 2007	Percreta	3	1	9 wks	Abd pain	Yes; suspected MAP	Laparotomy, hysterectomy
Son et al., 2007	Increta	0	3	8 wks	Abd pain/syncope	Abd/pelvis computed tomography	Laparotomy, hysterectomy
Tanyi et al., 2008	Percreta	1	1	7 wks	VB/abd pain	No; threatened abortion	D&C/laparotomy, hysterectomy
Papadaskis et al., 2008[††]	Percreta	2	1	11 wks	VB	No; missed abortion	D&C/laparotomy, hysterectomy
Soleymani et al., 2009	Increta	0	0	11 wks	VB	Yes; suspected MAP	D&C/UAE, resolved
Yang et al., 2009	Increta	2	3	12 wks	VB	Yes; suspected MAP	UAE, resolved
Pont et al., 2010	Percreta	1	1	13 wks	Abd pain	n/a	Laparotomy, hysterectomy
Hanif et al., 2011	Percreta	2	2	12 wks	Abd pain/syncope	No; ectopic pregnancy	Laparotomy, hysterectomy
Shojai et al., 2012[††]	Increta	2	0	7 wks	n/a	No; missed abortion	D&C/laparotomy, hysterectomy
Shaamash et al., 2014	Accreta	2	0	11 wks	VB/abd pain	Yes; suspected MAP versus molar changes	D&C/laparotomy, hysterectomy

[§]Cesarean delivery; [†]dilation and curettage; [*]vaginal bleeding; [**]uterine artery embolization; [#]gestational age; [^]unknown or not reported; [††]failed medical management with misoprostol.

continued trials of medical management could still be within reason with strict precautions. Providers need to consider clinical nuances, patient treatment preferences, and compliance with treatment regimen.

However, failed medical management raises concern, especially in patients with risk factors for a MAP. This should trigger further evaluation with a thorough repeat formal TVUS to rule out a MAP and have radiology look closer at the placenta to myometrial interaction and morphology. Relaying identifiable risk factors and pertinent clinical findings to radiology is important to assist in their assessment. Ultrasound is the primary modality for diagnosing a MAP [11]; a MAP is more difficult to diagnosis in the first trimester with much lower accuracies compared to second and third trimesters [1, 12]. On ultrasound, some features indicative of a MAP include thinning or nonvisualization of the myometrium overlying the placenta, presence of placental lacunae (irregular shaped vascular spaces) with turbulent flow, loss of retroplacental clear space, interruption of the interface between the bladder and myometrium, and hypervascularization of the placental-myometrial interface [5, 11–14]. Measurement of the smallest anterior myometrial thickness in a sagittal view combined with the number of prior cesarean deliveries has been shown to significantly increase the prediction of a MAP [13]. In addition, patients with risk factors for a MAP should have imaging of the anterior myometrium and bladder with a high-frequency transducer. A similar approach should be taken if a placenta previa or loss of the retroplacental clear space is detected.

Vascular findings have also been described in a MAP. Placental lacunae and indistinct intraplacental channels with turbulent flow have the highest sensitivity for a MAP [11, 15]. These should not be confused with vascular lakes, which are more round and have laminar flow. While retroplacental hypervascularity can occur with a MAP, disruption of flow may be seen at the site of invasion [16]. Moreover, multiple enlarged vessels can surround the myometrium in cases of placenta percreta, which may also be associated with an irregular vascular bladder wall [14]. Upon review of our patient's TVUS images with our radiology team after they were aware of the diagnosis, they retrospectively noted potential features that were indicative of a MAP (Figure 2).

Magnetic resonance imaging (MRI) may be used when an ultrasound is not definitive or if the placenta is posterior [16]. MRI protocols include a form of T2-weighted imaging, where the placenta is distinct from the myometrium and homogeneous, except for a thin septae. MRI findings of a MAP include uterine bulging, heterogeneous placenta, thick T2-dark intraplacental bands, and focal disruption of the myometrium. However, myometrial thinning can be misleading and may be normal. In cases of placenta percreta, direct invasion or tenting of the bladder may be present [14].

In patients with a concern for a first trimester MAP, their management needs to entail extensive counseling regarding therapeutic options with a definitive (hysterectomy) or conservative (leave placenta in situ) management depending on patients fertility goals [5, 11]. Preoperative counseling for these patients ought to include the potential for a hysterectomy, risk of a hemorrhage requiring blood transfusions,

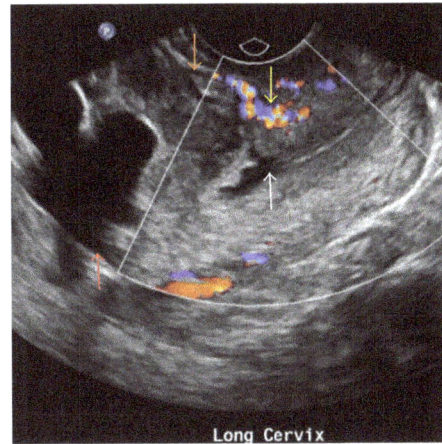

FIGURE 2: Longitudinal grayscale and color Doppler image of the lower uterine segment and cervix demonstrates endometrial fluid (red arrow) and an irregular, heterogeneously hypoechoic placenta (orange arrow) with blood supply from cervical vessels (yellow arrow) extending into the anterior myometrial wall and over the internal cervical os (white arrow).

and maternal death in order for patients to have realistic expectations about the various outcomes [5, 11]. If there is a high suspicion for a first trimester MAP, presurgical planning along with a multidisciplinary approach is essential to help prevent complications at the time of surgery; appropriate specialties need to be consulted and the operating room should be appropriately prepped (e.g., blood products and necessary instruments) [3, 5]. A prior study has recommended focusing on patient education to help increase the detection of first trimester MAPs; at the time of discharge after a cesarean delivery, it is important to discuss with patients that in future pregnancies an early prenatal visit with TVUS to rule out a MAP should be performed [4].

Being adequately prepared in the OR with appropriate hospital resources is essential. Our patient was scheduled for a routine minor procedure in an outpatient ambulatory surgical center but necessitated transfer to the main hospital for higher level of care. In patients with risk factors and possible concern for a MAP, it is critical that these surgeries be performed in a tertiary hospital setting where sufficient resources are available if any complications arise [11].

MAPs represent a life-threatening concern and pose additional risk when patients are not diagnosed until the time of surgery. In patients with failed medical management for a missed abortion, assessment of MAP risk factors is critical and considered to further guide management. Communicating pertinent information to radiology better equips them in their ultrasound investigation and may place additional focus on detecting MAPs earlier and prevent unanticipated discoveries peripartum [12]. Early diagnosis of a MAP allows providers to coordinate a multidisciplinary treatment approach and thoroughly counsel patients on options and expectations. Ensuring adequate resources and personnel at a tertiary hospital is necessary to provide the highest quality of care and improve outcomes.

Consent

Written consent was obtained from the patient.

References

[1] A. H. Shaamash, W. M. Houshimi, E.-M. M. El-Kanzi, and A. E. Zakaria, "Abortion hysterectomy at 11 weeks' gestation due to undiagnosed placenta accreta (PA): A case report and a mini review of literatures," *Middle East Fertility Society Journal*, vol. 19, no. 3, pp. 147–152, 2014.

[2] M. P. Buetow, "Sonography of placenta percreta during the first trimester," *American Journal of Roentgenology*, vol. 179, no. 2, p. 535, 2002.

[3] R. Shojai, P. Roblin, and L. Boubli, "Failed early medical abortion: Beware of the uterine scar! Case report," *The European Journal of Contraception and Reproductive Health Care*, vol. 17, no. 3, pp. 237–239, 2012.

[4] I. E. Timor-Tritsch and A. Monteagudo, "Unforeseen consequences of the increasing rate of cesarean deliveries: early placenta accreta and cesarean scar pregnancy. A review," *American Journal of Obstetrics & Gynecology*, vol. 207, no. 1, pp. 14–29, 2012.

[5] F. Moretti, M. Merziotis, Z. M. Ferraro, L. Oppenheimer, and K. Fung Kee Fung, "The importance of a late first trimester placental sonogram in patients at risk of abnormal placentation," *Case Reports in Obstetrics and Gynecology*, vol. 2014, pp. 1–4, 2014.

[6] S. Wu, M. Kocherginsky, and J. U. Hibbard, "Abnormal placentation: twenty-year analysis," *American Journal of Obstetrics & Gynecology*, vol. 192, no. 5, pp. 1458–1461, 2005.

[7] C. S. Shellhaas, S. Gilbert, M. B. Landon et al., "The frequency and complication rates of hysterectomy accompanying cesarean delivery," *Obstetrics & Gynecology*, vol. 114, no. 2, pp. 224–229, 2009.

[8] American College of Obstetricians and Gynecologists, "ACOG Practice Bulletin No. 150 Early Pregnancy Loss," *Obstetrics & Gynecology*, vol. 125, no. 5, pp. 1258–1267, 2015.

[9] F. T. Kraus, W. Raymond, M. D. Redline, and J. Deborah, *Placental Pathology (Atlas of Nontumor Pathology)*, DC Am. Regist. Pathol., Washington, Wash, USA, 2004.

[10] N. Papadakis and C. J. Christodoulou, "Placenta percreta presenting in the first trimester: review of the literature," *Clin. Exp. Obstet. Gynecol*, vol. 35, no. 2, pp. 98–102, 2007.

[11] American College of Obstetricians and Gynecologists, "ACOG Practice Bulletin No. 529: placenta accreta," *Obstet. Gynecol*, vol. 1, no. 120, pp. 207–211, 2012.

[12] J. J. Stirnemann, E. Mousty, G. Chalouhi, L. J. Salomon, J.-P. Bernard, and Y. Ville, "Screening for placenta accreta at 11-14 weeks of gestation," *American Journal of Obstetrics & Gynecology*, vol. 205, no. 6, pp. 547–e6, 2011.

[13] M. W. F. Rac, E. Moschos, C. E. Wells, D. D. McIntire, J. S. Dashe, and D. M. Twickler, "Sonographic finDings of morbidly adherent placenta in the first trimester," *Journal of Ultrasound in Medicine*, vol. 35, no. 2, pp. 263–269, 2016.

[14] W. C. Baughman, J. E. Corteville, and R. R. Shah, "Placenta accreta: Spectrum of US and MR imaging findings," *RadioGraphics*, vol. 28, no. 7, pp. 1905–1916, 2008.

[15] J. I. Yang, H. Y. Kim, H. S. Kim, and H. S. Ryu, "Diagnosis in the first trimester of placenta accreta with previous Cesarean section," *Ultrasound in Obstetrics & Gynecology*, vol. 34, no. 1, pp. 116–118, 2009.

[16] Y.-J. Chen, P.-H. Wang, W.-M. Liu, C.-R. Lai, L.-P. Shu, and J.-H. Hung, "Placenta accreta diagnosed at 9 weeks' gestation," *Ultrasound in Obstetrics & Gynecology*, vol. 19, no. 6, pp. 620–622, 2002.

22

Undetected Severe Fetal Myelosuppression following Administration of High-Dose Cytarabine for Acute Myeloid Leukemia: Is More Frequent Surveillance Necessary?

Jessica Parrott and Marium Holland

Division of Maternal Fetal Medicine, Department of Obstetrics and Gynecology, University of Kansas School of Medicine,
3901 Rainbow Boulevard, Kansas City, KS 66160, USA

Correspondence should be addressed to Jessica Parrott; jparrott3@kumc.edu

Academic Editor: Erich Cosmi

Background. Cytarabine use during pregnancy carries a 5–7% risk of neonatal cytopenia. We report two cases of fetal myelosuppression following high-dose cytarabine administration for acute myeloid leukemia (AML). *Case 1.* A 36-year-old G9P6 diagnosed with AML at 21 weeks was monitored for fetal anemia weekly and growth monthly. At 33 weeks (after 2 cycles), BPP was 2/10 and MCA PSV was elevated at 1.51 MoM. Urgent cesarean section was performed. The infant had an initial pH of 6.78 and pancytopenia (hematocrit 13.3%, platelets 3 K/UL, and white blood cell count 2.0 K/UL). Initially transfusion dependent, the neonate had count recovery by 3 weeks. *Case 2.* A 30-year-old G4P3 with AML at 26 weeks was monitored for fetal anemia twice weekly and growth monthly. At 34 weeks (after cycle 1), she was admitted with neutropenic fever. The fetal MCA PSV was borderline at 1.48 MoM. It improved to 1.38 MoM at 35 weeks but the fetal tracing worsened. At delivery the fetus was found to have a hematocrit of 30%, but with normal platelet and WBC. The fetus did not require any transfusions. *Conclusion.* Cytarabine use during pregnancy may cause neonatal myelosuppression. We recommend monitoring for fetal anemia with MCA Dopplers twice weekly.

1. Introduction

Leukemia in pregnancy is found in approximately 1 of every 75,000–100,000 pregnancies with acute myeloid leukemia (AML) accounting for greater than two-thirds of these. An estimated 75% of acute leukemias will be diagnosed in the second or third trimester of pregnancy [1]. Treatment via chemotherapy in the second and third trimester demonstrates increased risks of intrauterine growth restriction (IUGR), intrauterine fetal death (IUFD), neonatal sepsis or death, and neonatal cytopenias (5–7%) [2]. Due to the potential fetal risks of growth restriction and anemia, obstetric management typically includes serial ultrasounds to monitor growth and fetal well-being. Currently however, there are no recommendations as to the frequency with which middle cerebral artery (MCA) Dopplers should be performed to monitor for fetal anemia. We present two cases of AML diagnosed in the second trimester of pregnancy, both of which received HIDAC chemotherapy. The first was

complicated by near-fatal fetal pancytopenia and metabolic acidosis necessitating early delivery and the second complicated by isolated fetal anemia.

2. Case 1

A 36-year-old gravida 9 para 6 at 21 weeks and 2 days presented with progressive fatigue and malaise. She was found to have anemia (hemoglobin 9.1 gm/dl), thrombocytopenia (platelets 78 k/UL), and 6% circulating blasts on peripheral smear. Bone marrow biopsy confirmed diagnosis of acute myeloid leukemia (FAB classification M2) showing 8% blasts with evidence of dysplasia and hypercellular marrow. FISH was positive for t(8; 21); PML/RaRa and C-KIT were negative. After obtaining a baseline echo, she was started on induction chemotherapy, 7 + 3 (cytarabine 100 mg/m^2 /day continuous infusion for 7 days + daunorubicin 90 mg/m^2/day intravenous days 1–3). The mother had a biphasic nadir at 7–9 days and at 15–24 days. She was found to be platelet refractory

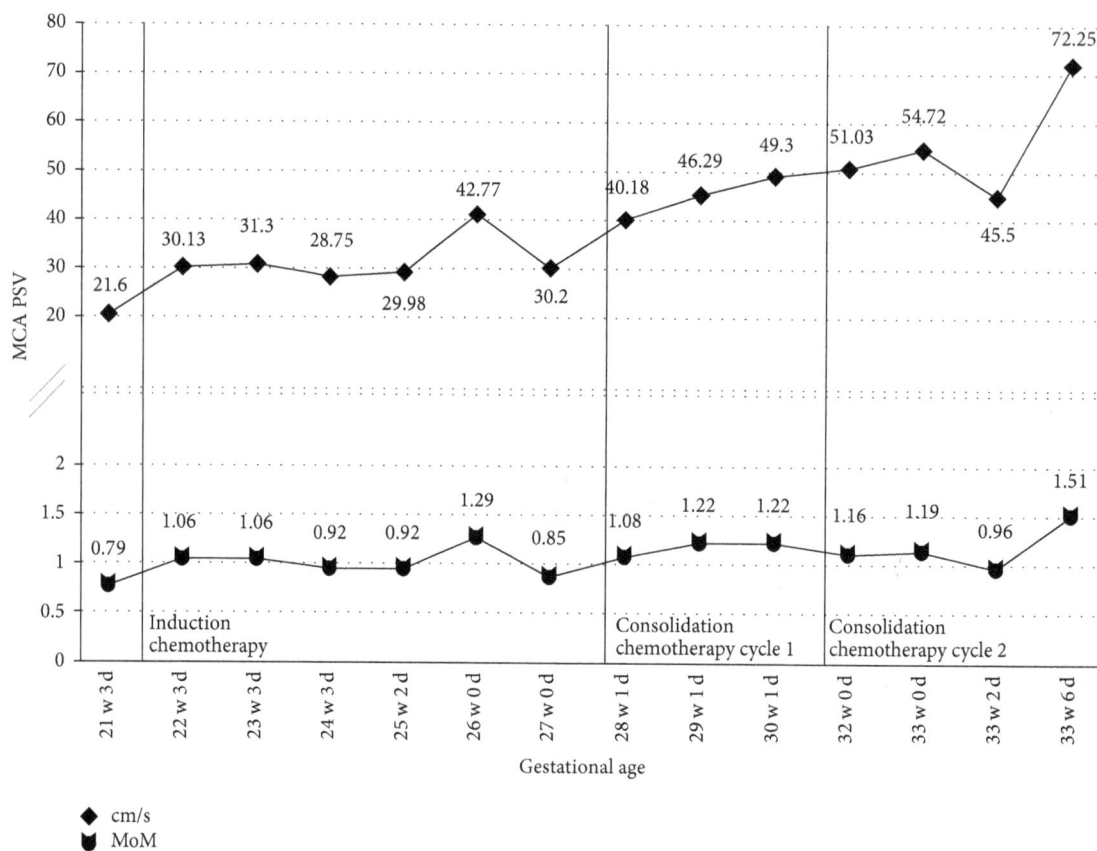

FIGURE 1: MCA PSV measurements for Case 1. Vertical lines indicate the time of chemotherapy administration. PSV cm/s, peak systolic velocity measurement; MoM, multiples of mean of PSV measurement for corresponding gestational age.

with a positive platelet antibody and required HLA-matched platelets; thus, she remained inpatient until count recovery. Repeat bone marrow biopsy showed both morphologic and multiphase flow cytometry remission. She subsequently was admitted at 27 weeks and 6 days and underwent cycle 1 of consolidation therapy with high-dose cytarabine 3 g/m^2/day continuous infusion for 6 days. At 31 weeks 6 days, she was admitted for cycle 2 of high-dose cytarabine.

The fetus was monitored twice daily with nonstress tests while being admitted to the hospital for chemotherapy. The pregnancy was followed with serial growth ultrasounds every 4 weeks with weekly Doppler ultrasounds of both the middle cerebral artery (MCA) and umbilical artery. Figure 1 shows the MCA peak systolic velocity (PSV) trend from 21 weeks until delivery. She was treated with dexamethasone IV twice daily for 3 days for fetal lung maturity at 23 weeks. Her pregnancy was complicated by gestational diabetes diagnosed at 27 weeks that was managed with insulin. She had excellent glycemic control during pregnancy with fasting values less than 85 mg/dL and postprandial values less than 110 mg/dL. At 32 weeks, the daily fetal monitoring had moderate variability but the fetus never demonstrated 15 × 15 reactivity. Thus, BPPs were performed every 2–4 days, which were either 6/10 (−2 breathing, −2 NST) or 8/10 (−2 NST).

At 33 weeks and 6 days (cycle day 15), the fetus appeared to rapidly decompensate over the course of the day. BPP in the morning was 6/10 (−2 breathing, −2 NST). Throughout the day, the fetal heart rate became progressively less reassuring with minimal variability. Repeat BPP in the afternoon was 2/10 (+2 for amniotic fluid index), with centralized MCA peak index (<2.5%) and elevated MCA PSV (1.51 MoM). There was no ultrasound evidence of fetal hydrops or cardiac decompensation. The umbilical artery and ductus venosus Dopplers were normal. Shortly thereafter, the fetal heart rate tracing appeared to become sinusoidal; this resolved, however there was absent to minimal variability with prolonged decelerations. The decision was made to proceed with delivery. Given the extreme maternal pancytopenia with a platelet count of 11 k/UL, a joint decision with haematology was made to delay delivery until after infusion of a loading dose of aminocaproic acid (Amicar, Akorn) and 1 pack of platelets prior to cesarean section. She also received 2 units of packed red blood cells at this time. Cesarean section was performed under general anesthesia 2 hours later with a continuous aminocaproic acid infusion and platelet infusion. Prior to induction of anesthesia the fetal heart rate was 125–130 bpm with absent variability, however initial Apgar was 0 and there was no detectable heart rate. Extensive neonatal resuscitation was performed, requiring intubation, chest compressions, and endotracheal tube epinephrine. Blood gas of the umbilical artery was pH 6.78, with a pCO$_2$ tension of 84 mm Hg, pO$_2$ tension of 27 mm Hg, and base deficit of 20.9, respectively. There was no evidence of placental abruption at the time of delivery and placental pathology showed focal mild chronic inflammation and chronic infarct without chorioamnionitis or funisitis. Initial labs in the neonatal ICU showed pancytopenia with hematocrit of 13.3%, platelets 3 K/UL and white blood cell count of 2.0 K/UL, On exam, the infant was pale, hypotensive, and with scattered petechiae and bruising. To stabilize the infant, he required transfusions of packed red blood cells, platelets, and fresh frozen plasma for severe pancytopenia; dopamine infusion for hypotension and poor perfusion; surfactant for respiratory distress; and bicarbonate for persistent acidosis.

The infant's pancytopenia slowly resolved over the first 3 weeks, requiring a total of 3 blood transfusions and 7 platelet transfusions. There was no evidence of malformations. Postnatal echocardiogram showed severe septal wall hypertrophy, right ventricle hypertrophy, and hyperdynamic left ventricular function with mid-cavity obliteration at the level of the papillary muscles. Pediatric cardiology was consulted and treated the infant with propranolol. Serial echocardiograms showed slow resolution of cardiac hypertrophy and improvement in left ventricular function with normalization around 1 month of life. Immediate postnatal head ultrasound was negative for intraventricular hemorrhage. Seizure-like activity and concern for encephalopathy was noted initially but EEG was negative. Head MRI however at approximately 2 weeks of life showed numerous microhemorrhagic foci predominantly involving the cerebellum as well as a small subacute subarachnoid hemorrhage. The infant's immediate postnatal course was also complicated by oliguria with acute renal failure and tubular necrosis; max creatinine was 6.17 mg/dL at 2 weeks of life. At 2 months of life, the creatinine had improved to 1.5 mg/dL.

The mother tolerated the surgery well with a total blood loss of 1500 cc. She received aminocaproic acid and oxytocin infusion for 24 hours after surgery with no bleeding complications. Her postoperative course was complicated by a wound infection. The incision was opened 1.5 cm just inferior to the umbilicus and was allowed to heal by secondary intention and oral antibiotic therapy. She has since completed her consolidation chemotherapy and is currently in remission.

3. Case 2

A 30-year-old G4P3003 at 26 weeks pregnant presented to urgent care with nonspecific symptoms and fatigue. Laboratory evaluation revealed pancytopenia. She established prenatal care and repeat labs showed persistent pancytopenia, raising concern for a haematologic malignancy. A subsequent bone marrow biopsy confirmed acute myelogenous leukemia. She was admitted to the hospital and started on induction chemotherapy, 7 + 3 (cytarabine 100 mg/m^2/day continuous infusion for 7 days + daunorubicin 90 mg/m^2/day intravenous days 1–3). Maternal fetal medicine was also consulted on admission. She was counseled on the risks and her pregnancy was followed with serial growth ultrasounds and weekly Doppler ultrasounds (see Figure 2) to monitor for fetal growth restriction and fetal anemia. She tolerated the chemotherapy well and subsequently received high-dose

cytarabine for consolidation therapy (cytarabine 3 g/m^2/day continuous infusion for 6 days).

At 34 2/7 weeks, she was admitted for neutropenic fever (cycle 1, day 19). Fetal monitoring was nonreactive but with moderate variability, occasional variable decelerations. The patient's hemoglobin was 5.8 with platelet count of 39 K/UL. She received platelet and blood transfusions with subsequent improvement in fetal tracing. At 34 5/7 weeks, the fetal MCA PSV was noted to have risen to a borderline value, at 1.48 MoM (previously always within normal limits). Fetal growth was normal at the 33rd percentile. At 34 6/7 weeks, the fetal MCA PSV improved (1.28 MoM) but the fetal tracing worsened with decreased variability and increase in the number of variable decelerations. At 35 0/7 weeks, the MCA PI was now centralized with a MCA PSV of 1.38 MoM; a biophysical profile was found to be 6/10, and with continued worsening in the fetal tracing, the decision was made to proceed with delivery.

She underwent an uncomplicated repeat cesarean section with no bleeding complications. Her postoperative course was unremarkable. The infant was born with anemia (hematocrit 30%) but did not require any blood transfusions. The platelet count (274 K/UL) and white blood cell count (7.7 K/UL) were normal at birth. The infant was discharged on hospital day 7. The patient is currently undergoing workup for a bone marrow transplant.

4. Comment

AML in pregnancy is a rare entity, with most of our data coming from case reports. In 2015, the British Journal of Haematology published guidelines for diagnosis and management of AML in pregnancy based on the compiled data available. AML is diagnosed and treated by the same guidelines used in nonpregnant individuals [3]. The recommended treatment consists of induction chemotherapy with cytarabine and an anthracycline (typically daunorubicin) to achieve complete remission, followed by consolidation therapy with high-dose cytarabine or hematopoietic stem cell transplantation [1]. Due to increased maternal mortality, decreased survival time, and reduced remission rates with delay in therapy, the recommendation is to proceed with treatment [1].

We know that both cytarabine and daunorubicin cross the placental barrier; however, with a higher molecular weight and hydrophilic properties, daunorubicin has an incomplete transfer. Cytarabine has low protein binding and wide tissue distribution, including the amniotic cavity [4]. Chemotherapy in the first trimester is associated with an increased risk of congenital malformations and risk of miscarriage (approximately 20%) and it is therefore recommended that the pregnancy be terminated prior to treatment when diagnosis occurs in the first trimester. Administration of cytarabine in the second and third trimesters carries a risk of IUGR (~13%), IUFD (~6%), preterm birth, and neonatal cytopenias [1–3]. It is unknown whether treatment with an anthracycline during pregnancy has potential cardiotoxicity to the fetus as it does in adults. Limited studies using daunorubicin with long-term follow-up of these children have shown no cardiac damage [1]. Leukemia itself also has an impact on perinatal

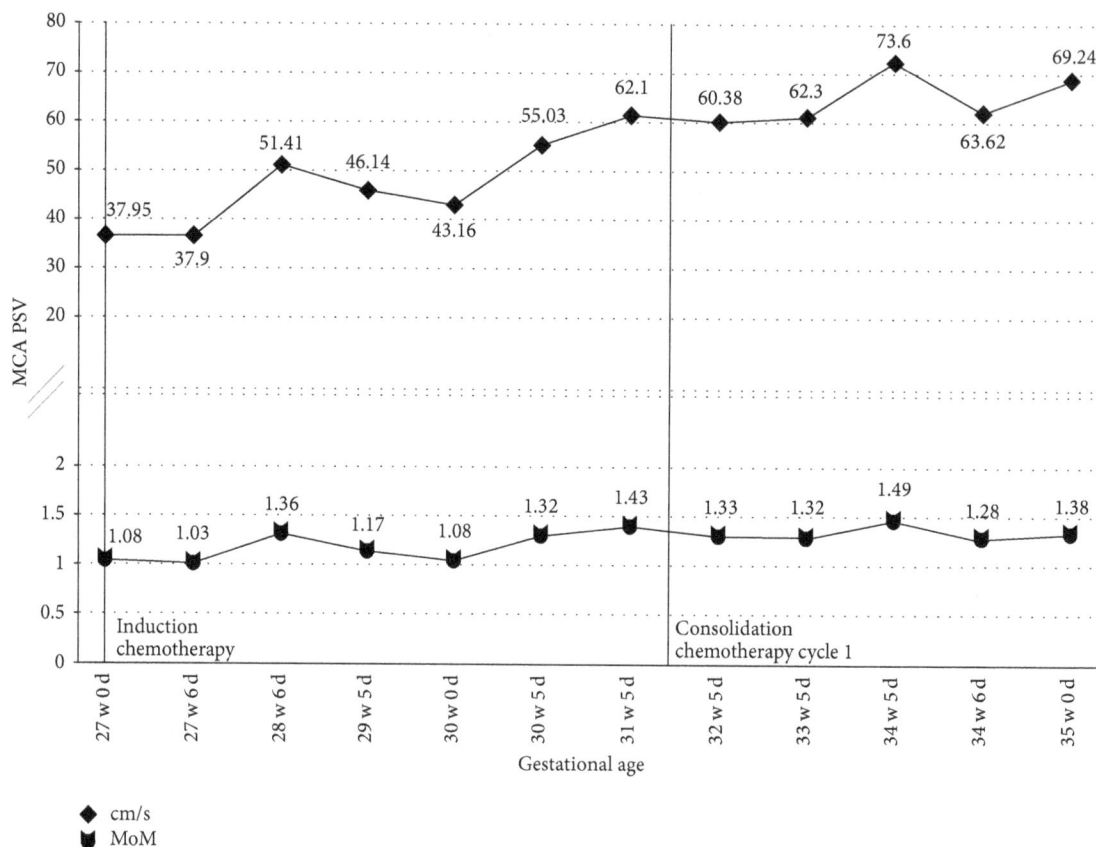

FIGURE 2: MCA PSV measurements for Case 2. Vertical lines indicate the time of chemotherapy administration. PSV cm/s, peak systolic velocity measurement; MoM, multiples of mean of PSV measurement for corresponding gestational age.

outcome, despite treatment. There are known associations of spontaneous abortion, prematurity, IUGR, and IUFD [2]. This increased risk of fetal death is not completely understood. Postulated etiologies include maternal anemia, disseminated intravascular coagulation and leukemic cells affecting blood flow, and nutrient and/or oxygen exchange in the intervillous spaces of the placenta [3].

Here we present one case complicated by severe neonatal pancytopenia and a second complicated by moderate neonatal anemia. Two studies examining the maternal and neonatal outcomes of pregnant women with AML [5] or those receiving chemotherapy treatments [2] report a 5–7% risk of neonatal cytopenias. All of these cases received cytarabine either alone or in combination with 1 or more chemotherapeutic agents [2, 5]. With immature liver and kidneys, neonates have a limited capacity to metabolize and eliminate drugs which is part of the reason we do not recommend administering chemotherapy after 35 weeks [1]. So although each case describes a transient myelosuppression, it may last 3-4 weeks which can place the neonate at substantial risk for complications such as sepsis [2, 5–8]. Thus, while the overall risk of neonatal cytopenias is low, it can have a profound effect leading to multiple transfusions and potential complications.

Utilizing MCA peak systolic velocity (PSV), fetal anemia can be diagnosed via noninvasive methods. Studies have demonstrated that a threshold of 1.5 MoM is suggestive of

moderate to severe fetal anemia [9]. In 2014, a study evaluated the use of MCA Dopplers for monitoring of fetal anemia when chemotherapy is administered to pregnant women with ovarian, cervical, or breast cancer. They measured the MCA PSV one day before and the third day after chemotherapy. No severe range fetal anemia was diagnosed but they found a number of cases of mild fetal anemia which supports the use of MCA Dopplers in monitoring pregnancies treated with chemotherapy [9]. The 2015 guidelines published in the British Journal of Haematology recommend serial ultrasounds every 4 weeks for growth and fetal well-being to monitor for growth restriction. They do not, however, comment on monitoring for fetal anemia [3]. In contrast, a 2014 review article published in the European Journal of Haematology recommends checking for fetal anemia before and after chemotherapy but does not provide any guidance as to when this should be performed [1]. Clearly, the data supports monitoring for fetal anemia but guidance is needed regarding timing and frequency.

For our first case, we decided to screen for fetal anemia weekly with MCA Dopplers on ultrasound. Despite this frequency of monitoring, it was the fetus developing a metabolic acidosis as demonstrated by the nonreassuring fetal heart rate tracing that prompted us to repeat the MCA Dopplers and discover the fetal anemia. If we had been monitoring at an increased frequency, such as twice weekly, we might have noticed an increasing trend or caught the anemia at an earlier date and been able to intervene at that time, possibly preventing the neonatal hypoxic event and severe pancytopenia seen at birth. With our second case, we chose to monitor the MCA Dopplers twice weekly. At the time of delivery mild to moderate neonatal anemia was present but did not require any interventions.

In both cases, there was never any ultrasound evidence of hydrops fetalis or cardiac decompensation. The umbilical artery and ductus venosus Doppler studies were normal throughout the entire pregnancy for both women. The Doppler interrogations were all performed with the same methodology; however, the person performing each ultrasound was not always the same. We do not believe that this would have contributed to any difference in findings. It is not unreasonable to suspect that the more significant fetal compromise seen in the first case could be related to receiving 2 cycles of consolidation therapy with the high-dose cytarabine compared to the 1 cycle received in the second case; however, there is no current literature to support this theory.

While the risk of neonatal cytopenia is low, the impact can be significant as evidenced by this case. We have a non-invasive method for screening for fetal anemia that should be utilized with pregnant women receiving chemotherapy. With medications that induce a prolonged period of maternal myelosuppression, such as cytarabine, we would recommend monitoring the pregnancy with serial ultrasounds and MCA Dopplers at least twice weekly during the period of maternal myelosuppression. If there is concern for progression of fetal anemia and development of hydrops fetalis, the frequency of monitoring should be increased and delivery may need to be considered.

References

[1] X. Thomas, "Acute myeloid leukemia in the pregnant patient," *European Journal of Haematology*, vol. 95, no. 2, pp. 124–136, 2015.

[2] E. Cardonick and A. Iacobucci, "Use of chemotherapy during human pregnancy," *Lancet Oncology*, vol. 5, no. 5, pp. 283–291, 2004.

[3] S. Ali, G. L. Jones, D. J. Culligan et al., "Guidelines for the diagnosis and management of acute myeloid leukaemia in pregnancy," *British Journal of Haematology*, vol. 170, no. 4, pp. 487–495, 2015.

[4] D. C. Doll, Q. S. Ringenberg, and J. W. Yarbro, "Managment of cancer during pregancy," *Archives of Internal Medicine*, vol. 148, no. 9, pp. 2058–2064, 1988.

[5] A. Chang and S. Patel, "Treatment of Acute Myeloid Leukemia During Pregnancy," *Annals of Pharmacotherapy*, vol. 49, no. 1, pp. 48–68, 2015.

[6] D. M. Biener, G. Gossing, A. Kuehnl, M. Cremer, and J. W. Dudenhausen, "Diagnosis and treatment of maternal acute myeloid leukemia during pregnancy imitating HELLP syndrome," *Journal of Perinatal Medicine*, vol. 37, no. 6, pp. 713-714, 2009.

[7] N. A. Murray, D. Acolet, M. Deane, J. Price, and I. A. Roberts, "Fetal marrow suppression after maternal chemotherapy for leukaemia.," *Archives of Disease in Childhood - Fetal and Neonatal Edition*, vol. 71, no. 3, pp. F209–F210, 1994.

[8] K. Matsuo, K. Shimoya, S. Ueda, K. Wada, M. Koyama, and Y. Murata, "Idarubicin administered during pregnancy: Its effects on the fetus," *Gynecologic and Obstetric Investigation*, vol. 58, no. 4, pp. 186–188, 2004.

[9] M. J. Halaska, M. Komar, R. Vlk et al., "A pilot study on peak systolic velocity monitoring of fetal anemia after administration of chemotherapy during pregnancy," *European Journal of Obstetrics Gynecology and Reproductive Biology*, vol. 174, no. 1, pp. 76–79, 2014.

Unilateral Atraumatic Expulsion of an Ectopic Pregnancy in a Case of Bilateral Ectopic Pregnancy

Victoria Sampson, Oluremi Mogekwu, Ammar Ahmed, and Farida Bano

Department of Obstetrics and Gynaecology, Queen's Hospital, Romford, UK

Correspondence should be addressed to Victoria Sampson; victoriasampson1@gmail.com

Academic Editor: A. O. Awonuga

Ectopic pregnancy occurs in 1-2% of pregnancies. The fallopian tube is the most common site; however, bilateral tubal ectopic pregnancy is an extremely rare phenomenon, seen in approximately 1/200,000 pregnancies. It is usually the result of assisted reproductive techniques (ART). Ultrasound (USS) and serial beta-hCG levels have shown poor efficacy for accurate diagnosis. Laparoscopy is the diagnostic gold standard. The majority of cases are managed surgically with bilateral salpingectomy. A 26-year-old female presented to our early pregnancy unit with pain and vaginal bleeding at 5-week gestation after IVF. USS was inconclusive and her b-hCG levels rose with worsening pain; therefore, a decision was made for diagnostic laparoscopy. Although there was a clear right sided ectopic pregnancy, the left tube was swollen and therefore a methylene blue dye test was carried out to confirm blockage. Atraumatic milking, to expose the dye, expelled necrotic tissue which histology confirmed to be a second ectopic pregnancy. She made a good recovery with falling beta-hCG levels and left tubal preservation. As the use of ART increases, bilateral ectopic pregnancies will become more common. Novel and established techniques should be used to help confirm the diagnosis and assist in tubal preservation.

1. Introduction

Ectopic pregnancies (EPs) constitute 1-2% of all pregnancies [1] and are a leading cause of first-trimester maternal mortality [2]. Ectopic pregnancy describes implantation of a blastocyst outside of the uterine cavity. The fallopian tubes are the most common site, accounting for 95% of EPs [3]. Key risk factors include previous EP, known tubal damage, pelvic inflammatory disease, presence of an intrauterine device, smoking, assisted reproductive techniques (ART), and extremes of maternal age [2, 4].

Bilateral tubal ectopic pregnancies (BEPs) are a very rare form of ectopic pregnancy [5], and incidence has been reported as 1 in 725 to 1 in 1580 of ectopic pregnancies equating to approximately 1 in 200,000 pregnancies [6].

The majority of cases are diagnosed intraoperatively; traditional diagnostic methods such as serial beta-human chorionic gonadotrophin levels (beta-hCG) or transvaginal ultrasound have shown poor efficacy when applied to BEPs [5]. Management is typically with bilateral salpingectomy.

We present a case of bilateral ectopic pregnancy in which diagnosis was assisted by the use of methylene blue dye test. It was managed with unilateral salpingectomy and preservation of the remaining fallopian tube following atraumatic expulsion of the contralateral ectopic pregnancy during tubal insufflation.

2. Case Report

A 26-year-old Caucasian woman presented to our early pregnancy unit with five-week amenorrhea, sudden onset of abdominal pain, and vaginal bleeding for one week. On initial assessment, her vital signs were stable. She achieved conception via in vitro fertilization (IVF) on her fourth attempt; two blastocysts were implanted 36 days prior to presentation. She had one live child aged 4 years delivered vaginally and three early recurrent miscarriages. There was no further significant medical history.

Investigation with a transvaginal ultrasound scan (TVUS) showed an endometrial thickness of 2.5 mm with

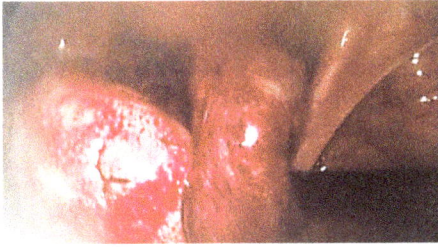

FIGURE 1: Left hematosalpinx.

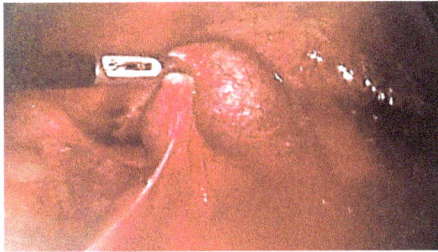

FIGURE 2: Right tubal ectopic pregnancy.

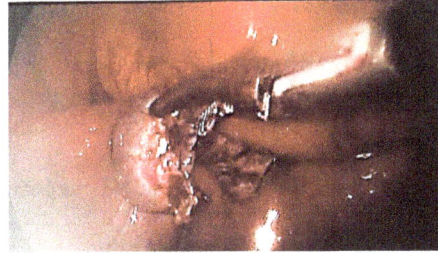

FIGURE 3: Right fallopian tube after salpingectomy.

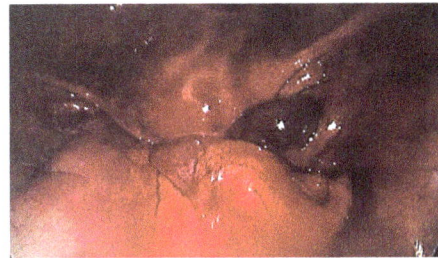

FIGURE 4: Laparoscopic picture of the tissue from the left fallopian tube.

interrupted midline echo, and no free fluid was noted. A diagnosis of pregnancy of unknown location was made but a complete miscarriage was suspected. Subsequently, serum beta-hCG and serum progesterone levels were checked to correlate with the clinical picture. She was offered pain relief and she was advised of admission due to her pain, both of which she declined. The patient was advised to return in 48 hours for repeat blood tests. A normal rise in serum beta-hCG levels from 618 IU/L to 1290 IU/L over a 48-hour interval was noted.

A repeat TVUS was carried out at this stage. This showed an endometrial thickness of 4.7 mm, and a likely ectopic pregnancy on the left measuring 16 mm × 19 mm was noted. The patient was informed about the findings and was counseled accordingly. Risks and benefits of laparoscopy ± salpingectomy versus methotrexate were discussed with the patient and she decided to opt for surgery.

A diagnostic laparoscopy was carried out; there was a mild hemoperitoneum. The left fallopian tube appeared edematous and dilated indicating a possible hematosalpinx or ectopic pregnancy (Figure 1). Simultaneously, there was a definite right ectopic pregnancy (Figure 2), and as a result a right salpingectomy was carried out, without any complications (Figure 3).

Given the uncertainty regarding the left tube, a methylene blue dye test was carried out on the left tube and a small amount of blue spillage was noted. The left fallopian tube was then maneuvered with atraumatic forceps, in a milking motion, until a necrotic-looking tissue was released at the level of the left fimbria (Figure 4).

Good hemostasis was achieved and the total blood loss was estimated to be 250 ml. Both tissue samples were sent for histology. The patient had an uneventful recovery and was discharged home with the plan to return for follow-up in one weeks' time for repeat serum beta-hCG and ultrasound scan. Follow-up of this nature was planned due to the uncertainty

of the content of the remaining tube; histology results would not be available for a minimum of two weeks. If there was a contralateral ectopic pregnancy, resolution of b-hCG would assist in excluding residual trophoblastic tissue. As this case had not been encountered previously, the repeat ultrasound was completed mainly for reassurance.

The following week, blood tests confirmed an optimal decline of beta-hCG levels and ultrasound scan was normal. Histology report confirmed the presence of chorionic villi and decidua in both tissue samples, confirming the diagnosis of bilateral ectopic pregnancy. The patient made an uneventful recovery.

3. Discussion

Any ectopic pregnancy is a potential medical emergency. Late or misdiagnosis can result in serious complications such as tubal rupture, hemorrhagic shock, and death [7]; yet, timely diagnosis, especially of bilateral tubal ectopic pregnancy, has proven to be particularly challenging.

Unlike unilateral ectopic pregnancies, measurement of serum beta-hCG levels for bilateral cases is neither a sensitive nor a reliable diagnostic marker given the presence of two pregnancies [8]. Furthermore, the efficacy of preoperative ultrasound in diagnosing BEPs is also poor with only a couple of successful cases known [9]; most cases identify one ectopic pregnancy or the patient presents in an unstable condition. Our case reiterates this difficulty with the initial ultrasound scan confirming an ectopic pregnancy on the left but was unable to visualize the ectopic pregnancy on the right, but intraoperatively the right sided ectopic pregnancy was much clearer. The current established method of diagnosing the second ectopic pregnancy is by direct inspection of the contralateral tube intraoperatively. Despite this, there have been cases of missed bilateral ectopic pregnancies resulting in a second emergency surgery following contralateral rupture [10].

Regarding unilateral EP, salpingectomy (tube removal) and salpingostomy (ectopic removal with tubal preservation) are the two surgical options. As tubal damage is the biggest risk factor for recurrence, salpingectomy is the preferred surgical management if the contralateral tube appears normal [11]. Salpingostomy can be considered if there are concerns about tubal factor infertility; it has been thought that salpingostomy was the preference over salpingectomy in order to preserve fertility [12]. Cheng et al. performed a meta-analysis comparing the fertility outcomes after salpingostomy versus salpingectomy; they included two randomized controlled trials and eight cohort studies. They found that the two RCTs did not indicate a significant difference between the two groups whereas the cohort studies suggest an increased intrauterine pregnancy (IUP) rate in the salpingostomy group. However, when excluding 2 of the cohort studies, they saw no significant difference between the IUP rates of the two treatment options [13].

BEPs pose management dilemmas as both tubes are damaged, resulting in a high risk of recurrence. In the literature, the majority of cases are managed with bilateral salpingectomy [14, 15]. There have been cases of successful conservative surgery [6] but also cases associated with persistent symptoms requiring further surgery or treatment with methotrexate [16, 17].

In our case, the patient was already undergoing IVF treatment, bypassing the need for tubal preservation. Women undergoing fertility treatment with tubal disease secondary to hydrosalpinx or tubal factor infertility have been shown to have a lower success rate of IVF compared to other causes of infertility [18]. This has led to the thought that sapling fluid can be embryotoxic by preventing implantation or being detrimental to the embryo development [18, 19]. A Cochrane review including 9 studies looked at the effect of surgical intervention in tubal factor infertility; the review found strong evidence for salpingectomy or tubal occlusion prior to IVF treatment in the case of hydrosalpinx [19], which is therefore a recommended practice [20]. Therefore, an argument could be made to offer all women with BEPs, secondary to IVF, bilateral salpingectomies in the hope of improving future outcomes. For our patient, the low index of suspicion for BEPs meant the option of bilateral salpingectomy was not considered especially as the diagnosis was not confirmed until the histology result was available.

Assisted reproductive techniques are a known risk factor for ectopic pregnancies [21]; the risk varies according to the technique employed with intrafallopian transfers conferring the highest risk [22, 23], a technique which has fallen out of practice. Regarding intrauterine transfers, midfundal techniques reduced the risk of ectopic pregnancy by 75% when compared to the deep fundal technique [22]. A large multicenter trial showed that the risk with ART is significantly higher if there is preexisting tubal factor infertility [24]. The rates of ectopic pregnancy secondary to ART have decreased over the past decade, likely secondary to improvements in techniques. Reduction in the number of embryos transferred has also contributed to the reduced risk [25]. Zhu et al. found that, of the 16 case reports of bilateral ectopic pregnancy since 2008, 43% were associated with assisted reproduction [26]. This figure is slightly less than previous literature reviews quoting 50% and 64%, respectively [27, 28]. Some cases thought to be spontaneous have revealed intraoperative signs of concealed ovarian induction [5]. Risk factors for spontaneous BEPs are similar to those for unilateral EPs and there are no established differences in their clinical presentation [5, 16].

As demonstrated, BEPs are difficult from a diagnostic and management perspective. In the absence of clinical guidance, new and innovative ideas are required to establish the best practice in these rare cases. Methylene blue tubal insufflation is commonly used at laparoscopy to identify tubal obstruction in cases of subfertility. Our case represents a novel approach in using methylene blue to assist the diagnosis of a contralateral ectopic pregnancy where intraoperative inspection was inconclusive.

An unexpected outcome was the atraumatic expulsion of the pregnancy resulting in the preservation of the tube. Complete removal of the ectopic pregnancy was confirmed by resolution of the b-hCG levels. For this to be considered a treatment option for other women, functionality of the tube must be established with a subsequent spontaneous intrauterine pregnancy. This must be weighed up against the risk of a recurrent ectopic pregnancy. Further cases are needed to ascertain trends.

In conclusion, as the use of assisted reproductive techniques increases, bilateral ectopic pregnancies will become more common. A high index of suspicion should be used in high risk cases with extra care taken to evaluate the contralateral tube. Both novel and established techniques should be used to ensure accurate diagnosis of which tubal insufflation may assist as not only diagnostic but also potential treatment option.

Ethical Approval

IRB/Ethics Committee ruled that approval was not required for this study.

References

[1] X.-L. Chen, Z.-R. Chen, Z.-L. Cao et al., "The 100 most cited articles in ectopic pregnancy: a bibliometric analysis," *SpringerPlus*, vol. 5, no. 1, article no. 1815, 2016.

[2] H. Rogers, "MBRRACE - Confidential enquiries into maternal death," *The practising midwife*, vol. 19, no. 4, pp. 33–36, 2016.

[3] C. Chanana, N. Gupta, I. Bansal et al., "Different sonographic faces of ectopic pregnancy," *Journal of Clinical Imaging Science*, vol. 7, no. 1, p. 6, 2017.

[4] W. M. Ankum, B. W. J. Mol, F. Van der Veen, and P. M. M. Bossuyt, "Risk factors for ectopic pregnancy: a meta-analysis," *Fertility and Sterility*, vol. 65, no. 6, pp. 1093–1099, 1996.

[5] S. K. Jena, S. Singh, M. Nayak, L. Das, and S. Senapati, "Bilateral simultaneous tubal ectopic pregnancy: a case report, review of

literature and a proposed management algorithm," *Journal of Clinical and Diagnostic Research*, vol. 10, no. 3, pp. QD01–QD03, 2016.

[6] S. Hoffmann, H. Abele, and C. Bachmann, "Spontaneous Bilateral Tubal Ectopic Pregnancy: Incidental Finding during Laparoscopy - Brief Report and Review of Literature," *Geburtshilfe und Frauenheilkunde*, vol. 76, no. 4, pp. 413–416, 2016.

[7] F. L. De Graaf and C. Demetroulis, "Bilateral tubal ectopic pregnancy: diagnostic pitfalls," *The British Journal of Clinical Practice*, vol. 51, no. 1, pp. 56–58, 1997.

[8] M. Arab, S. N. Kazemi, Z. Vahedpoorfard, and A. Ashoori, "A rare case of bilateral ectopic pregnancy and differential diagnosis of gestational trophoblastic disease," *Journal of Reproduction and Infertility*, vol. 16, no. 1, pp. 49–52, 2015.

[9] L. Sentilhes, P.-E. Bouet, T. Jalle, F. Boussion, C. Lefebvre-Lacoeuille, and P. Descamps, "Ultrasound diagnosis of spontaneous bilateral tubal pregnancy," *Australian and New Zealand Journal of Obstetrics and Gynaecology*, vol. 49, no. 6, pp. 695-696, 2009.

[10] R. M. Tabachnikoff, M. O. Dada, R. J. Woods, D. Rohere, and C. P. Myers, "Bilateral tubal pregnancy. A report of an unusual case," *JRM-The Journal of Reproductive Medicine*, vol. 43, no. 8, pp. 707–709, 1998.

[11] T. Tulandi, "Randomised controlled trial: Salpingectomy for tubal ectopic pregnancy is appropriate in the presence of healthy-looking contralateral tube," *Evidence-Based Medicine*, vol. 19, no. 5, p. 177, 2014.

[12] J. Li, K. Jiang, and F. Zhao, "Fertility outcome analysis after surgical management of tubal ectopic pregnancy: A retrospective cohort study," *BMJ Open*, vol. 5, no. 9, Article ID e007339, 2015.

[13] X. Cheng, X. Tian, Z. Yan et al., "Comparison of the Fertility Outcome of Salpingotomy and Salpingectomy in Women with Tubal Pregnancy: A Systematic Review and Meta-Analysis," *PLOS ONE*, vol. 11, no. 3, p. e0152343, 2016.

[14] M. Sheeba and G. Supriya, "Spontaneous bilateral tubal gestation: a rare case report," *Case Reports in Obstetrics and Gynecology*, vol. 2016, pp. 1–4, 2016.

[15] E. D. Abi Khalil, S. M. Mufarrij, G. N. Moawad, and I. S. Mufarrij, "Spontaneous bilateral ectopic pregnancy: a case report," *Journal of Reproductive Medicine*, vol. 61, no. 3, pp. 306–308, 2016.

[16] J. Andrews and S. Farrell, "Spontaneous bilateral tubal pregnancies: a case report," *Journal of Obstetrics and Gynaecology Canada*, vol. 30, no. 1, pp. 51–54, 2008.

[17] Y. Zhang, J. Chen, W. Lu, B. Li, G. Du, and X. Wan, "Clinical characteristics of persistent ectopic pregnancy after salpingostomy and influence on ongoing pregnancy," *Journal of Obstetrics and Gynaecology Research*, vol. 43, no. 3, pp. 564–570, 2017.

[18] M. Noventa, S. Gizzo, C. Saccardi et al., "Salpingectomy before assisted reproductive technologies: a systematic literature review," *Journal of Ovarian Research*, vol. 9, no. 1, 2016.

[19] N. Johnson et al., "Surgical treatment for tubal disease in women due to undergo in vitro fertilisation," 2017.

[20] National Collaborating Centre for Women's and Children's, *National institute for health and clinical excellence: guidance, in fertility: assessment and treatment for people with fertility problems*, Royal College of Obstetricians & GynaecologistsNational Collaborating Centre for Women's and Children's Health, London, UK, 2013.

[21] M. Polat, F. K. Ü. Boynukalın, İ. Yaralı, and H. Yaralı, "Bilateral ectopic pregnancy following ICSI," *BMJ case reports*, vol. 2014, 2014.

[22] A. Nazari, H. A. Askari, J. H. Check, and A. O'Shaughnessy, "Embryo transfer technique as a cause of ectopic pregnancy in in vitro fertilization," *Fertility and Sterility*, vol. 60, no. 5, pp. 919–921, 1993.

[23] H. B. Clayton, L. A. Schieve, H. B. Peterson, D. J. Jamieson, M. A. Reynolds, and V. C. Wright, "Ectopic pregnancy risk with assisted reproductive technology procedures," *Obstetrics and Gynecology*, vol. 107, no. 3, pp. 595–604, 2006.

[24] C. Li, W.-H. Zhao, Q. Zhu et al., "Risk factors for ectopic pregnancy: a multi-center case-control study," *BMC Pregnancy and Childbirth*, vol. 15, no. 1, article no. 187, 2015.

[25] K. M. Perkins, S. L. Boulet, D. M. Kissin, and D. J. Jamieson, "Risk of ectopic pregnancy associated with assisted reproductive technology in the United States, 2001–2011," *Obstetrics and Gynecology*, vol. 125, no. 1, pp. 70–78, 2015.

[26] B. Zhu, G.-F. Xu, Y.-F. Liu et al., "Heterochronic bilateral ectopic pregnancy after ovulation induction," *Journal of Zhejiang University: Science B*, vol. 15, no. 8, pp. 750–755, 2014.

[27] J. F. De Los Ríos, J. D. Castañeda, and A. Miryam, "Bilateral ectopic pregnancy," *Journal of Minimally Invasive Gynecology*, vol. 14, no. 4, pp. 419–427, 2007.

[28] H. H. Bustos-lopez, G. Rojas-poceros, J. Barron-vallejo, S. Cintora-zamudio, A. Kably-ambe, and R. F. Valle, "Conservative laparoscopic treatment of bilateral ectopic pregnancy: two case reports and review of the literature," *Journal of Gynecologic Surgery*, vol. 14, no. 1, pp. 39–45, 1998.

24

Postpartum Treatment of a Herniation of the Anterior Uterine Wall due to Remains of Placenta Increta

Anis Haddad ⓘ,[1] **Olfa Zoukar** ⓘ,[1] **Houda Mhabrich** ⓘ,[2] **Awatef Hajjeji,**[1] **and Raja Faleh**[1]

[1]*Department of Obstetrics and Gynecology, Fattouma Bourguiba Teaching Hospital of Monastir. Rue 1er Juin 1955, 5000 Monastir, Tunisia*
[2]*Department of Radiology, Fattouma Bourguiba Teaching Hospital of Monastir. Rue 1er Juin 1955, 5000 Monastir, Tunisia*

Correspondence should be addressed to Anis Haddad; dr.haddadanis@gmail.com

Academic Editor: Kyousuke Takeuchi

In recent years, the incidence of placenta accreta and associated complications has increased significantly. The authors report the case of a pregnant woman in the 5th month of pregnancy for premature rupture of the membranes. The placenta was inserted low. The evolution was marked spontaneous work followed by the expulsion of the fetus. The delivery of the placenta was haemorrhagic and incomplete. Ultrasonic testing showed a placental fragment integrated in the thickness of the myometrium. Conservative treatment with methotrexate was published a few days later and MRI showed that the anterior uterine sac was filled with blood clots associated with pelvic effusion. A laparotomy was then performed to resect the pouch and the one-piece fragment. The follow-up was uneventful.

1. Introduction

Placenta accreta or abnormally adherent placenta remains a source of concern to any obstetrician despite the progress made in terms of both diagnosis and management during delivery and the postpartum period. Because of the dramatic increase in its incidence in the last few decades, together with the rise in caesarean delivery rates and the still-high maternal morbid-mortality rates, much more vigilance is required. Furthermore, a rescue hysterectomy has a significant psychological impact, mainly because of early permanent loss of fertility. This is why there is a tendency to opt for a conservative treatment whenever possible.

Many authors [1, 2] reported, in isolated cases or limited series, different techniques for uterine preservation. This treatment, whose feasibility and success often remain unpredictable, exposes patients to various morbidities that can pose diagnostic and management problems as was the case we report here. This case consists of an unusual complication of placenta accreta diagnosed in the second trimester of pregnancy and manifested as anterior uterine herniation that was conservatively managed.

2. Observation

A 26-year-old woman, fourth parity second gesture two abortion (G4 P1 A2), was referred to our hospital for a 24-hour history of premature rupture of membranes. She was at 22 weeks of gestation with a normal pregnancy. She had a history of prior cesarean section due to severe preeclampsia at 34 weeks of amenorrhea (WA) three years earlier, a spontaneous miscarriage, and a medication-induced termination of pregnancy without complications. Apart from this, she had no other significant past medical history.

On admission, the clinical examination showed a clear amniotic fluid flow, a spaced out uterine contraction pattern, and a one-centimeter dilated and 50% effaced cervix. An ultrasonographic examination revealed an ongoing viable pregnancy, anamnios and a low-lying anterior placenta with multiple lacunae (Figure 1). The biological findings were suggestive of chorioamnionitis given a CRP at 55.9 mg / ml and a WBC at 16850/ mm^3 and that was why the prescription of antibiotic therapy was justified.

The evolution was marked by the expulsion of the fetus after 4 hours and the complete retention of the placenta despite an oxytocin infusion already on for 6 hours without

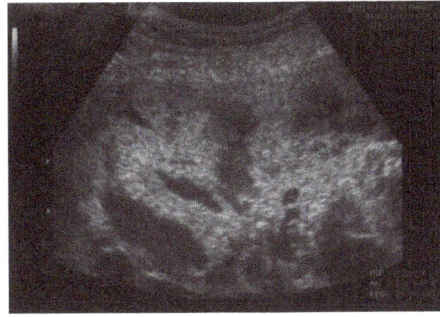

FIGURE 1: Ultrasonography appearance of a lacunary placenta.

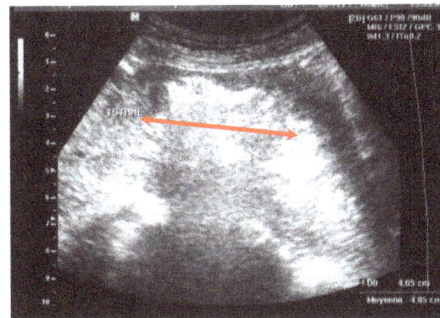

FIGURE 2: Ultrasonography aspect of the placenta increta fragment.

any bleeding. The fetal weight was 560 grams. The patient was then transferred to the operating room for uterine revision under general anesthesia. This was difficult and haemorrhagic due to an abnormally adherent placenta. The initial amount of blood lost was about 1200 ml. To control bleeding, a Sulprostone infusion was required in addition to 4 packed red blood cells and 4 fresh frozen plasma bags. An ultrasound performed immediately postabortion revealed only a 3 cm isthmic and echoic image suggestive of a retained placenta increta (Figure 2). Therefore, a medical treatment based on methotrexate was recommended in the absence of bleeding.

Given the patient's favorable initial evolution, she was discharged on the 5th day with an ultrasound control scheduled in about ten days. The ultrasound showed a swelling of the isthmic region in the form of a hernial sac containing a heterogeneous echoic image of 7 cm along its long axis. There was no associated abdominal effusion. A further exploration by pelvic MRI confirmed previous uterine herniation and revealed a content that was suggestive of an organized hematoma. It also led to a suspected uterine scar dehiscence with possible loss of substance at this level (Figure 3). After the abortion, the placenta remained intrauterine for almost two hours and did not deliver. Accordingly, a laparotomy was decided to resect this sac along with the redundant placenta increta fragment and repair, if possible, this fragile zone. Otherwise, a total hysterectomy would be the ultimate solution.

A surgical exploration revealed an unruptured isthmic hernial pocket, covered by the peritoneum and traversed by multiple dilated veins (Figure 4). Conducting a transverse

hysterotomy to open the hernial sac enabled us to easily detach the vesicouterine peritoneum and to evacuate the hematoma (Figure 5). The walls of the sac were then resected along with the increta placental fragments and then a hysterorrhaphy was performed without difficulty by separate points (Figure 6).

Subsequent follow-up was uneventful without any abnormal bleeding. A pelvic ultrasound was normal and there was an insignificant β-HCG level. The histopathological examination of the resection specimen confirmed the increta character of the placenta. A hysterosalpingogram performed 6 months later showed a normal uterine cavity without isthmocele.

3. Discussion

Our case illustrates well the progressive continuation of a fragment of placenta increta left in place after delivery in the second trimester of pregnancy on a cicatricial uterus despite the medical treatment with methotrexate. This fragment was at the origin of an anterior and isthmic uterine sacculoform neoformation.

In recent decades there has been a rise in the incidence of placenta accreta and its variants (increta and percreta) coinciding with an increasing number of caesarean sections worldwide [3, 4]: currently estimated between 1/2500 [5] and 1/500 [6] deliveries.

Several risk factors are described in the literature, the most important of which are caesarean section scars and curettage [3]. These two factors were present in our patient.

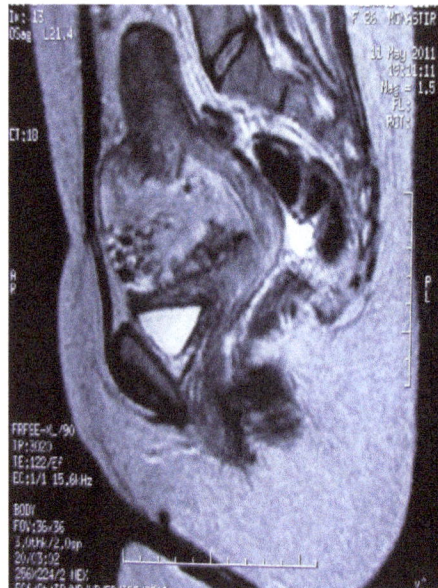

FIGURE 3: MRI aspect of the anterior uterine sacculation containing the placenta increta fragment with blood clots.

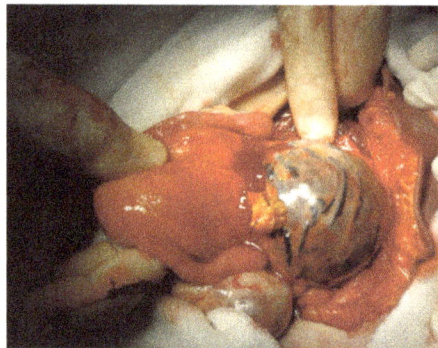

FIGURE 4: Operative view of anterior uterine sacculation.

Despite its low incidence, placenta increta continues to be the most feared complication in obstetrics as it is one of the main causes of maternal and fetal/neonatal morbidity and mortality [7, 8].

The ideal management of this complication remains uncertain although much progress has already been made [2]. Ideally, the diagnosis should be made antenatally by medical imaging for women at high risk, which enables health care providers to plan the delivery more effectively and reduce morbidity. Unfortunately, in many cases, especially during the first or second trimester, diagnosis is made only on account of the unusual resistance of the placenta to detachment when attempting a uterine revision [9, 10].

Conventionally, the recommended management consists in a caesarean hysterectomy or hysterectomy scheduled as soon as the diagnosis is retained after the delivery of the fetus, in the presence of a multidisciplinary and experienced team [11]. However, in a recent review of the literature, Rossi et al. found that this procedure, albeit radical, was associated with 53% of maternal morbidity and 3% of maternal mortality [12].

Since the publication of the first case managed conservatively by Arulkumaran et al. in 1986 [13] leaving the placenta in situ and combining chemotherapy with methotrexate as adjuvant therapy, many teams [1, 2, 7, 9] have been performing conservative management preserving the uterus and subsequent fertility. Several methods have been reported about isolated cases or limited series without consensual attitudes [1, 2, 9]. Undoubtedly, this current conservative trend has been facilitated by advances in many parameters: bleeding control by selective embolization and vascular ligation techniques, transfusion of blood and coagulation factors, improved resuscitation, and medical imaging allowing more and more cases of this anomaly to be diagnosed antenatally. In fact, prior awareness of the existence of this pathology allows for better planning and management by bringing together the necessary material and human resources for the smooth running of the treatment.

Although medical imaging is useful for antenatal diagnosis, findings suggestive of placenta increta are not always obvious. In a recent and extensive review of 167 placenta accreta

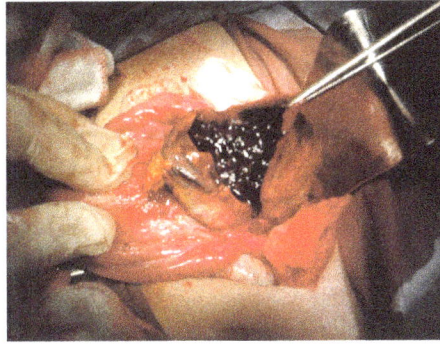

FIGURE 5: Operative view of the opening of the sac containing placenta increta and blood clots.

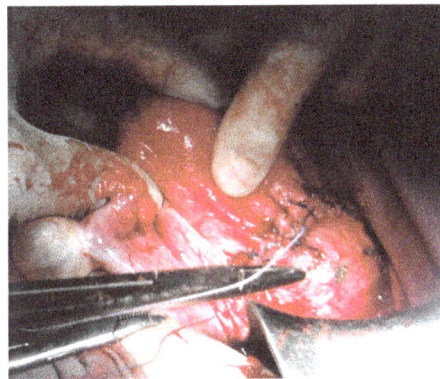

FIGURE 6: Operative view of the hysterorrhaphy after resection of the sac and its contents.

cases, only 44% of them were suspected on ultrasound [8]. In another series, it was only 24% [14]. The diagnosis seems to be more difficult during the early stages of pregnancy, probably due to the paucity of ultrasound signs. Indeed, for Yu M et al. [15], the diagnosis was suspected only in one case among the 31 identified in the second trimester. Although placenta accreta is rare in the 2nd trimester, it is not exceptional. Rashbaum et al. estimated the prevalence of clinical placenta accreta at 0.04% among second trimester abortions [16].

Ultrasound diagnosis of placenta accreta is suspected when there is at least one of the following signs: placental lacunae, obliteration of the retroplacental clear space, interruption of bladder boundaries, andmyometrial thickness less than 1 mm [17]. In our case there was only the first sign and it was interpreted as a subchorionic hematoma.

The MRI is not a first intention in screening, but it is of great help in the presence of technical difficulties with ultrasound (posterior placenta, obese women, etc.) or to make an extra uterine lesional assessment when placenta percreta is suspected [17]. It is the examination of choice for the diagnosis of a uterine herniation while at the same time specifying its anatomical structure and its content [18].

Uterine herniation is a rare and specific complication of pregnancy in which a weakened part of the uterus is transformed into a pouch or hernial sac whose wall contains all the usual uterine layers [19]. Cases reported in the literature include a history of uterine surgery and curettage, uterine malformation, or excessive enzymatic digestion during

trophoblast implantation [18, 19]. An association between placenta accreta and uterine herniation has already been suggested [19]. In most cases, the placenta is in the sac and infiltrates the myometrium [19]. The ultrasound diagnosis of the sac is sometimes difficult and remains unknown until delivery, which must be done by caesarean section because of a high risk of uterine rupture [18].

Elsewhere, the retention of a placenta increta fragment is manifested by the delayed onset, in relation to the abortion date, of a heterogeneous echogenic uterine mass. This interval varies from 2 weeks for Ju et al. [20] to 3 years for Lim et al. [21].

This abnormal placentation also predisposes, as described in our observation, to premature delivery and premature rupture of membranes [4, 22]. In the present case, a possible implantation of the egg on the scar of an old caesarean section already weakened by 2 curettages was at the origin of the abnormal invasion of the myometrium and thus the uterine herniation.

Several therapeutic options for conservative treatment are described in the literature [1, 7, 9]. They include surgical treatment and adjuvant therapy. The former can be summarized as the attempt to systematically extract, whenever possible, the maximum of the placenta during delivery or to keep it in situ. Whenever required and when the patient's condition allows, particularly in case of a stable hemodynamic state, a radiological uterine arterial embolization or bilateral vascular ligation of the hypogastric arteries can be helpful [23]. Keeping the placenta in situ seems to be associated with a lower risk of maternal morbidity and secondary hysterectomy, but with a higher predisposition to the risk of sepsis [7].

The adjuvant therapy was based primarily on the administration of a 50 mg/m^2 body surface area dose of methotrexate to promote placental resorption or its secondary delivery. The median timerequired for complete spontaneous resorption of the placenta was 13.5 weeks (range: 4-60 weeks) in the Sentilhes et al. [8] review. For Timmermans et al., this treatment failed only in 5 out of 22 cases [9].

Overall, Sentilhes et al. found a conservative treatment failure rate of 22%. In these cases a hysterectomy was performed either immediately or secondarily given the extent or recurrence of bleeding or for severe sepsis [8].

In our case, despite the prescription of methotrexate, the placental fragment left in place was a source of endometritis and a progressive increase in the volume of the hernial sac probably due to the pressure exerted by bleeding. An exploratory laparotomy was then carried out on the 18th day for fear of imminent uterine rupture and to control the infection. Indeed the excision of the increta fragment allowed us to repair the weakened uterine zone and to control the infection.

Other authors reoperated on their patients to complete the resection of an evolutive placenta increta fragment by laparotomy [24], hysteroscopy [25], or curettage [26]. Recently Kent et al. [27] demonstrated the feasibility of laparoscopic resection of the sac.

4. Conclusion

The trophoblastic invasion of a pregnancy implanted on a cicatricial uterus is a situation that has been on the rise in recent years due to the increase in obstetric scars. This invasion may be the source of an abnormal placentation that causes weakening of the isthmic region, which becomes thin, and an abnormal adherence of the placenta. These abnormalities may in turn be responsible for obstetric morbidity caused by premature rupture of the membranes, late abortion, severe postabortion or postpartum hemorrhage, and placental retention. The retention of a fragment of placenta increta after abortion may remain poorly symptomatic initially and may cause, by an excess of pressure on an already thinned and weakened area, an anterior bulge like a hernia sac. Thus a mass made of placenta and embedded blood is made and can be complicated by infection, rupture, and hemorrhage. The diagnosis is guided by systematic ultrasound which should check, in addition to uterine emptiness, the condition of the lower segment to search in the thickness of the uterine wall of an evocative heterogeneous echogenic image. The MRI is a more precise imaging procedure for identifying herniation and its content. To treat this mass, two approaches can be adopted on a case-by-case basis according to the state of the patient and the radiological workup of the lesion. The first treatment modality is medical, based on methotrexate injections and regular monitoring until the involution of the mass. The second is surgical, aiming at either extracting the increta fragment by curettage or better by hysteroscopy or resecting the hernia and its contents followed by complete reconstruction of the lower segment. It seems that the latter solution is the safest and can be performed by laparotomy or laparoscopy. Arterial embolization may be associated with this treatment.

Conservative management of uterine herniation due to placenta accreta should be considered as the first-line approach for women who desire future fertility. Otherwise, hysterectomy may be the ultimate life-saving solution in case of failure of conservative approaches or if required by the workup of the lesion.

References

[1] M. Bennett and L. Townsend, "Conservative Management of Clinically Diagnosed Placenta Accreta Following Vaginal Delivery," *Obstetric Anesthesia Digest*, vol. 31, no. 1, pp. 65-66, 2011.

[2] T. Endo, T. Hayashi, A. Shimizu et al., "Successful uterus-preserving surgery for treatment of chemotherapy- resistant placenta increta," *Gynecologic and Obstetric Investigation*, vol. 69, no. 2, pp. 112–115, 2010.

[3] T. Hung, W. Shau, C. Hsieh, T. Chiu, J. Hsu, and T. Hsieh, "Risk Factors for Placenta Accreta," *Obstetrics & Gynecology*, vol. 93, no. 4, pp. 545–550, 1999.

[4] S. Matsuzaki, S. Matsuzaki, Y. Ueda et al., "A Case Report and Literature Review of Midtrimester Termination of Pregnancy Complicated by Placenta Previa and Placenta Accreta," *American Journal of Perinatology Reports*, vol. 05, no. 01, pp. e006–e011, 2015.

[5] Committee on Obstetric Practice, "ACOG committee opinion," in *Int J Gynaecol Obstet*, vol. 77, pp. 169-170, American College of Obstetricians and Gynecologists, 2002.

[6] S. Wu, M. Kocherginsky, and J. U. Hibbard, "Abnormal placentation: twenty-year analysis," *American Journal of Obstetrics & Gynecology*, vol. 192, no. 5, pp. 1458–1461, 2005.

[7] G. Kayem, C. Davy, F. Goffinet, C. Thomas, D. Cléent, and D. Cabrol, "Conservative versus extirpative management in cases of placenta accreta," *Obstetrics & Gynecology*, vol. 104, no. 3, pp. 531–536, 2004.

[8] L. Sentilhes, C. Ambroselli, and G. Kayem, "Maternal outcome after conservative treatment of placenta accreta," *Obstetrics Gynaecology*, vol. 115, no. 3, pp. 526–534, 2010.

[9] S. Timmermans, A. C. van Hof, and J. J. Duvekot, "Conservative management of abnormally invasive placentation," *Obstetrical & Gynecological Survey*, vol. 62, no. 8, pp. 529–539, 2007.

[10] G. Son, J. Kwon, H. Cho et al., "A case of placenta increta presenting as delayed postabortal intraperitoneal bleeding in the first trimester," *Journal of Korean Medical Science*, vol. 22, no. 5, pp. 932–935, 2007.

[11] Y. Oyelese and J. C. Smulian, "Placenta previa, placenta accreta, and vasa previa," *Obstetrics & Gynecology*, vol. 107, no. 4, pp. 927–941, 2006.

[12] A. C. Rossi, R. H. Lee, and R. H. Chmait, "Emergency postpartum hysterectomy for uncontrolled postpartum bleeding: A systematic review," *Obstetrics & Gynecology*, vol. 115, no. 3, pp. 637–644, 2010.

[13] S. Arulkumaran, C. S. A. Ng, I. Ingemarsson, and S. S. Ratnam, "Medical Treatment of Placenta Accreta with Methotrexate," *Acta Obstetricia et Gynecologica Scandinavica*, vol. 65, no. 3, pp. 285-286, 1986.

[14] E. Clouqueur, C. Rubod, A. Paquin, L. Devisme, and P. Deruelle, "Placenta accreta: diagnosis and management in a French type-3 maternity hospital," *J Gynecol Obstet Biol Reprod*, vol. 37, no. 5, pp. 499–504, 2008.

[15] M. Yu, X. Y. Liu, Q. Dai, Q. C. Cui, Z. Y. Jin, and J. H. Lang, "Diagnosis and treatment of placenta accreta in the second trimester of pregnancy," *Zhongguo Yi Xue Ke Xue Yuan Xue Bao*, vol. 32, no. 5, pp. 501–504, 2010.

[16] W. K. Rashbaum, E. Jason Gates, J. Jones, B. Goldman, A. Morris, and W. D. Lyman, "Placenta accreta encountered during dilation and evacuation in the second trimester," *Obstetrics & Gynecology*, vol. 85, no. 5, pp. 701–703, 1995.

[17] E. Thia W H, S. Lee L, H. Tan K, and K. Tan L, "Ultrasonographical features of morbidly-adherent placentas," *Singapore Med J*, vol. 48, no. 9, pp. 799–803, 2007.

[18] E. M. Gottschalk, J.-P. Siedentopf, I. Schoenborn, S. Gartenschlaeger, J. W. Dudenhausen, and W. Henrich, "Prenatal sonographic and MRI findings in a pregnancy complicated by uterine sacculation: Case report and review of the literature," *Ultrasound in Obstetrics & Gynecology*, vol. 32, no. 4, pp. 582–586, 2008.

[19] D. E. DeFriend, P. A. Dubbins, and P. M. Hughes, "Sacculation of the uterus and placenta accreta: MRI appearances.," *British Journal of Radiology*, vol. 73, no. 876, pp. 1323–1325, 2000.

[20] W. Ju and S. C. Kim, "Placenta increta after first-trimester dilatation and curettage manifesting as an unusual uterine mass: Magnetic resonance findings," *Acta Radiologica*, vol. 48, no. 8, pp. 938–940, 2007.

[21] S. Lim, S. Ha, K. Lee, and J. Lee, "Retained placenta accreta after a first-trimester abortion manifesting as an uterine mass," *Obstetrics & Gynecology Science*, vol. 56, no. 3, pp. 205–207, 2013.

[22] P. Rajiah, K. L. Eastwood, M. L. D. Gunn, and M. Dighe, "Uterine diverticulum," *Obstetrics & Gynecology*, vol. 113, no. 2, pp. 525–527, 2009.

[23] Y. Y. Cheng, J. I. Hwang, S. W. Hung et al., "Angiographic embolization for emergent and prophylactic management of obstetric hemorrhage: a four-year experience," *J Chin Med Assoc*, vol. 66, no. 12, pp. 727–734, 2003.

[24] J. A. Schnorr, J. S. Singer, E. J. Udoff, and P. T. Taylor, "Late uterine wedge resection of placenta increta," *Obstetrics & Gynecology*, vol. 94, no. 5, pp. 823–825, 1999.

[25] J. A. Greenberg, J. D. Miner, and S. K. O'Horo, "Uterine artery embolization and hysteroscopic resection to treat retained placenta accreta: A case report," *Journal of Minimally Invasive Gynecology*, vol. 13, no. 4, pp. 342–344, 2006.

[26] L. Zhong, D. Chen, M. Zhong, Y. He, and C. Su, "Management of patients with placenta accreta in association with fever following vaginal delivery," *Medicine*, vol. 96, no. 10, p. e6279, 2017.

[27] A. Kent, F. Shakir, and H. Jan, "Demonstration of laparoscopic resection of uterine sacculation (niche) with uterine reconstruction," *Journal of Minimally Invasive Gynecology*, vol. 21, no. 3, p. 327, 2014.

25

21-Year-Old Pregnant Woman with MODY-5 Diabetes

Anastasia Mikuscheva, Elliot McKenzie, and Adel Mekhail

Department of Gynecology and Obstetrics, Dunedin University Hospital, Dunedin, New Zealand

Correspondence should be addressed to Anastasia Mikuscheva; a.mikuscheva@gmail.com

Academic Editor: John P. Geisler

The term "Maturity-Onset Diabetes of the Young" (MODY) was first described in 1976 and is currently referred to as monogenic diabetes. There are 14 known entities accounting for 1-2% of diabetes and they are frequently misdiagnosed as either type 1 or type 2 diabetes. MODY-5 is an entity of monogenic diabetes that is associated with genitourinary malformations and should be considered by obstetricians in pregnant women with a screen positive for diabetes, genitourinary malformations, and fetal renal anomalies. Correct diagnosis of monogenic diabetes has implications on managing patients and their families. We are reporting a case of a 21-year-old pregnant woman with a bicornuate uterus, fetal renal anomalies, and a family history of diabetes that were suggestive of a MODY-5 diabetes.

1. Introduction

Monogenic beta-cell diabetes is thought to be responsible for approximately 2% of all diabetes cases diagnosed before the age of 45 years [1]. Approximately 80% of cases are misdiagnosed as either type 1 or type 2 diabetes, reflecting lack of physician awareness and/or access to genetic testing [2]. Clues to the diagnosis of monogenic forms of diabetes include lack of typical characteristics of type 1 diabetes (no pancreatic autoantibodies, low or no insulin requirement five years after diagnosis, persistence of stimulated C-peptide of 4200 pmol/L, absence of diabetic ketoacidosis) or type 2 diabetes (lack of obesity, hypertension, dyslipidemia), in the presence of a strong family history [1].

Renal cysts and diabetes syndrome (RCAD) or Maturity-Onset Diabetes of the Young type 5 (MODY-5) is a form of monogenic diabetes caused by a mutation in the gene coding for the transcription factor hepatocyte nuclear factor 1-beta (HNF1B) [3]. HNF1B is critical for the development of the kidney and pancreas. In humans, mutations in HNF1B lead to congenital anomalies of the kidney and urinary tract, pancreas atrophy, pancreatic endocrine and exocrine deficiency, and genital malformations. [4]. The majority of HNF1 mutation carriers have extrarenal phenotypes with diabetes being the most common.

The gene was first described as causing Maturity-Onset Diabetes of the Young type 5 [5]; however, it is more commonly associated with renal disease. Diabetes usually presents in early adulthood with a median age of 20 years (range 15 days to 61 years) and frequently requires insulin treatment [6]. Renal abnormalities are frequently detected on antenatal ultrasound scans from as early as 17 weeks of gestation. Patients with a HNF1B mutation have renal function that ranges from normal to dialysis dependent or transplanted [7].

Genital tract malformations in HNF1B disease were first reported by Lindner et al. [8] in 1999; subsequently, a range of uterine malformations have been described that include bicornuate uterus, uterus didelphys, rudimentary uterus, and vaginal atresia [9].

It is important to establish in a subject with a uterine and renal abnormality whether they have a HNF1B mutation because of the 50% chance of having transmitted this to any of their existing children or to any future pregnancies. Their children will be identified as being at increased risk of the development of any of the features of the HNF1B phenotype [10].

2. Case Report

Miss A. was a 21-year-old fit and well woman without a prior documented significant medical or surgical history,

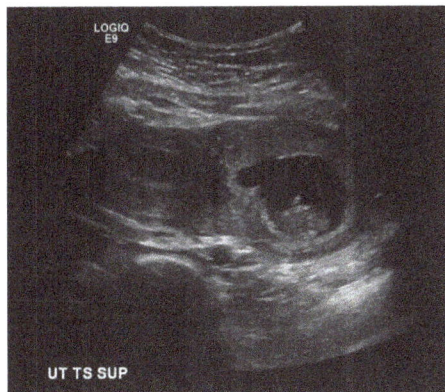

FIGURE 1: Bicornuate uterus at 9 + 5-week dating scan.

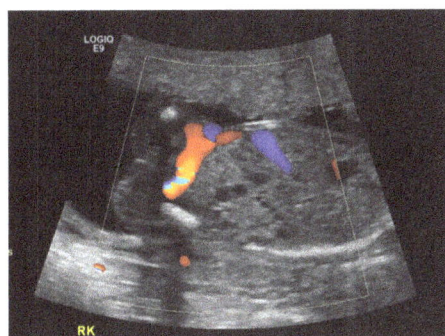

FIGURE 2: Multicystic dysplastic right kidney in the fetus at 19-week GA.

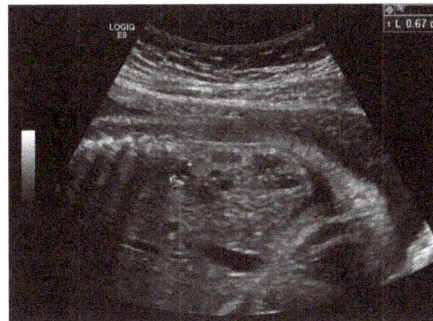

FIGURE 3: Multicystic dysplastic right kidney at 27 + 6 weeks.

who was referred to our antenatal clinic by her midwife because a bicornuate uterus was discovered on the dating scan (Figure 1) of her spontaneously conceived first pregnancy. Physical examination was normal. Full blood count and liver function tests were normal. She was negative for HIV, hepatitis B, Chlamydia, and syphilis. An HbA1C, routinely done in New Zealand for diabetes screening, was mildly elevated at 41 mmol/mol. Because of this result the patient was referred to the combined endocrine clinic and blood sugar monitoring was commenced. She had persistent hyperglycemia and investigations to exclude type I diabetes were performed. The anti-GAD antibodies and Islet Cell Cytoplasmic autoantibodies came back negative. She was started on insulin treatment as blood sugars were higher than 8 mmol/l on regular testing. Renal function tests showed normal sodium, potassium, urea, and creatinine levels. Given the uterine malformation a renal scan of Miss A.'s kidneys was performed at the fetal anatomy scan and no abnormality was detected. Given the normal renal ultrasound result no other renal imaging of the patient's kidneys was performed. The anatomy scan however showed a right multicystic dysplastic kidney in the fetus with no other abnormality (Figure 2). A repeat anatomy scan at 28 weeks showed a shrinking right kidney from 4 cm to 2.5 cm as well as a prominent in size and slightly echogenic left kidney (Figure 3).

At 21 weeks when Miss A. was hospitalized for an unprovoked episode of a minor antepartum hemorrhage, MODY-5 was suspected for the first time given her unexplained early onset diabetes and uterine malformation. Her renal function tests repeated during that hospitalization confirmed the presence of hyperuricemia (0.37 mmol/L) and a hypomagnesaemia of 0.4 mmol/L was discovered. Other biochemical tests were normal.

She was referred to the geneticist for counseling and testing MODY associated gene disorders, which came back positive for a heterozygous deletion of the hepatocyte nuclear factor 1-beta (HNF1B) gene and confirmed the diagnosis. Subsequently pancreas elastase was measured to test exocrine pancreas function which was fortunately normal. The patient's family history is strongly positive for diabetes and renal cysts have been diagnosed in her maternal cousin and her child.

Due to the diabetes diagnosis growth scans of the female fetus were performed every 4 weeks. The fetus remained in breech position during the course of the pregnancy. At 29 + 5 weeks of gestation a polyhydramnios of 31 cm was noted. At 32 weeks the patient presented to our unit with threatened preterm labor and was started on Betamethasone intramuscularly for lung maturation and Nifedipine orally for tocolysis. She was discharged after 48 hours when she had settled. At this point the baby was on the 96th centile of the Australasian Society of Ultrasound in Medicine ASUM charting for growth with an estimated fetal weight of 2.34 kg. The amniotic fluid index had reduced to 21. She represented after 5 days with premature prelabor rupture of membranes and went into spontaneous labor and the baby was delivered vaginally from breech position.

The baby girl was born alive, with APGARS 2-3-6, and a birth weight of 2105 g. The physical examination was normal. She was admitted to the neonatal intensive care unit of our hospital where she remained for 5 weeks with an uncomplicated course. However, at one week postpartum a neonatal ultrasound scan confirmed an absent right kidney and the presence of a bicornuate uterus (Figure 4) in the neonate; no other abnormality was seen. The dysplastic right kidney had been completely resorbed. Genetic testing was arranged and showed a heterozygous deletion of the HNF1B gene. An elevated creatinine of 71 umol/L was found in

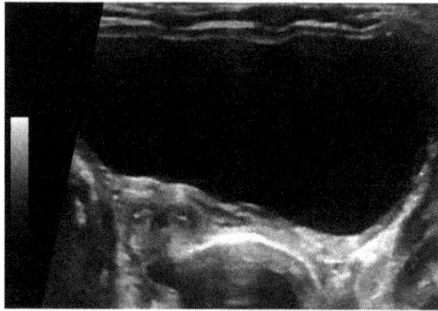

FIGURE 4: Neonatal bicornuate uterus 1 week postpartum.

the neonate on laboratory testing. This is attributed to the premature birth as retesting after 6 weeks showed a normal kidney function.

3. Discussion

Oram at al. showed that there is a high prevalence of HNF1B mutations in women with both uterine and renal abnormalities. In contrast, no mutations were found in any woman who had an isolated uterine abnormality. They concluded that HNF1B testing should be offered to women who have renal anomalies in addition to uterine anomalies but not routine screening of all women with a uterine abnormality [10]. In our case, mild renal impairment was present through hyperuricemia and hypomagnesaemia even though renal morphologic abnormalities were not detected on ultrasound. We suggest that genetic testing should be offered to young female patients with uterine abnormalities and otherwise unexplained diabetes even in the absence of kidney abnormalities on imaging if kidney impairment is present on laboratory functions.

The diagnosis is important as sometimes monogenic diabetes can be difficult to manage and can lead to microangiopathic complications. Diagnosing the disease in a patient will permit genetic counseling and genetic testing of family members where diagnosis is suspected.

The renal implications of MODY-5 can be variable ranging from very mild impairment with morphologically normal kidneys and renal impairment evident on renal functions tests only [4], like in our patient's case, to end stage renal disease requiring renal replacement therapy.

In our case, serial renal scanning of the fetus showed atrophy of the multidysplastic right kidney which probably implies a progressive loss of function in utero over time compensated by the prominence of the contralateral functioning kidney. Apart from the multicystic dysplastic kidney visualized at the anatomy scan possible implications for the fetus include oligo/anhydramnios in case of kidney function deterioration in utero, IUGR, and low birth weight and neonatal cholestatic jaundice [11]. In view of these potentially severe complications genetic testing in the mother and postnatally in the baby is important to confirm the diagnosis and thus anticipate potential difficulties.

4. Conclusion

The optimal care for pregnant patients with MODY-5 due to HNF1B mutations is multidisciplinary and involves obstetricians, endocrinologists, geneticists, nephrologists, and pediatricians. Obstetrician should be aware of this condition due to its possible implications in maternal and fetal morbidity and arrange for genetic testing in patients with early onset diabetes that is not type I diabetes and genitourinary malformations. In our case while the mother's kidneys appear structurally normal on ultrasound an impaired renal function was discovered on further testing. Despite the more common association of MODY-5 with renal malformation we think that genetic testing is also warranted in cases where genital malformations are diagnosed and renal impairment is only present on laboratory testing.

References

[1] R. Murphy, S. Ellard, and A. T. Hattersley, "Clinical implications of a molecular genetic classification of monogenic β-cell diabetes," *Nature Clinical Practice Endocrinology & Metabolism*, vol. 4, no. 4, pp. 200–213, 2008.

[2] S. BM, Maturity-onset diabetes of the young (MODY)- how many cases are we missing.pdf.

[3] E. Barbacci, A. Chalkiadaki, C. Masdeu et al., "HNF1β/TCF2 mutations impair transactivation potential through altered coregulator recruitment," *Human Molecular Genetics*, vol. 13, no. 24, pp. 3139–3149, 2004.

[4] L. Heidet, S. Decramer, A. Pawtowski et al., "Spectrum of HNF1B mutations in a large cohort of patients who harbor renal diseases," *Clinical Journal of the American Society of Nephrology*, vol. 5, no. 6, pp. 1079–1090, 2010.

[5] Y. Horikawa, N. Iwasaki, M. Hara et al., "Mutation in hepatocyte nuclear factor-1β gene (TCF2) associated with MODY," *Nature Genetics*, vol. 17, no. 4, pp. 384–385, 1997.

[6] E. L. Edghill, C. Bingham, S. Ellard, and A. T. Hattersley, "Mutations in hepatocyte nuclear factor-1β and their related phenotypes," *Journal of Medical Genetics*, vol. 43, no. 1, pp. 84–90, 2006.

[7] C. Bingham, S. Ellard, L. Allen et al., "Abnormal nephron development associated with a frameshift mutation in the transcription factor hepatocyte nuclear factor-1β," *Kidney International*, vol. 57, no. 3, pp. 898–907, 2000.

[8] T. H. Lindner, P. R. Njølstad, Y. Horikawa, L. Bostad, G. I. Bell, and O. Søvik, "A novel syndrome of diabetes mellitus, renal dysfunction and genital malformation associated with a partial deletion of the pseudo-POU domain of hepatocyte nuclear factor-1β," *Human Molecular Genetics*, vol. 8, no. 11, pp. 2001–2008, 1999.

[9] C. Bingham, S. Ellard, T. R. P Cole et al., "Solitary functioning kidney and diverse genital tract malformations associated with hepatocyte nuclear factor-1β mutations," *Kidney International*, vol. 61, no. 4, pp. 1243–1251, 2002.

[10] R. A. Oram, E. L. Edghill, J. Blackman et al., "Mutations in the hepatocyte nuclear factor-1β (HNF1B) gene are common with combined uterine and renal malformations but are not

found with isolated uterine malformations," *American Journal of Obstetrics & Gynecology*, vol. 203, no. 4, 364 pages, 2010.

[11] D. Beckers, C. Bellanné-Chantelot, and M. Maes, "Neonatal cholestatic jaundice as the first symptom of a mutation in the hepatocyte nuclear factor-1β gene (HNF-1β)," *Journal of Pediatrics*, vol. 150, no. 3, pp. 313-314, 2007.

26

Hysterectomy with Fetus In Situ for Uterine Rupture at 21-Week Gestation due to a Morbidly Adherent Placenta

Katerina Pizzuto ⓘ,[1,2] **Cory Ozimok,**[1,3] **Radenka Bozanovic,**[1,4] **Kathleen Tafler,**[1,2] **Sarah Scattolon,**[1,2] **Nicholas A. Leyland** ⓘ,[2] **and Michelle Morais** ⓘ[1,2]

[1]*School of Medicine, McMaster University, 1280 Main St. West, Hamilton, Ontario L8S4K1, Canada*
[2]*Department of Obstetrics and Gynecology, McMaster University, 1280 Main St. West, Hamilton, Ontario L8S4L8, Canada*
[3]*Department of Radiology, McMaster University, 1200 Main St. West, Hamilton, Ontario L8N3Z5, Canada*
[4]*Department of Pathology, McMaster University, 1200 Main St. West, Hamilton, Ontario L8N 3Z5, Canada*

Correspondence should be addressed to Katerina Pizzuto; katerina.pizzuto@medportal.ca

Academic Editor: John P. Geisler

Background. Uterine rupture due to a morbidly adherent placenta is a rare obstetrical cause of acute abdominal pain in the pregnant patient. We present a case to add to the small body of published literature describing this diagnosis. *Case.* A 32-year-old G5T2P1A1L2 with multiple prior cesarean sections presented at 21^{+3} weeks' gestation with abdominal pain and presyncope. Ultrasound showed a large volume of complex intraabdominal free fluid and a heterogenous placenta with irregular lacunae and increased vascularity extending to the posterior bladder wall. Exploratory laparotomy identified a uterine defect and a hysterectomy was performed due to significant bleeding. Pathology confirmed a diagnosis of placenta percreta. *Conclusion.* Early recognition and management of uterine rupture due to a morbidly adherent placenta are essential to prevent catastrophic hemorrhage.

1. Introduction

Pregnant patients commonly present with abdominal pain. Diagnosis can be challenging as the differential for both obstetric and nonobstetric causes can be extensive, and the physical examination can be altered when a gravid uterus is present. Two rare obstetric causes of acute abdominal pain include uterine rupture and intra-abdominal hemorrhage due to a morbidly adherent placenta. As the rate of cesarean sections increases, these severe complications may become more frequent and should be included in the differential diagnosis for abdominal pain in pregnancy. This case report aims to contribute to the small body of published literature describing these rare complications of pregnancy.

2. Case

A 32-year-old G5T2P1A1L2, at 21 weeks and 3 days of gestation, was brought to Labour and Delivery Triage at a tertiary care centre by ambulance. The patient had noted abdominal pain that she felt may be bowel related. After attempting to have a bowel movement, she experienced a presyncopal episode that prompted her to call for an ambulance.

Upon arrival, the maternal heart rate was 71, respiratory rate was 18, oxygen saturation was 98% on room air, and blood pressure was 80/40 mmHg. The fetal heart rate was auscultated to be normal at 145 beats per minute. The patient arrived with an intravenous line in situ and was receiving a fluid bolus. She appeared to be in pain but was awake and oriented. On history, the patient did not endorse any change to her bowel habits, fever, nausea, or vomiting. She did not have any vaginal bleeding, contraction-like pain, rupture of membranes, or abnormal vaginal discharge. Her past obstetrical history was significant for a therapeutic abortion, a classical cesarean section for a stillborn infant after preterm premature rupture of membranes and cord prolapse, an elective cesarean section at term, and a subsequent elective cesarean section at term with an incidental finding of uterine dehiscence at the time of surgery. She was otherwise healthy.

In her current pregnancy, she had been referred to the Maternal Fetal Medicine service for investigation of a suspected abnormally adherent placenta, possibly placenta

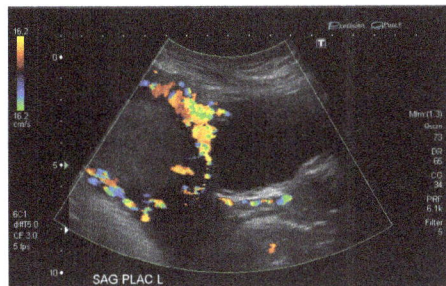

FIGURE 1: Doppler ultrasound in the sagittal plane at midline in the pelvis demonstrates turbulent peripheral vascularity in the placenta extending across the myometrium to the posterior wall of the bladder. The bladder contour is otherwise smooth; however, the finding remains highly suggestive of placenta percreta. No defect in the uterine wall could be identified, but given the large volume of hemorrhagic ascites, an emergency diagnostic laparoscopy was subsequently performed.

increta or placenta percreta. This was identified at the time of her anatomy ultrasound, when a complete anterior placenta previa was noted, along with concerning findings including loss of the placental-myometrial interface, multiple large and irregularly shaped lacunae, significant vascularity within the myometrium abutting the bladder wall, and a marginal placental abruption measuring 37.5 x 57.6 x 9.5mm. The fetus was appropriately grown and anatomic survey was normal.

Repeat vital signs continued to be stable. Blood pressure improved to 92/51 with an ongoing fluid bolus. The abdomen was soft and tender throughout, with most pain in the right lower quadrant; however, the uterus itself was nontender. In addition, there was rebound tenderness and voluntary guarding.

Laboratory investigations initially revealed a hemoglobin of 87 g/L, leukocytes of 12.0 x 10^9 per liter, and platelets of 154 x 10^9/L. AST was 13 U/L ALT 7 U/L and Kleihauer-Betke was negative. The patient was known to be anemic, with a hemoglobin of 92 g/L approximately one month prior. An abdominal ultrasound done emergently identified a normal liver, biliary tree, common bile duct, spleen, aorta, kidneys, and gallbladder. There was no evidence of hydronephrosis or renal stone. The appendix was not visualized. There was no evidence of ovarian torsion. There was free fluid throughout the abdomen with low-level echoes concerning for blood. In the left flank there was a large heterogeneous mass-like echogenic area without internal vascularity, measuring 14 x 10 cm, concerning an intra-abdominal hematoma. An obstetrical ultrasound identified a single live intrauterine gestation. The placenta was again noted to be heterogeneous with multiple irregularly shaped lacunae, and the border between the myometrium and placenta was difficult to identify along the anterior wall, as shown in Figure 1. There was increased vascularity at the placental base and along the myometrial-bladder interface. Attempts were made to assess the integrity of the uterine wall, but visualization was limited due to the fluid in the extrauterine spaces of the pelvis. There was no clear area of uterine dehiscence identified.

Blood work was repeated several hours after the initial measurements, once the suspicion of intra-abdominal hemorrhage was reported on ultrasound. Repeat hemoglobin was stable at 87 g/L, leukocytes rose to 15.6 g/L and platelets were relatively stable at 144 x 10^9/L. Coagulation studies showed a normal INR and PTT of 0.9 and 30 s, respectively, but fibrinogen was relatively low for the pregnancy state at 2.7 g/L. There was no further deterioration of clotting factors throughout the intraoperative course. The patient's vital signs remained stable, with continued slightly low blood pressure. Despite the stable hemoglobin, given the ultrasound findings suggestive of intra-abdominal hemorrhage and hematoma, along with the clinical finding of an acute surgical abdomen, the patient was taken to the operating room for an exploratory laparotomy via Pfannenstiel incision. The main concern was for bleeding due to either uterine rupture and/or bleeding from placenta percreta. The patient was counseled extensively regarding this possibility and the current previable gestation. Consent was obtained to proceed with hysterectomy if these concerns were confirmed intraoperatively.

Upon entry into the peritoneal cavity there was a significant amount of old and new blood, which was immediately evacuated. A small defect on the anterior surface of the uteruswas actively bleeding; it was felt to be the source of the hemoperitoneum. This focal area of the uterine wall was very thin, revealing placenta extending through the level of the serosa. Internal iliac ligation and hysterectomy were performed with the fetus in situ, due to the active bleeding. The estimated blood loss was 2.5 liters, most of which was noted in the abdomen at the beginning of the surgical procedure from prior blood loss. The patient received 3 units of packed red blood cells, 2 units of fresh frozen plasma, and 10 units of cryoprecipitate and 1L of Ringer's Lactate intraoperatively.

Fresh surgical specimens were forwarded to pathology, including bilateral fallopian tubes, the cervix, and the uterus containing the fetus and placenta. The uterine cornua and fallopian tubes, as well as peritoneal reflections, were anatomically normally in position. The serosal surface was intact, except for a 1.0 x 0.6 cm variegated, slightly ragged area, at the midline of the anterior wall, approximately equidistant from the fundus and cervix (Figure 2).

A subchorionic blood clot, continuous with a retroplacental hemorrhage, was noted. A brick-like color indicated that bleeding was remote. Cross-sections of the uterus demonstrated placental infiltration directly under the serosa, with a variegated appearance of the clotted blood admixed with infarcted tissue. Representative sections from the deepest point of placental invasion demonstrated retroplacental hematoma directly abutting serosal uterine surface with adjacent nonviable villi. Overall gross and microscopic findings confirmed the clinical diagnosis of placenta percreta with retroplacental hematoma.

3. Discussion

Placenta accreta is defined as an abnormally adherent placenta that invades and is inseparable, from the uterine wall.

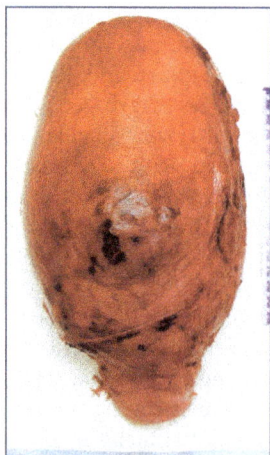

Figure 2: Intact hysterectomy specimen. Anterior wall demonstrates softened tumescence, with patchy hemorrhagic and congested appearance.

The term placenta increta is used when the chorionic villi invade only the myometrium, whereas placenta percreta describes invasion through the myometrium and serosa and occasionally into adjacent organs [1]. The incidence of placenta accreta has been steadily increasing over time and is approximately 1 in 533 pregnancies [2]. Several risk factors have been identified for the development of placenta accreta, including previous cesarean delivery, advanced maternal age, high gravidity, multiparity, previous uterine curettage, and placenta previa [3]. This patient had several of the above-listed risk factors. Placenta accreta is most commonly associated with hemorrhage in the third stage of labour, and there is a high incidence of significant postpartum hemorrhage necessitating hysterectomy [3, 4].

Accurate prenatal diagnosis of placental accreta is vital in order to facilitate appropriate antenatal management, delivery planning, and appropriate patient counseling. Ultrasound is the standard modality for assessing the placenta, but MRI has also proven useful [5]. The normal placenta in the second trimester is homogeneous in echotexture and is separated from the more hypoechoic myometrium by a thin subplacental clear space [6]. Doppler imaging demonstrates regular continuous retroplacental myometrial blood flow. Findings on ultrasonography that can be seen in the spectrum of morbidly adherent placenta include thinning of the myometrium, loss of the subplacental clear space, disruption of the serosa-bladder wall interface, presence of an exophytic mass beyond the uterine serosa, increased retroplacental vascularity, increased vascularity along the bladder wall, and placental lacunae [7]. A heterogenous appearing placenta due to the presence of lacunae, which appear as vascular structures demonstrating turbulent flow on Doppler, has the highest sensitivity, ranging from 78 to 93% after 15-week gestational age. Specificity of this finding is only 78.6% [6]. MRI can be useful in equivocal cases and in the setting of a posterior placental position [5]. Findings diagnostic of placenta accreta include abnormal uterine bulging, heterogenous signal intensity, and T2 dark intraplacental bands [6].

In cases of percreta, placental tissue may be seen extending across the myometrium into surrounding structures; tenting of the bladder wall is highly suggestive of invasion. It has been shown that, although less sensitive compared to US, MRI offers the advantage of more accurate determination of the depth and topography of placental invasion [8]. Many authors advocate a two-step approach for assessing high risk patients, beginning with a second trimester ultrasound at 18-20 weeks and further evaluation with MRI if there are suspicious or inconclusive findings [6, 7, 9].

Uterine rupture or intra-abdominal hemorrhage prior to delivery is a rare complication of placenta accreta. This is the first Canadian case report describing uterine rupture associated with a morbidly adherent placenta in the second trimester. This is also the first reported case of a hysterectomy being performed with fetus in situ for uterine rupture. Unfortunately, our patient presented at a gestational age remote from viability. Prior to surgery, a long discussion with the patient revealed that she did not wish conservative treatment, but rather she preferred definitive management in the case of intra-abdominal hemorrhage due to either uterine rupture or placenta percreta. Due to active hemorrhage intraoperatively, in order to preserve maternal health and well-being and in accordance with the patient's wishes, we felt it was most prudent not to attempt conservative management to prolong the pregnancy. Conservative measures could be considered with guarded optimism in patients wishing to attempt pregnancy preservation.

There is only one case reported by Aboulafia et al. that describes successful conservative management of a patient with a similar presentation [8]. This patient presented at 23 weeks placental tissue protruding through the serosa; thus, the uterus was oversewn to cover the exposed placental tissue. She was managed as an inpatient with daily nonstress tests and the pregnancy was successfully prolonged until 32 weeks when she underwent an elective cesarean section and curettage to remove the densely adherent placenta and no hysterectomy was required [10]. The two other cases of attempted conservative management were unsuccessful. In the case described by Hibczuk, there was a uterine defect identified with placental tissue visible through the uterine serosa, and this area was oversewn and no hysterectomy was performed [11]. This patient clinically deteriorated and required a subsequent hysterectomy. Similarly, in the case reported by Hornemann, an area of extrauterine placental tissue and bleeding was identified and coagulated [8]. Postoperatively, the patient continued to have ongoing hemorrhage and was taken back for a hysterectomy. Based on this literature, we concluded that conservative measures may be ineffective to control bleeding and would possibly leave the uterus and placenta in a compromised condition to support an ongoing pregnancy. Given our patient's wishes for definitive management and the finding of active bleeding from the placental site, we felt it prudent to proceed with hysterectomy as planned preoperatively.

In terms of definitive management, a hysterectomy is most commonly performed. Given that significant hemorrhage can occur during this procedure, adjunct procedures can be used to minimize blood loss including internal iliac balloon occlusion and internal iliac ligation. Internal iliac artery occlusion with a balloon has been shown to significantly reduce the blood loss and risk of hysterectomy in patients undergoing nonemergency cesarean section for morbidly adherent placenta [12]. In an emergency setting, it may be challenging to coordinate a balloon occlusion preoperatively, and this service may not be available in all centres. A surgical alternative to balloon occlusion is internal iliac ligation. Camuzcuoglu et al. describe several cases where internal iliac ligation is helpful and safe in the surgical management of patients with placenta previa and/or percreta to reduce blood loss and risk of reoperation [13]. Historically, internal iliac ligation used to be reserved for intractable bleeding refractory to other surgical management, but its utility has expanded to be used both prophylactically and therapeutically in a number of clinical scenarios with excessive hemorrhage including the treatment of uterine atony, invasive placentation, and uterine laceration [14]. The rare complications of internal iliac ligation can include injury to the iliac vein or ureter, inadvertent external iliac artery ligation, and the development of vesical, perineal, or gluteal necrosis [15]. We do recognize that there is a failure rate of internal iliac ligation and that it can be unsuccessful at stopping hemorrhage in some cases [16]. In this subset of patients, one may consider internal aortic compression as a means of temporizing blood loss while hysterectomy is performed [17]. In this patient, she did have significant blood loss documented at 2.5L, but much of the blood loss occurred prior to the hysterectomy from the area of rupture and can be attributed to the preexisting intraabdominal hemorrhage. In our experience, during cases where there is a significant amount of blood in the operative field and ongoing active bleeding, an internal iliac ligation performed at the outset of the procedure can decrease active bleeding, clearing the operative field while allowing the surgeon to proceed with the remainder of the procedure more expeditiously.

In summary, there have been case reports describing pregnant patients presenting with acute onset of abdominal pain and a surgical abdomen found to have uterine rupture due to morbidly adherent placenta. This is the first Canadian case report, and the first report to describe a hysterectomy performed with fetus in situ where the diagnosis of hemorrhage due to uterine rupture and morbidly adherent placenta was suspected preoperatively. It is important to consider this rare but morbid and severe diagnosis when seeing an obstetrical patient with acute abdominal pain.

References

[1] F. Cunningham, L. Kenneth, B. Steven, and Y. Catherine, *Williams Obstetrics*, vol. 24e, Mcgraw-hill, 2014.

[2] S. Wu, M. Kocherginsky, and J. U. Hibbard, "Abnormal placentation: twenty-year analysis," *American Journal of Obstetrics & Gynecology*, vol. 192, no. 5, pp. 1458–1461, 2005.

[3] N.-H. Morken and H. Henriksen, "Placenta percreta - Two cases and review of the literature," *European Journal of Obstetrics & Gynecology and Reproductive Biology*, vol. 100, no. 1, pp. 112–115, 2001.

[4] A. Mehrabadi, J. A. Hutcheon, S. Liu et al., "Maternal Health Study Group of the Canadian Perinatal Surveillance System. Contribution of placenta accreta to the incidence of postpartum hemorrhage and severe postpartum hemorrhage," *Obstetrics & Gynecology*, vol. 125, no. 4, pp. 814–821, 2015.

[5] K. M. Elsayes, A. T. Trout, A. M. Friedkin et al., "Imaging of the placenta: a multimodality pictorial review," *RadioGraphics*, vol. 29, no. 5, pp. 1371–1391, 2009.

[6] W. C. Baughman, J. E. Corteville, and R. R. Shah, "Placenta accreta: Spectrum of US and MR imaging findings," *RadioGraphics*, vol. 28, no. 7, pp. 1905–1916, 2008.

[7] S. Ayati, L. Pourali, M. Pezeshkirad et al., "Accuracy of color doppler ultrasonography and magnetic resonance imaging in diagnosis of placenta accreta: A survey of 82 cases," *International Journal of Reproductive BioMedicine*, vol. 15, no. 4, pp. 225–230, 2017.

[8] A. Hornemann, M. K. Bohlmann, K. Diedrich et al., "Spontaneous uterine rupture at the 21st week of gestation caused by placenta percreta," *Archives of Gynecology and Obstetrics*, vol. 284, no. 4, pp. 875–878, 2011.

[9] C. R. Warshak, R. Eskander, A. D. Hull et al., "Accuracy of ultrasonography and magnetic resonance imaging in the diagnosis of placenta accreta," *Obstetrics & Gynecology*, vol. 108, no. 3, pp. 573–581, 2006.

[10] Y. Aboulafia, O. Lavie, S. Granovsky-Grisaru, O. Shen, and Y. Z. Diamant, "Conservative surgical management of acute abdomen caused by placenta percreta in the second trimester," *American Journal of Obstetrics & Gynecology*, vol. 170, no. 5, pp. 1388-1389, 1994.

[11] V. Hlibczuk, "Spontaneous uterine rupture as an unusual cause of abdominal pain in the early second trimester of pregnancy," *The Journal of Emergency Medicine*, vol. 27, no. 2, pp. 143–145, 2004.

[12] D. Meng-jun, J. Guang-xin, L. Jian-hua, Z. Yu, C. Yun-yan, and Z. Xue-bin, "Pre-cesarean prophylactic balloon placement in the internal iliac artery to prevent postpartum hemorrhage among women with pernicious placenta previa," *International Journal of Gynecology & Obstetrics*, 2018.

[13] A. Camuzcuoglu, M. Vural, N. G. Hilali et al., "Surgical management of 58 patients with placenta praevia percreta," *Wiener Klinische Wochenschrift*, vol. 128, no. 9-10, pp. 360–366, 2016.

[14] I. Sziller, P. Hupuczi, and Z. Papp, "Hypogastric artery ligation for severe hemorrhage in obstetric patients," *Journal of Perinatal Medicine*, vol. 35, no. 3, pp. 187–192, 2007.

[15] Y. Simsek, E. Yilmaz, E. Celik et al., "Efficacy of internal iliac artery ligation on the management of postpartum hemorrhage and its impact on ovarian reserve," *Journal of Turkish Society of Obstetric and Gynecology*, vol. 9, no. 3, pp. 153–158, 2012.

[16] S. K. Chattopadhyay, B. Deb Roy, and Y. B. Edrees, "Surgical control of obstetric hemorrhage: hypogastric artery ligation or hysterectomy?" *International Journal of Gynecology and Obstetrics*, vol. 32, no. 4, pp. 345–351, 1990.

[17] M. Belfort, J. Zimmerman, G. Schemmer, R. Oldroyd, R. Smilanich, and M. Pearce, "Aortic Compression and Cross Clamping in a Case of Placenta Percreta and Amniotic Fluid Embolism: A Case Report," *American Journal of Perinatology Reports*, vol. 1, no. 01, pp. 033–036, 2011.

27

Benign Metastasizing Leiomyoma of the Uterus: Rare Manifestation of a Frequent Pathology

Maria Inês Raposo (ID),[1,2] **Catarina Meireles** (ID),[3] **Mariana Cardoso**,[2] **Mariana Ormonde** (ID),[2] **Cristina Ramalho**,[1] **Mónica Pires**,[1] **Mariana Afonso**,[3] **and Almerinda Petiz**[1]

[1]Department of Gynecology, Francisco Gentil Portuguese Oncology Institute, Porto, Portugal
[2]Department of Gynecology, Hospital of Divino Espírito Santo of Ponta Delgada, EPER, São Miguel, Azores, Portugal
[3]Department of Pathology, Francisco Gentil Portuguese Oncology Institute, Porto, Portugal

Correspondence should be addressed to Maria Inês Raposo; minesraposo@hotmail.com

Academic Editor: Erich Cosmi

Benign Metastasizing Leiomyoma (BML) is a rare condition with few cases reported in the literature. It is usually incidentally diagnosed several years after a primary gynecological surgery for uterine leiomyoma. Differential diagnosis of BML is complex requiring an extensive work-up and exclusion of malignancy. Here, we report two cases of BML based on similarity of histopathological, immunohistochemical, and genetic patterns between lung nodules and uterine leiomyoma previously resected, evidencing the variability of clinical and radiological features of BML. We highlight the importance of 19q and 22q deletions as highly suggestive of BML. These findings are particularly relevant when there is no uterine sample for review.

1. Introduction

Uterine leiomyoma is the most common gynecological tumor [1–4]. BML is a rare variant [1–13] characterized by multiple leiomyomatous lesions in distant locations, most commonly the lungs [3–11]. Less frequently involved areas are lymph nodes, inferior vena cava, heart, brain, bones, abdomen, retroperitoneum, pelvis, breast, esophagus, liver, appendix, trachea, skin, muscle, and parametria [14, 15]. The antagonistic terminology of BML reflects the coexistence of benign appearance with a biological behavior suggesting malignancy [2, 3, 8, 16]. When multiple pulmonary nodules are incidentally detected in women with history of surgery for uterine leiomyoma, clinicians should be aware of this potential diagnosis [5, 11, 13].

The incidence of BML remains unclear [6]. Since its first publication by Steiner, in 1939 [18], approximately 150 cases have been published [1]. Due to the rarity of this condition, the pathophysiology and management remains controversial [2, 4]. The literature is scarce on studies regarding the cytogenetic evaluation [7].

Here we report two clinical cases of BML diagnosed in the Portuguese Oncology Institute of Porto (Table 1). Our aim is to review its diagnostic challenges, focusing on clinical, radiological, and anatomopathological findings. We also intend to determine the implications of cytogenetic study of this rare condition. Table 2 summarizes the case reports regarding pulmonary BML recently published in the literature.

2. Case Presentation

2.1. Case 1. A 49-year-old, premenopausal, asymptomatic woman, with past clinical history significant for total hysterectomy 10 years earlier due to a leiomyoma of the uterus, presented with a miliary pattern in a routine chest radiography as in computed tomography (CT) scan (Figure 1). We performed a Positron Emission Tomography (PET) scan that showed weak fluorodeoxyglucose (FDG) uptake in lung nodules. She underwent CT-guided biopsy of a pulmonary nodule which revealed spindle cells consistent with smooth muscle differentiation, without cellular atypia, necrosis, or mitotic figures. Immunohistochemical examination was

TABLE 1: Clinical cases.

Case	Age	Respiratory symptoms	Primary surgery for leiomyoma	Radiology	Final diagnosis	Microscopy and Immunohistochemistry	Cytogenetic evaluation	Treatment	Follow-up
1	49	Asymptomatic	Total hysterectomy, 10 years ago	Miliary pattern PET: weak FDG uptake	CT-guided biopsy	Smooth muscle tumor, SMA+, desmin +, hormonal receptors+, low Ki-67	Lung tumor: 19q13 and 22q12 deletions	Bilateral salpingo-oophorectomy and Letrozole.	9 months, stable
2	48	Cough	Total hysterectomy, 13 years ago	Multiple pulmonary nodules PET: weak FDG uptake	CT-guided biopsy	Smooth muscle tumor, SMA+, desmin +, hormonal receptors+, low ki-67	Lung tumor and primary leiomyoma: 19q13 and 22q12 deletions	Bilateral salpingo-oophorectomy	6 months, stable

PET= positron emission tomography; FDG= Fluorodeoxyglucose; CT= computed tomography; SMA=smooth muscle actin.

TABLE 2: Pulmonary BML case reports.

Refer	Age	Respiratory symptoms	Primary surgery for leiomyoma	Radiology	Final diagnosis	Microscopy and Immunohistochemistry	Cytogenetic evaluation	Treatment	Follow-up
Nurettin et al. [1]	41	Dyspnea	Myomectomy, 10 years ago	Multiple pulmonary nodules PET: no FDG uptake	VATS biopsy	Smooth muscle tumor, SMA+, desmin +, hormonal receptors+, low ki-67	Not applicable	Bilateral salpingo-oophorectomy, total hysterectomy and Progesterone	5 years, stable
Ma et al. [3]	45	Asymptomatic	Myomectomy, 11 years ago	Multiple pulmonary nodules PET: abnormal FDG uptake	Aspiration Biopsy	Smooth muscle tumor, SMA+, desmin +, hormonal receptors+, ki-67=1%	Not applicable	Pulmonary wedge resection	5 months, stable
Chen et al. [5]	32	Chest tightness and labored breathing	Myomectomy, 1 month earlier	Miliary nodules	Thoracoscopic Biopsy	Spindle cells, SMA+, desmin +, hormonal receptors+	Not applicable	Tamoxifen	3 months, stable
Lee et al. [8]	52	Asymptomatic	Vaginal hysterectomy, 10 years ago	Multiple lung cavitations and nodules PET: no FDG avid	Needle Biopsy	Spindle cells, SMA+, desmin +, hormonal receptors+	Not applicable	GnRH Agonist	15 months, stable
Ras et al. [9]*	53	Asymptomatic	Myomectomy, 26 years earlier	Multiple pulmonary nodules	Thoracotomy Biopsy	Bland smooth muscle cells, desmin +, hormonal receptors+, low ki-67	Not applicable	Subtotal hysterectomy, bilateral salpingo-ooforectomy, removal of the tumors from parametria and appendectomy and pulmonary wedge resection by thoracotomy	Not applicable

TABLE 2: Continued.

Refer	Age	Respiratory symptoms	Primary surgery for leiomyoma	Radiology	Final diagnosis	Microscopy and Immunohistochemistry	Cytogenetic evaluation	Treatment	Follow-up
Ottlakan et al. [10]	36	Asymptomatic	Hysterectomy, 7 years earlier	Multiple pulmonary nodules	Core Biopsy	Smooth muscle cells, SMA+	Lung nodules: 19q22q deletion	Pulmonary wedge resection and cautery resection, through mini-thoracotomy (seven procedures)	Many recurrences
Patré et al. [11]*	76	Acute respiratory distress	Total hysterectomy, 4 years earlier	Multiple pulmonary nodules and pleural effusion	Surgical biopsy	Spindle cells, SMA+, desmin +, hormonal receptors+, caldesmon+	Not applicable	Resection of pulmonary nodules, removal of trochanteric lesion and aromatase inhibitors	45 months, stable
Khan et al. [14]	47	Shortness pf breath and chest pain	Cervical hysterectomy, 3 years prior	Multiple pulmonary nodules PET: mild FDG uptake	CT guided biopsy and VATS biopsy	Smooth muscle tumor, SMA+, desmin +, hormonal receptors+, HMB45-, CD34-, EMA-	Lung nodules: Loss of 19 and 22 and deletion of 1p	VATS wedge resection and anastrozole	12 months, stable
Bakkensen et al. [15]*	46	Asymptomatic	Total hysterectomy, 7 years ago	Multiple pulmonary nodules PET: no FDG uptake	CT guided biopsy	Bland spindle cells, SMA+, desmin +, hormonal receptors+	Not applicable	Bilateral salpingo-ooforectomy, resection of pelvic mass, opportunistic appendectomy and letrozole	2 years, stable
Zhong et al. [17]*	51	Asymptomatic	Myomectomy, 26 years earlier	Multiple pulmonary nodules PET: abnormal FDG uptake	CT guided biopsy	Spindle-shaped cells, SMA+, desmin+, hormonal receptors+, CD34-, S100-, HMB45-, Ki-67<20%	Not applicable	Removal of lumbar spine tumor and Tamoxifen	5 months, stable

*BML of other sites; PET= positron emission tomography; FDG= fluorodeoxyglucose; VATS=video-assisted thoracoscopic surgery; CT= computed tomography; SMA=smooth muscle actin.

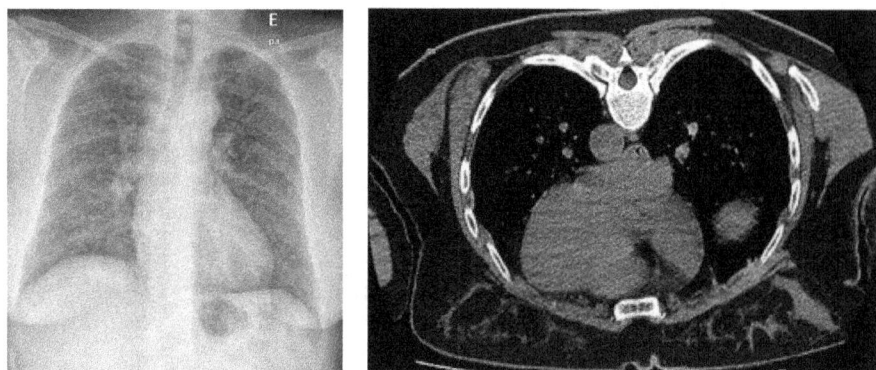

FIGURE 1: Chest radiography and CT images of patient 1.

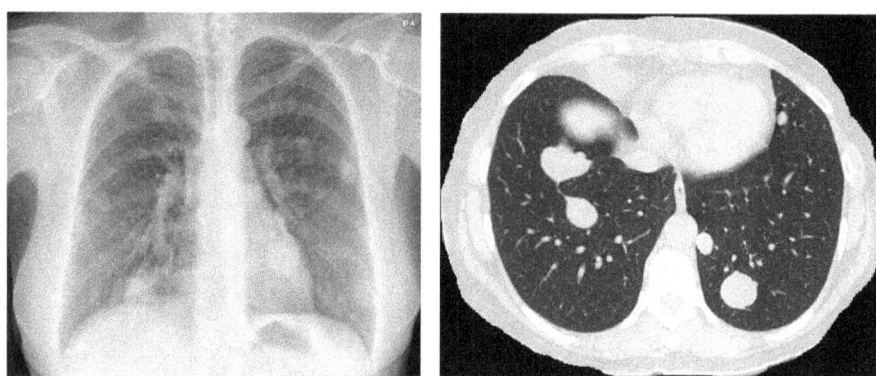

FIGURE 2: Chest radiography and CT images of patient 2.

positive for smooth muscle actin (SMA), desmin, estrogen, and progesterone receptors and was negative for HBM-45, CK7, and S100. The proliferative index, assessed with Ki-67 index, was low. Cytogenetic evaluation of lung tumor tissue showed 19q and 22q terminal deletions. Cytogenetic analysis of previous leiomyoma was not performed due to insufficient pathological material. After diagnosing BML, patient underwent bilateral salpingo-oophorectomy followed by Letrozole therapy. At 9 months follow-up, there was no further development of the disease.

2.2. Case 2. A 48-year-old premenopausal woman was referred because of persistent cough. Her past clinical history included a hysterectomy 13 years earlier for uterine leiomyoma. Chest radiography and CT revealed multiple pulmonary bilateral nodules (Figure 2) with no FDG uptake in the PET scan. CT-guided biopsy of a pulmonary nodule was performed and the resected uterine leiomyoma was reviewed. Both specimens showed identical histopathology of a low grade, benign appearing, and smooth muscle tumor (Figure 3). The immunohistochemical profile of BML is indistinguishable from that of the primary uterine tumor with positivity for SMA, desmin, estrogen, and progesterone receptors (Figure 4) and negativity for HMB-45, CD31, CD34, and EMA. The staining for ki-67 showed low mitotic activity. Cytogenetic analysis revealed shared profile between both samples, including 19q and 22q terminal deletions (Figure 5). Since these findings were consistent with BML, surgical

castration was performed. After 6 months of follow-up, the remaining lesions were stable.

3. Discussion

BML is found primarily in reproductive aged women [2, 5, 11], as in the presented cases. The mean age at diagnosis is 47,3 years [6]. The course of the disease correlates with the level of reproductive hormones [5]. Several theories have been proposed along the years regarding the etiology of BML, including [5–10] hematogenous spread of uterine leiomyoma; in situ proliferation of smooth muscle induced by hormonal stimulation; metastasis of low-grade uterine leiomyosarcoma previously subdiagnosed; peritoneal seeding after surgery for uterine leiomyoma and metaplastic transformation. Since most cases of BML occur from 8,8 to 15 years after gynecological surgery [2, 5, 6, 8], we hypothesize that surgically induced vascular spread is the most likely cause [1, 10]. In addition, we agree with the majority of researchers who consider that BML is clonally derived from uterine leiomyoma [3–8]. The exclusive occurrence in women with history of uterine leiomyoma, the positivity for hormonal receptors, and the susceptibility to antihormonal therapy favor this origin [4, 13]. Overlapping in histopathological, immunohistochemical, and cytogenetic findings between pulmonary and uterine lesions suggests their association [6, 7].

Main clinical symptoms of BML vary depending on the organs involved [15]. Regarding pulmonary BML, patients

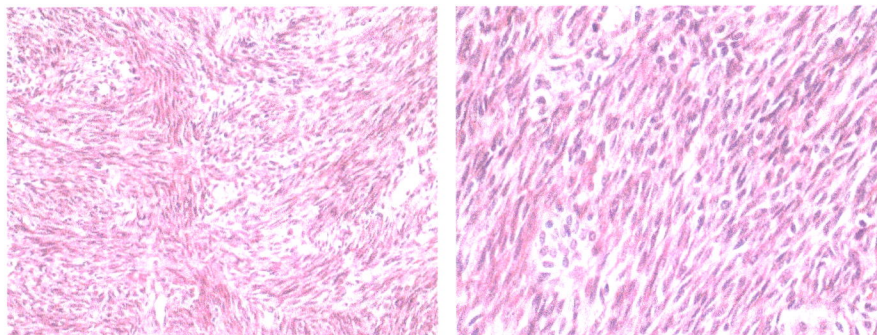

FIGURE 3: Histopathologic examination of BML and uterine leiomyoma of patient 2.

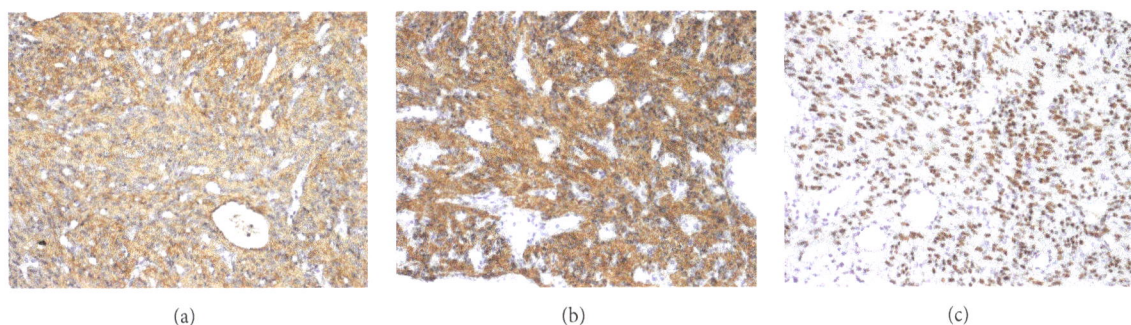

(a)   (b)   (c)

FIGURE 4: Immunohistochemical staining of BML and uterine leiomyoma of patient 2. (a) SMA, (b) Desmin, and (c) Hormonal Receptors.

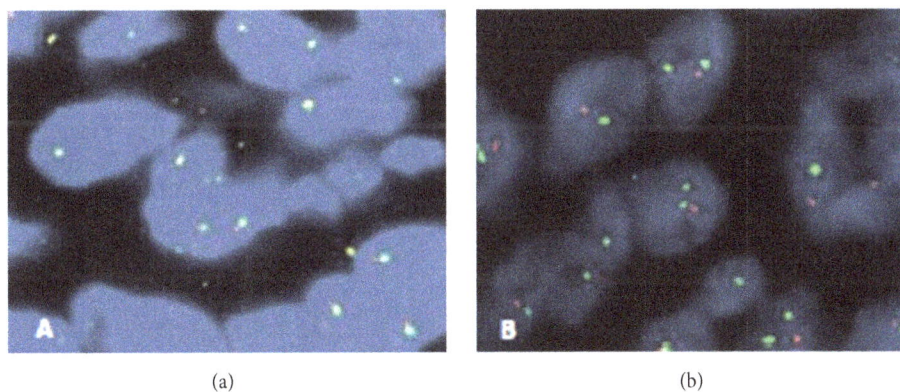

(a)   (b)

FIGURE 5: Cytogenetic study of BML and uterine leiomyoma of patient 2, using *"Fluorescence In Situ Hybridization" (FISH),* with probes *LSI EWSR1 (22q12) Dual Color, Break Apart Rearrangement Probe, Abbott,* and *ZytoLight SPEC 19q13/19q13 Dual Color Probe, Zytovision. (a)* 22q12 deletion and (b) 19q13 deletion.

are usually asymptomatic [2, 5, 8, 13] and the disease is an incidental finding, as we described in patient 1. Only one-third of patients develop respiratory symptoms, such as cough, hemoptysis, dyspnea, thoracalgia, and respiratory failure [3]. Hemothorax and pneumothorax have also been reported [4, 6].

Imaging findings are not specific for pulmonary BML [4, 5]. Multiple bilateral well-circumscribed pulmonary nodules are found in the majority of patients [1, 2, 8]. Another rarely reported features are solitary pulmonary nodule, interstitial lung disease, cystic lesions, cavitary lung nodules, and miliary pattern [5, 8, 11]. Radiologic findings of extrapulmonary BML are rarer and less well characterized in the literature.

However, both pulmonary and extra-pulmonary nodules of BML show weak or absent FDG uptake on PET [15]. This allows exclusion of metastasis from uterine sarcoma or extrathoracic malignant tumors [1, 2].

Histopathological confirmation is required for definitive diagnosis of BML [1, 5]. These lesions reveal a smooth muscle phenotype with low mitotic activity, limited vascularization and lacks of anaplasia and necrosis [4–8, 10–13]. Its immunohistochemical features include positivity for smooth muscle actin, desmin, caldesmon, calponin, vimentin [1, 2], and hormonal receptors (estrogen and progesterone receptors) [1, 5]. Low ki-67 index [1, 5] and negativity for HMB-45 [4] are useful for ruling out uterine leiomyosarcoma and lymphangioleiomyomatosis, respectively. It is extremely important to differentiate BML from uterine leiomyosarcoma since follow-up and treatment are distinct [5, 8, 13].

Recent genetic studies confirm a shared profile between BML and uterine tumor [6, 7, 12]. The present study contributes to the individualization of BML as a genetically distinct entity, since both patients had 19q and 22q terminal deletions in pulmonary tissue, as previously described by *Nucci M. et al.* [12]. This cytogenetic profile was found in 3% of uterine leiomyomas, suggesting that BML arises from a biologically distinct minority of leiomyomas [12, 14]. Consequently, these mutations could be used as a marker for uterine leiomyomas with potential to develop BML. Given the rarity of this disease, we do not recommend performing a genetic screening test for all women undergoing surgery due to uterine leiomyoma [6]. However, from our standpoint, searching for 19q and 22q terminal deletions in lung nodules of women with past history of gynecological surgery has a determinant role in the differential diagnosis of BML. Therefore, this genetic study becomes even more useful for BML diagnosis when uterine specimen is unavailable or insufficient for retrospective review [12].

Since BML treatment is not standardized [1, 2, 4] it should be individualized for each patient depending on the metastasis sites [17]. If the disease is resectable, *en bloc* removal of lesions should be attempted [15, 16]. For pulmonary BML, although primary option consists in surgical excision of the maximum possible number of pulmonary nodules, it may not be technically feasible. Alternative therapies include surgical castration by bilateral oophorectomy, chemical castration [1, 2, 5, 10, 11], or combined therapy [2]. Some researchers advocate expectant treatment in climacteric women [2]. BML usually has an indolent evolution [2, 4] and favorable prognosis [11, 13]. According to the literature, after the excision of intrapulmonary lesions the median survival rate is 94 months [3, 13]. The patients described were re-examined every three months using a pulmonary CT. Although their pulmonary lesions remained stable, an extended follow-up is required to track disease progression.

4. Conclusion

A multidisciplinary approach is crucial for the diagnosis of BML in women with pulmonary smooth muscle neoplasia and history of uterine leiomyoma. The striking resemblance of BML to uterine fibroids should lead to correct diagnosis. When primary uterine tumor cannot be reassessed, the presence of 19q and 22q terminal deletions in lung nodules is strongly predictive of BML [10, 12], promoting proper treatment and surveillance for this benign condition. In the future, new cytogenetic markers may optimize BML diagnosis [7, 9]. Further studies are necessary to clarify the etiology of BML and standardize its management.

Consent

Informed consent has been obtained from the women described for publication of the present clinical cases.

Disclosure

This work was previously presented as a poster at the 25th World Congress on Controversies in Obstetrics, Gynaecology, and Infertility (COGI) in 2017.

References

[1] N. AKA, "Benign Pulmonary Metastasizing Leiomyoma of the Uterus," *Journal of Clinical and Diagnostic Research*, 2016.

[2] S. Chen, Y. Zhang, J. Zhang et al., "Pulmonary benign metastasizing leiomyoma from uterine leiomyoma," *World Journal of Surgical Oncology*, vol. 11, article no. 163, 2013.

[3] H. Ma and J. Cao, "Benign pulmonary metastasizing leiomyoma of the uterus: A case report," *Oncology Letters*, vol. 9, no. 3, pp. 1347–1350, 2015.

[4] J. Miller, M. Shoni, C. Siegert, A. Lebenthal, J. Godleski, and C. McNamee, "Benign metastasizing leiomyomas to the lungs: An institutional case series and a review of the recent literature," *The Annals of Thoracic Surgery*, vol. 101, no. 1, pp. 253–258, 2016.

[5] S. Chen, R.-M. Liu, and T. Li, "Pulmonary benign metastasizing leiomyoma: A case report and literature review," *Journal of Thoracic Disease*, vol. 6, no. 6, pp. E92–E98, 2014.

[6] E. Barnas, M. Ksiazek, R. Ras, A. Skret, J. Skret-Magieroo, and E. Dmoch-Gajzlerska, "Benign metastasizing leiomyoma: A review of current literature in respect to the time and type of previous gynecological surgery," *PLoS ONE*, vol. 12, no. 4, 2017.

[7] K. T. Patton, L. Cheng, V. Papavero et al., "Benign metastasizing leiomyoma: clonality, telomere length and clinicopathologic analysis," *Modern Pathology*, vol. 19, no. 1, pp. 130–140, 2006.

[8] S. R. Lee, Y.-I. Choi, S. J. Lee et al., "Multiple cavitating pulmonary nodules: Rare manifestation of benign metastatic leiomyoma," *Journal of Thoracic Disease*, vol. 9, no. 1, pp. E1–E5, 2017.

[9] R. Raś, M. Książek, E. Barnaś et al., "Benign metastasizing leiomyoma in triple location: lungs, parametria and appendix," *Menopausal Review*, vol. 2, pp. 117–121, 2016.

[10] A. Ottlakan, B. Borda, G. Lazar, L. Tiszlavicz, and J. Furak, "Treatment decision based on the biological behavior of pulmonary benign metastasizing leiomyoma," *Journal of Thoracic Disease*, vol. 8, no. 8, pp. E672–E676, 2016.

[11] J. Pastré, K. Juvin, B. Grand, L. Gibault, J. Valcke, and D. Israël-Biet, "Pulmonary benign metastasizing leiomyoma presented as acute respiratory distress," *Respirology Case Reports*, vol. 5, no. 2, 2017.

[12] M. R. Nucci, R. Drapkin, P. D. Cin, C. D. M. Fletcher, and J. A. Fletcher, "Distinctive cytogenetic profile in benign metastasizing leiomyoma: pathogenetic implications," *The American Journal of Surgical Pathology*, vol. 31, no. 5, pp. 737–743, 2007.

[13] Rokana Taftaf, Sandra Starnes, Jiang Wang et al., "Benign Metastasizing Leiomyoma: A Rare Type of Lung Metastases—Two Case Reports and Review of the Literature," *Case Reports in Oncological Medicine*, vol. 2014, Article ID 842801, 4 pages, 2014.

[14] M. Khan, A. Faisal, H. Ibrahim, T. Barnes, and G. M. Van-Otteren, "Pulmonary benign metastasizing leiomyoma: A case

report," *Respiratory Medicine Case Reports*, vol. 24, pp. 117–121, 2018.

[15] J. B. Bakkensen, W. Samore, P. Bortoletto, C. C. Morton, and R. M. Anchan, "Pelvic and pulmonary benign metastasizing leiomyoma: A case report," *Case Reports in Women's Health*, vol. 18, p. e00061, 2018.

[16] Y. Kim, K. J. Eoh, J. Lee et al., "Aberrant uterine leiomyomas with extrauterine manifestation: intravenous leiomyomatosis and benign metastasizing leiomyomas," *Obstetrics & Gynecology Science*, vol. 61, no. 4, p. 509, 2018.

[17] D. Zong, W. He, J. Li, H. Peng, P. Chen, and R. Ouyang, "Concurrent benign metastasizing leiomyoma in the lung and lumbar spine with elevated standardized uptake value level in positron-emission tomography computed tomography," *Medicine*, vol. 97, no. 27, p. e11334, 2018.

[18] P. Steiner, "Metastasizing Fibroleiomyoma of The Uterus - Report of a case and review of the literature," *American Journal of Pathology*, vol. 15, no. 1, 1939.

28

Selective Reduction of a Heterotopic Cesarean Scar Pregnancy Complicated by Septic Abortion

Joan Tymon-Rosario[1] **and Meleen Chuang** ⓘ[1,2]

[1]*Montefiore Medical Center, Department of Obstetrics & Gynecology and Women's Health, Bronx, NY, USA*
[2]*Albert Einstein College of Medicine, Bronx, NY, USA*

Correspondence should be addressed to Meleen Chuang; mechuang@montefiore.org

Academic Editor: Cem Ficicioglu

Background. Heterotopic pregnancy involving the implantation of an ectopic pregnancy into a prior cesarean scar with a concurrent intrauterine pregnancy is a rare and potentially life-threatening condition with minimal information in the literature to guide treatment and management options. *Case.* A 40-year-old G5P3103 at 12 weeks and 3 days with a history of two cesarean deliveries was diagnosed with a live heterotopic pregnancy containing a cesarean scar ectopic and an intrauterine pregnancy. After selective reduction of the cesarean scar gestation with potassium chloride (KCl), the patient presented ten days later to the emergency department with septic abortion and sepsis. The patient underwent bilateral uterine artery embolization followed by ultrasound guided uterine evacuation with dilation and curettage, which was complicated by intraoperative hemorrhage and persistent bacteremia. The patient had resolution of her bacteremia after total abdominal hysterectomy. *Conclusion.* Conservative management of uterine infection resulting from selective reduction of a heterotopic pregnancy cesarean scar pregnancy may be considered; however, severe septicemia and persistent bacteremia may necessitate definitive surgical management.

1. Introduction

A heterotopic pregnancy refers to the presence of simultaneous pregnancies at two different implantation sites, with the majority of ectopic pregnancies located in the fallopian tube. The literature to date involves discussion of the management of the more "traditional" heterotopic pregnancies with successful results. There is growing number of case reports of cesarean scar pregnancy with concurrent intrauterine pregnancies with variable clinical outcomes. Given the rise in cesarean sections and usage of assisted reproductive techniques over the past decades, this clinical conundrum will continue to increase in incidence. The rarity of a heterotopic pregnancy with one gestation being cesarean scar pregnancy (CSP) inherently limits evidence based recommendations on management options as well as all the potential adverse outcomes of various treatment options. We report a unique clinical circumstance of the implantation of an ectopic pregnancy into a prior cesarean scar with a concurrent intrauterine pregnancy and the subsequent complications that arose

after selective reduction that ultimately necessitated hysterectomy.

2. Case

A 40-year-old G5P3103 at 12 weeks and 3 days with a history of two prior cesarean sections and known heterotopic pregnancy consisting of cesarean scar pregnancy and intrauterine pregnancy (Figure 1) presented ten days after successful selective reduction of cesarean scar pregnancy with potassium chloride (KCl) injection in the ultrasonography unit.

The patient reported two days of fevers prior to her presentation with new onset vaginal bleeding. After her initial visit after selective reduction, she was treated with Nitrofurantoin for a urinary tract infection at urgent care. She presented two days after urgent care to our emergency department (ED) with pain and ultrasonographic evaluation that demonstrated no fetal heartbeat and discharge home for

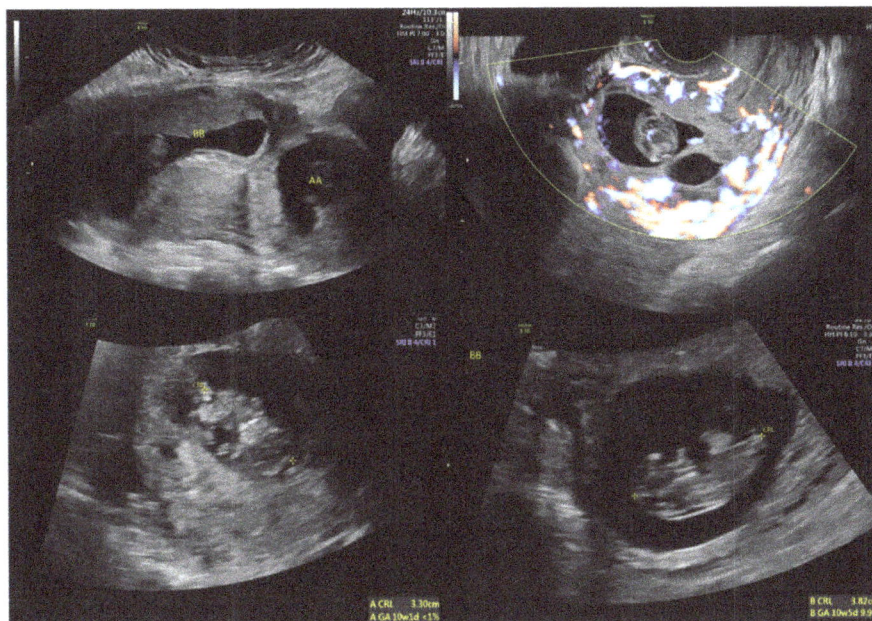

FIGURE 1: Sonographic imaged before selective reduction of cesarean scar pregnancy with potassium chloride (KCl injection). Upper left demonstrates cesarean scar pregnancy (AA) and intrauterine pregnancy (BB). Upper right demonstrates that cesarean scar pregnancy in close proximity to serosal edge of the uterus. Lower right and left demonstrate live pregnancy of Twin A (cesarean scar pregnancy) and Twin B (intrauterine pregnancy).

follow-up with her provider for management options. Three days after ED visit, she represented with new onset fevers, chills, back pain, and scant vaginal bleeding. She denied any significant past medical history and her previous surgical procedure included gastric bypass surgery, two cesarean sections, and an endometrial ablation for heavy menses.

On physical examination, the patient was febrile, tachycardic, hypotensive, and being in septic shock. She had scant dark blood in the vaginal vault, a 16 week size uterus with fundal tenderness. Ultrasound confirmed presence of no fetal cardiac activities and presence of high vascular flow to the myometrium surrounding the cesarean scar pregnancy (Figure 2).

The patient was counseled on septic abortion and she underwent a complete infectious disease workup, including blood cultures, urine cultures, and chest x-ray, and was started on broad-spectrum antibiotics (ampicillin, gentamicin, and clindamycin). Initial urine culture demonstrated no growth and initial blood culture grew *Enterococcus faecalis*. The patient desired uterine preservation and underwent bilateral uterine artery embolization using absorbable gelfoam and scheduled dilation and curettage under sonographic guidance the following day. The procedure was complicated with intraoperative hemorrhage of 1000cc that resolved with uterotonic medications and blood transfusion. Final pathology was consistent with products of conception. Hospitalized postoperatively, she continued to have daily low- grade fevers while on antibiotics with persistent daily positive blood cultures with *Enterococcus faecalis*. Antibiotic regimen was changed based upon the sensitivities to ampicillin and ceftriaxone, a normal echocardiogram ruled out endocarditis,

and repeat transvaginal ultrasound demonstrated a large amount of heterogeneous avascular material in the lower uterine segment. The postoperative serum beta-hCG was 896 IU/L. CT scan of the abdomen and pelvis demonstrated a large high-density material within the endometrial cavity of lower uterine segment (Figure 3).

With concerns for persistent bacteremia, failed antibiotic therapy, and retained materials within the uterine cavity, the patient underwent a total abdominal hysterectomy and bilateral salpingectomy. The specimen was bivalved to show the entire uterine cavity with large amounts of blood clots, adherent placental tissue as well as a very thin anterior uterine segment (Figure 4).

Final pathology demonstrated products of conception with associated chronic and acute inflammation. Uterine culture obtained at hysterectomy demonstrated growth of *Enterococcus faecalis*, confirming the uterus as source of bacteremia. The patient had resolution of her fevers and negative blood cultures after the hysterectomy. Intravenous antibiotics were discontinued on postoperative day four and transitioned to a two-week course of Augmentin. She was discharged home with a two-week office follow-up. At her postoperative check and six-week visit she recovered fully.

3. Discussion

Selective reduction of heterotopic cesarean scar pregnancies via abortifacient injection, embryo aspiration, or both has been shown in the literature to be effective with multiple case reports citing success [1–5]. There are three case reports describing the successful management of a heterotopic CSP

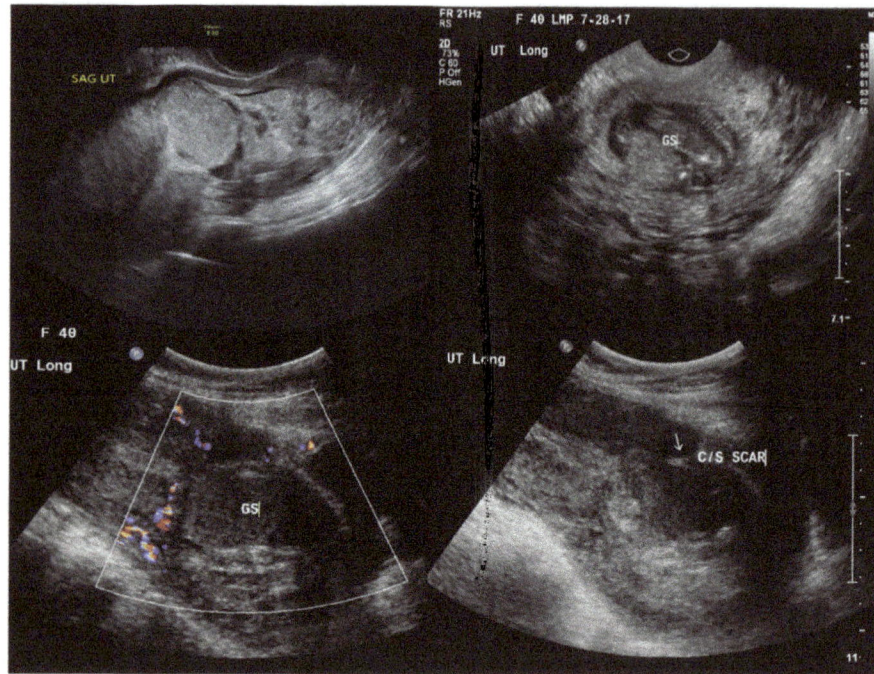

FIGURE 2: Sonographic findings when patient presented to the emergency room initially with the heterotopic gestation with a C-section scar ectopic containing fetal parts without discernible heart rate and an abnormal appearing intrauterine gestational sac in the lower uterine segment containing only low-level echoes.

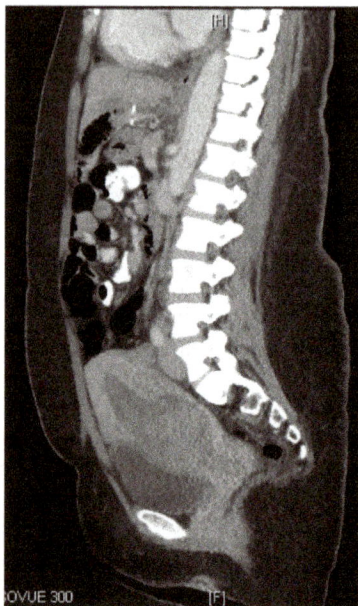

FIGURE 3: CT A/P with IV contrast with sagittal view demonstrating distention of the lower uterine segment of endometrial cavity.

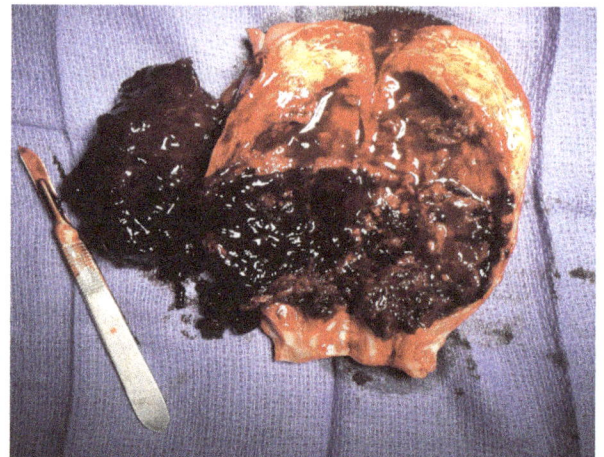

FIGURE 4: Bivalved uterus specimen shows anterior placenta adherent to lower uterine segment.

with selective reduction via potassium chloride injection of the cesarean scar pregnancy with preservation of the intrauterine gestation [1, 4, 6]. Hsieh et al. presented a successful case of embryo aspiration under sonographic guidance for selective embryo reduction in the setting of

a heterotopic cesarean scar pregnancy with a combined intrauterine pregnancy [5].

The successful selective reduction of a heterotopic cesarean scar pregnancy via ultrasound guided potassium chloride (KCl) injection has even been reported in the second trimester [6]. Our case presents complications that arose from conservative management of sepsis as a result of selective reduction of a heterotopic cesarean scar pregnancy with sepsis and postprocedure bacteremia. The usual complication expected from conservative management of cesarean scar pregnancies is hemorrhage requiring blood transfusion and hysterectomy secondary to a morbidly adherent placenta [2, 7]. Our patient chose selective reduction after being provided with the evidence of previous successful selective reductions as well as the associated risks such as miscarriage, infection, and heavy bleeding possibly necessity embolization or hysterectomy.

Other conservative options of CSP's besides medical management have previously been reported in the literature. These options include methotrexate followed by uterine curettage, wedge resection via laparotomy or laparoscopy, uterine artery embolization followed by subsequent dilation, and curettage or systemic methotrexate with hysteroscopic or resection [8–11].

While Yu et al. have previously demonstrated the successful selective reduction of a heterotopic cesarean scar pregnancy in the second trimester; our case report is unique in that it illustrates the subsequent development of septic abortion and attempted conservative management of such a complication. The persistent bacteremia from the retained products of conceptions after the curettage is a lesser known complication that has not been discussed in the literature. This case report demonstrates that septic abortion, sepsis, and bacteremia resulting from selective reduction of a heterotopic cesarean scar pregnancy are an important complication to consider. This potentially life-threatening complication requires diligent management with active patient counseling and reassessment of the patient's clinical status and if medical management ultimately fails hysterectomy is warranted.

Additional Points

Teaching Points. (1) Selective reduction may be an option to treat cesarean scar ectopic pregnancy for women desiring conservative management. (2) Septic abortion resulting from selective reduction of a heterotopic cesarean scar pregnancy is an important complication to consider. (3) Persistent bacteremia from retained products after surgical curettage of cesarean scar ectopic may necessitate definitive surgical management with hysterectomy.

References

[1] C.-N. Wang, C.-K. Chen, H.-S. Wang, H.-Y. Chiueh, and Y.-K. Soong, "Successful management of heterotopic cesarean scar pregnancy combined with intrauterine pregnancy after in vitro fertilization-embryo transfer," *Fertility and Sterility*, vol. 88, no. 3, pp. 706.e13–706.e16, 2007.

[2] A. H. Miyague, A. P. Chrisostomo, S. L. Costa, E. T. Nakatani, W. Kondo, and C. C. Gomes, "Treatment of heterotopic caesarean scar pregnancy complicated with post termination increase in size of residual mass and morbidly adherent placenta," *Journal of Clinical Ultrasound*, vol. 46, no. 3, pp. 227–230, 2018.

[3] Z. OuYang, Q. Yin, Y. Xu, Y. Ma, Q. Zhang, and Y. Yu, "Heterotopic cesarean scar pregnancy: Diagnosis, treatment, and prognosis," *Journal of Ultrasound in Medicine*, vol. 33, no. 9, pp. 1533–1537, 2014.

[4] L. J. Salomon, H. Hernandez, A. Chauveaud, S. Doumerc, and R. Frydman, "Successful management of a heterotopic Caesarean scar pregnancy: Potassium chloride injection with preservation of the intrauterine gestation: Case report," *Human Reproduction*, vol. 18, no. 1, pp. 189–191, 2003.

[5] B. C. Hsieh, J. L. Hwang, H. S. Pan et al., "Heterotopic caesarean scar pregnancy combined with intrauterine pregnancy successfully treated with embryo aspiration for selective embryo reduction: case report," *Hum Reprod*, vol. 19, pp. 285–287, 2004.

[6] H. Yu, H. Luo, F. Zhao, X. Liu, and X. Wang, "Successful selective reduction of a heterotopic cesarean scar pregnancy in the second trimester: A case report and review of the literature," *BMC Pregnancy and Childbirth*, vol. 16, no. 1, pp. 380–387, 2016.

[7] M. H. Vetter, J. Andrzejewski, A. Murnane, and C. Lang, "Surgical management of a heterotopic cesarean scar pregnancy with preservation of an intrauterine pregnancy," *Obstetrics & Gynecology*, vol. 128, no. 3, pp. 613–616, 2016.

[8] M. Kim, H. S. Jun, J. Y. Kim, S. J. Seong, and D. H. Cha, "Successful full-term twin deliveries in heterotopic cesarean scar pregnancy in a spontaneous cycle with expectant management," *Journal of Obstetrics and Gynaecology Research*, vol. 40, no. 5, pp. 1415–1419, 2014.

[9] J. S. Goldstein, V. S. Ratts, T. Philpott, and M. H. Dahan, "Risk of surgery after use of potassium chloride for treatment of tubal heterotopic pregnancy," *Obstetrics & Gynecology*, vol. 107, no. 2, pp. 506–508, 2006.

[10] M. Wang, Z. Yang, Y. Li et al., "Conservative management of cesarean scar pregnancies: a prospective randomized controlled trial at a single center," *International Journal of Clinical and Experimental Medicine (IJCEM)*, vol. 8, no. 10, pp. 18972–18980, 2015.

[11] P. Giampaolino, N. De Rosa, I. Morra et al., "Management of cesarean scar pregnancy: a single-institution retrospective review," *BioMed Research International*, vol. 2018, 9 pages, 2018.

29

Pelvic Inflammatory Disease: Possible Catches and Correct Management in Young Women

Chiara Di Tucci ⓘD, Daniele Di Mascio ⓘD, Michele Carlo Schiavi, Giorgia Perniola, Ludovico Muzii, and Pierluigi Benedetti Panici

Department of Gynecological and Obstetric Sciences, and Urological Sciences, University of Rome "Sapienza", Umberto I Hospital, Rome, Italy

Correspondence should be addressed to Chiara Di Tucci; chiara.ditucci@gmail.com

Academic Editor: Kyousuke Takeuchi

The incidence of adnexal masses increases exponentially with age and the most frequent causes in young women are physiologic cysts and pelvic abscesses with pelvic inflammatory disease (PID). Clinical examination can direct physicians to an appropriate management of adnexal mass, but the role of transvaginal ultrasound is crucial for diagnosis and treatment decision, even if it sometimes can be misleading, especially in young women. Ca 125, blood count, and CRP are useful to clarify suspected etiology of a pelvic mass, but specificity and positive predictive value are low because elevation of laboratory tests may occur in several benign conditions. In our work we present four cases of suspected pelvic masses. Despite guidelines for management of PID, the right timing to switch to surgical therapy is not clear. Therefore, the treatment decision should be based on a careful evaluation of various parameters such as signs symptoms and above all age. Moreover, we believe that, for a correct diagnosis and for the best fertility sparing treatment, it is also extremely important to refer to a gynecological oncology unit with an expert surgeon.

1. Introduction

The incidence of adnexal masses increases exponentially with age, and in 25-40-year-old women the prevalence of an adnexal lesion is reported to be about 7.8% [1]. The incidence of PID is particularly difficult to evaluate, because of high rates of subclinical PID, increasing rates of outpatient diagnosis, and inaccuracies in the diagnosis [2].

The most frequent benign gynecological causes are generally physiologic cyst [3], while the most frequent malignant causes in adolescent and young women are borderline ovarian tumors (BOT) and sex cord-stromal or germ cell tumors in 43% and 23% of women <35 years old [4]. Therefore, a right diagnosis and management of adnexal masses in these patients are extremely important and should be directed to identify the cause and preserve fertility as much as possible. Clinical examination based on symptoms and signs and laboratory tests may help physicians, but imaging significantly increases the accuracy of differential diagnosis [5]. Transvaginal ultrasound is the most commonly used imaging technique for preoperative characterization of any adnexal mass, with a sensitivity of 93% and a specificity of 81% when adopting the International Ovarian Tumor Analysis (IOTA) "Simple Rules" classification system [6]. Despite these excellent accuracy rates, when laparoscopic surgery is limited to women with cysts that appear benign, the rate of unexpected malignancy is 0-2.5% [7]. Furthermore, IOTA criteria cannot replace the gynecologist's skills, which are essential to improve overall survival rate, trying to preserve fertility at the same time. In this work, we present four cases of women with pelvic mass and the subsequent management, better describing the issues mentioned above.

2. Case One

A 31-year-old Italian patient came to our attention for pelvic pain in December 2016. She had no known previous history of sexually transmitted infections (STIs) nor known chronic disease under pharmacological treatment. She did not practice any contraceptive method and currently had a single sex partner with whom she had unprotected sex, trying to get pregnant. Last Pap smear (October 2016) reported

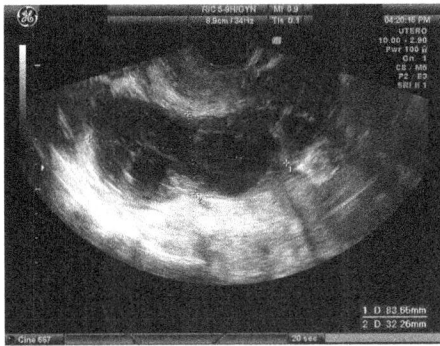

FIGURE 1: Case one: right adnexal mass.

mild inflammation and Doderlein's cytolysis. She had a regular 28-day menstrual cycle. In August 2015, she had been already admitted in another hospital for pelvic pain and she was treated with antibiotic therapy for a suspected pelvic inflammatory disease (PID). In October 2015 she had positive cervicovaginal swabs for Candida Albicans. In March 2016 she had negative Ca125 and AFP blood test (17.7 u/mL and 1.6 ng/mL, respectively). On physical examination, she referred pain in abdominal lower quadrants. During gynecological examination, we found leucorrhoea after the introduction of the speculum. She had low grade fever and blood tests showed hemoglobin level: 13.0 g/dL; total white blood cells: $4.63x10^9$/L; neutrophils: 44.6%; platelets: $231x10^9$/L and C-reactive protein (CRP) was positive (4 mg/dL; 0-0.5 mg/dL). Transvaginal ultrasound performed at the admission showed a normal sized uterus and a multilocular, solid, thick-walled structure with internal incomplete septa and color score 1 in both adnexal regions (65x58mm to the left and 83x32mm to the right) (Figure 1). Fluid and "sliding sign" were shown in the Pouch of Douglas. At laparoscopy, two voluminous adnexal masses, measuring about 7 cm, with exophytic vegetation and superficial vascularization, were seen bilaterally. Extemporaneous histological examination of biopsy showed the presence of serous BOT. A bilateral cystectomy and peritoneal staging were performed. Two weeks later, the final histological examination confirmed the previous diagnosis.

3. Case Two

A 24-year-old Italian patient was admitted to our hospital in February 2017 for severe pelvic pain progressively increasing in severity, bloating, and constipation. She had three sex partners and she did not practice any contraception. Last Pap smear (December 2016) was negative. She had regular menstrual cycle, with an increased flow (Heavy Menstrual Bleeding) and dysmenorrhea in the last three months. On physical examination, she presented abdominal pain, especially in lower quadrants. During gynecological examination, we did not find any pathological vaginal and cervical lesion and leucorrhoea was not present, but a pelvic neoformation of about 10 cm increasing in consistency was appreciated with the bimanual pelvic and digital rectal examination. She had no fever and inflammatory markers were normal

(total white blood cells: 4.63x109/L; neutrophils: 44.6%; CRP: negative). Transvaginal ultrasound showed a normal uterus and a multilocular solid mass of 90x30x40 mm with internal incomplete septa and color score 2 in left adnexal region. AFP, bHCG, and HE4 were negative, but Ca125 level was 834 u/mL, with a twofold increase in 15 days (400 u/mL at the beginning of February). The ultrasound examination skewed towards a pelvic inflammation, but we opted for an urgency laparoscopy, because of the woman's young age, pain, and the sudden Ca125 increase. After optical introduction, hydrosalpinx and widespread signs of pelviperitonitis were found. Drainage with removal of pus and multiple biopsies were performed. Histologic samples showed signs of flogosis. The patient was placed on doxycycline 100 mg twice a day for 7 days according to the Center for Disease Control and Prevention (CDC) guidelines for the management of PID [7]. She was educated on the method and the importance of preventing sexually transmitted diseases (STDs) and advised to treat her sexual partner with the same treatment.

4. Case Three

A 32-year-old Italian patient came to our attention for pelvic pain and fever in April 2017. She had been already admitted to our department for pelvic pain and she was treated with antibiotic therapy for a suspected PID. She had low grade fever and blood tests showed hemoglobin level: 11.8 g/dL; total white blood cells: $12.26\backslash x10^9$/L; neutrophils: 92.2%; platelets: $258x10^9$/L; CRP: 8.85 mg/dL (0-0.5 mg/dL). She had no known previous history of sexually transmitted infections (STIs). Last Pap smear (2016) was referred to be negative. One week after antibiotic therapy, we observed a slight decrease of CRP and remission of temperature, but also an increased pain in abdominal lower quadrants. Transvaginal ultrasound performed at the admission showed a normal uterus and, in the left adnexal region, a dilated, low-vascularized tube (43x29mm) attached to the left ovary (57x54x44mm) was shown. Right ovary was normal. No fluid was found in the Pouch of Douglas. The patient underwent diagnostic and operative laparoscopy: after having introduced the optic trocar, a mass with some colliquative areas in the left tubal corner of the uterus, measuring about 4 cm, was seen. The extemporaneous histological examination showed the presence of endometrial stromal sarcoma. Two weeks later, the final histological examination confirmed the previous diagnosis.

5. Case Four

In January 2018, a 22-year-old Italian patient came to our attention for pelvic pain associated with dysuria and pollakiuria, without fever or vaginal discharges. She had previous history of right ovariectomy for dermoid cyst in 2009.

Transvaginal ultrasound performed at the admission showed a normal uterus and a ground glass area (39x22 mm) in left adnexal region and a second dilated, low-vascularized, ground glass area, (80x28 mm) in the left ovary (20x10x15 mm) (Figures 2 and 3). No fluid was found in the Pouch of

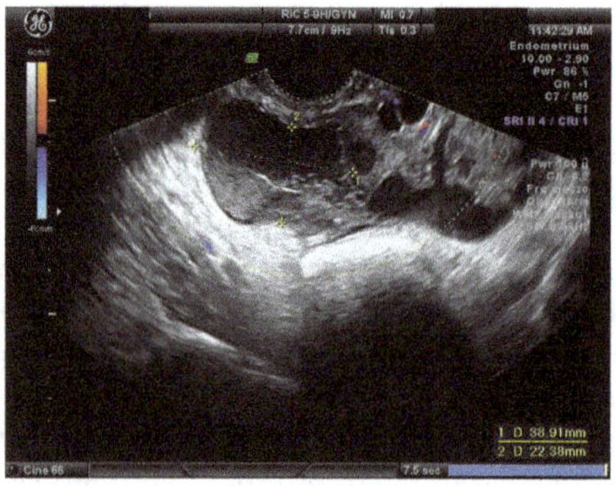

FIGURE 2: Case four: left adnexal mass (1).

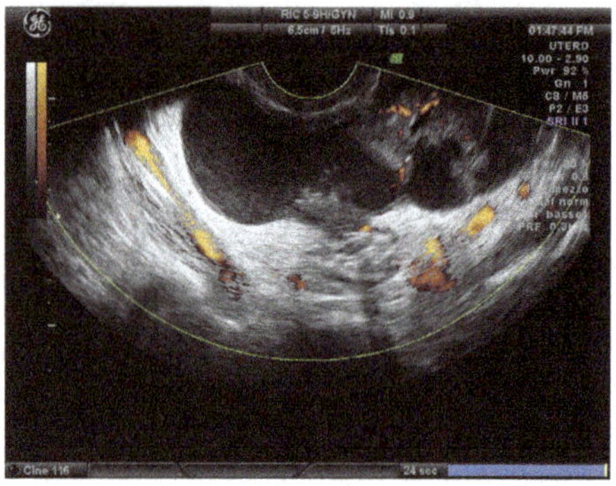

FIGURE 3: Case four: left adnexal mass (2).

Douglas. White blood cells were normal and CEA, CA19.9, and AFP were normal, but CRP was 10.800 microg/L, HE4 was 84.1, and Ca125 level was 463.6 u/mL. MRI described the presence of a formation with fluid content in the ovarian and paraovarian region with oval morphology of 35x15 mm; nearly MRI also revealed the presence of a formation with elongated morphology from the left ovary to the contralateral region adnexal. Antibiotic therapy was started, but then she undergone surgery, due to increase of CRP and pelvic pain persistence. After the introduction of the optic trocar, right salpinx presented with ectasia (hydrosalpinx), attached to the intestinal loops. Left adnexa presented an ovarian abscess. After having detected the ureters, the right tube was cleared. Drainage of the left adnexa abscess and lysis of adhesions were performed.

6. Discussion

Gynecological adnexal masses may origin from uterus, tubes, or ovaries and the goal of the evaluation is to tell benign conditions from malignant ones. During reproductive age, adnexal masses may present as symptoms that can guide the differential diagnosis, but sometimes symptoms can also lead to a misdiagnosis. For this reason, imaging may be helpful for diagnostic evaluation and treatment decision. Transvaginal ultrasound is the recommended imaging modality for a suspected or an incidentally identified pelvic mass, with good patient tolerability and cost-effectiveness [8]. Nevertheless, ultrasound examination sometimes can be misleading in

young women. In our first case, clinical symptoms, bilateral involvement, and inflammatory markers together with ultrasound examination led us to assume a diagnosis of PID, but we opted for surgery because of persistent pain despite medical treatment. Ca125, blood count, and CRP are useful to clarify suspected etiology of a pelvic mass and should be used to assess the possibility of malignancy. Nevertheless, specificity and positive predictive value of Ca125 levels are consistently higher in postmenopausal women compared with premenopausal women [9] and elevation of Ca125 levels in premenopausal women may occur in several conditions including fibroids, endometriosis, adenomyosis, pelvic infection, and nongynecologic diseases [10–12]. In our second case, the twofold Ca125 levels led us to hypothesize malignancy, even if women with benign conditions such as III/IV stage endometriosis can have Ca125 level elevation of 1,000 units/mL or greater, but ultrasound imaging directed us towards the hypothesis of a suspected infection. CDC guidelines suggest medical treatment as the first-line treatment of PID, but the patient's young age and the worsening pelvic pain led us to opting for surgical treatment to exclude malignant lesions and to try to preserve fertility [8]. There is some evidence for CRP to be an interesting marker of tumor bulk when associated with the clinical-pathological parameters, FIGO tumor stage, and postoperative residual tumor mass. In fact, elevated CRP serum levels independently predicted the presence of borderline and epithelium ovarian tumor in patients with suspicious adnexal masses and were reported to be of additional value to Ca125 in the preoperative differential diagnosis of adnexal masses [13]. In our first case too, the woman showed an elevated value of CRP. Young women with pelvic pain should be also screened for sexual transmitted disease to rule out infections that could lead to infertility, as recurrent PID is associated with an almost twofold increase in infertility [14]. In case of no response to medical therapy, patients should be directed to surgery to preserve fertility and to rule out the possibility of unexpected ovarian malignancy [7]. In our opinion, the presence of a gynecologic surgeon is mandatory, as it is significantly more likely to result in ovarian conservation [15], and the role of a gynecologic oncologist is associated with improved overall survival, in case of malignancies [16].

In our opinion, criteria for choosing medical therapy are mainly related to the absence of ascites, a moderate increase of Ca125, clinical and laboratory signs of infection such as pain, fever, leucorrhoea, CRP, and white blood cells. Conversely, surgery as a first-line treatment may be useful in case of ascites, rapid increase in Ca125, or ultrasound-suspected pelvic mass. In the event of failure to respond to medical treatment, we believe it is mandatory to direct the patient to laparoscopic surgery, as shown in Figure 4.

In case of ascites in combination with high levels of Ca125, laparoscopy with biopsies and cytological examination to confirm any diagnosis should precede laparotomy; diagnostic laparoscopy allows a comprehensive view of the surgical field, but it has its own risks: hemorrhagic, infectious, organ perforation, and aesthetical risks; furthermore, large masses could be broken with pelvic dissemination of suspect material, and this risk is strongly reduced with expert surgeons.

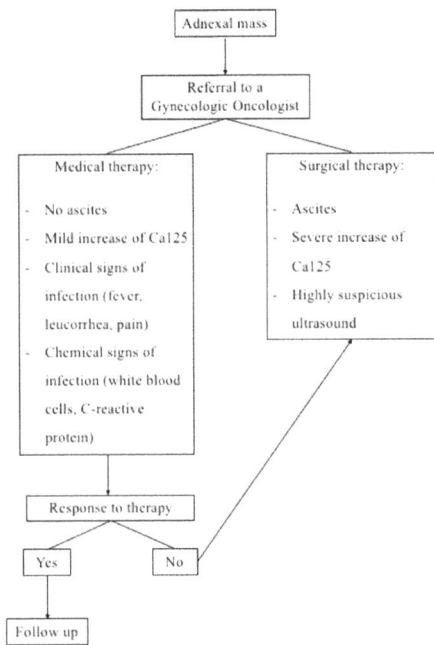

FIGURE 4: Flowchart.

In conclusion, despite guidelines for management of PID, the right timing to switch to surgical therapy is not clear. For this reason, other prospective studies are necessary to properly handle patients with suspected PID and to avoid pitfalls. Moreover, ultrasound diagnosis, biological markers, and laboratory tests have some limitations, particularly with early stage tumors, so future studies should focus on new molecules that may help the early diagnosis. Therefore, the treatment decision should be based on a careful evaluation of various parameters, above all age. Pelvic masses are generally benign in young women, but we believe it is extremely important to refer to a gynecological oncology unit for the correct diagnosis, for a presurgical oncofertility counseling and to obtain the best fertility sparing treatment.

References

[1] C. Borgfeldt and E. Andolf, "Transvaginal sonographic ovarian findings in a random sample of women 25-40 years old," *Ultrasound in Obstetrics & Gynecology*, vol. 13, no. 5, pp. 345–350, 1999.

[2] S. M. Lareau and R. H. Beigi, "Pelvic Inflammatory Disease and Tubo-ovarian Abscess," *Infectious Disease Clinics of North America*, vol. 22, no. 4, pp. 693–708, 2008.

[3] Evaluation and management of adnexal masses. Practice Bulletin No. 174. American College of Obstetricians and Gynecologists. Obstet Gynecol; 128: e210–e226, 2016.

[4] Overview of ovarian cancer incidence in England: incidence, mortality and survival. Trent Cancer Registry, the National Cancer Intelligence Network (NCIN) November 2012.

[5] American Institute of Ultrasound in Medicine. AIUM Practice Parameter for the performance of ultrasound of female pelvis. Laurel (MD): AIUM; 2014.

[6] J. Kaijser, A. Sayasneh, K. Van hoorde et al., "Presurgical diagnosis of adnexal tumours using mathematical models and scoring systems: a systematic review and meta-analysis," *Human Reproduction Update*, vol. 20, no. 3, pp. 449–462, 2014.

[7] L. Muzii, R. Angioli, M. Zullo, and P. B. Panici, "The unexpected ovarian malignancy found during operative laparoscopy: Incidence, management, and implications for prognosis," *Journal of Minimally Invasive Gynecology*, vol. 12, no. 1, pp. 81–89, 2005.

[8] Centers for Disease Control and Prevention (CDC). Sexually Transmitted Diseases Treatment Guidelines, 2015.

[9] K. Ushijima, K. Kawano, N. Tsuda et al., "Epithelial borderline ovarian tumor: Diagnosis and treatment strategy," *Obstetrics & Gynecology Science*, vol. 58, no. 3, pp. 183–187, 2015.

[10] J. Kaijser, T. Bourne, L. Valentin et al., "Improving strategies for diagnosing ovarian cancer: A summary of the International Ovarian Tumor Analysis (IOTA) studies," *Ultrasound in Obstetrics & Gynecology*, vol. 41, no. 1, pp. 9–20, 2013.

[11] T. Maggino, A. Gadducci, V. D'Addario et al., "Prospective multicenter study on ca 125 in postmenopausal pelvic masses," *Gynecologic Oncology*, vol. 54, no. 2, pp. 117–123, 1994.

[12] J. E. Dodge, A. L. Covens, C. Lacchetti et al., "Preoperative identification of a suspicious adnexal mass: A systematic review and meta-analysis," *Gynecologic Oncology*, vol. 126, no. 1, pp. 157–166, 2012.

[13] E. Reiser, S. Aust, V. Seebacher et al., "Preoperative C-reactive protein serum levels as a predictive diagnostic marker in patients with adnexal masses," *Gynecologic Oncology*, vol. 147, no. 3, pp. 690–694, 2017.

[14] RCOG. Green-Top Guideline no 62: Management of Suspected Ovarian Masses in Premenopausal Women. 2011.

[15] R. E. Bristow, A. C. Nugent, M. L. Zahurak, V. Khouzhami, and H. E. Fox, "Impact of Surgeon Specialty on Ovarian-Conserving Surgery in Young Females with an Adnexal Mass," *Journal of Adolescent Health*, vol. 39, no. 3, pp. 411–416, 2006.

[16] S. H. Rim, S. Hirsch, C. C. Thomas et al., "Gynecologic oncologists involvement on ovarian cancer standard of care receipt and survival," *World Journal of Obstetrics and Gynecology*, vol. 5, no. 2, pp. 187–196, 2016.

30

Standardized Digital Colposcopy with Dynamic Spectral Imaging for Conservative Patient Management

Angelika Kaufmann,[1] **Christina Founta,**[1,2] **Emmanouil Papagiannakis,**[3]
Raj Naik,[1] **and Ann Fisher**[1]

[1]*Northern Gynaecological Oncology Centre, Gateshead NHS Foundation Trust, Queen Elizabeth Hospital, Sheriff Hill, Gateshead NE9 6SX, UK*
[2]*Musgrove Park Hospital, Taunton & Somerset NHS Foundation Trust, Taunton TA1 5DA, UK*
[3]*DYSIS Medical Ltd, Edinburgh, UK*

Correspondence should be addressed to Ann Fisher; annfisher3@nhs.net

Academic Editor: Svein Rasmussen

Background. Colposcopy is subjective and management of young patients with high-grade disease is challenging, as treatments may impair subsequent pregnancies and adversely affect obstetric outcomes. Conservative management of selected patients is becoming more popular amongst clinicians; however it requires accurate assessment and documentation. Novel adjunctive technologies for colposcopy could improve patient care and help individualize management decisions by introducing standardization, increasing sensitivity, and improving documentation. *Case.* A nulliparous 27-year-old woman planning pregnancy underwent colposcopy following high-grade cytology. The colposcopic impression was of low-grade changes, whilst the Dynamic Spectral Imaging (DSI) map of the cervix suggested potential high-grade. A DSI-directed biopsy confirmed CIN2. At follow-up, both colposcopy and DSI were suggestive of low-grade disease only, and image comparison confirmed the absence of previously present acetowhite epithelium areas. Histology of the transformation zone following excisional treatment, as per patient's choice, showed no high-grade changes. *Conclusion.* Digital colposcopy with DSI mapping helps standardize colposcopic examinations, increase diagnostic accuracy, and monitor cervical changes over time, improving patient care. When used for longitudinal tracking of disease and when it confirms a negative colposcopy, it can help towards avoiding overtreatment and hence decrease morbidity related to cervical excision.

1. Introduction

In cytology-based cervical screening programs, women with high-grade cytology are directly referred for colposcopic examination [1, 2], to identify and treat precancerous changes of the cervix (cervical intraepithelial neoplasia, CIN) and prevent risk for progression to invasive cancer. High-grade CIN lesions identified colposcopically and/or histologically are conventionally excised. Furthermore, immediate treatment of women with high-grade cytology, even in the absence of high-grade colposcopic findings, is not unusual, as up to 84% of cases have been reported to have CIN2 or CIN3 on histology [3, 4].

However, excision of cervical tissue can result in cervical deficiency and increase the risk of miscarriage, preterm labour, preterm premature rupture of membranes [5, 6], and cervical stenosis. Furthermore, when the excision of dysplastic cells is incomplete, repeated treatment may be needed, increasing the risks. Considering that a large cohort of women undergo colposcopy during their childbearing years and that, in younger women, CIN2 has an up to 50% likelihood of regression [7–9], conservative management of CIN2 lesions is becoming increasingly popular amongst clinicians for selected patients [10].

In addition, sensitivity of colposcopy is known to be as low as 55–65% [11–13], punch biopsy has been reported to often miss the highest grade of disease [14], and there is evidence of considerable inter- and intraobserver disagreement between colposcopic assessments [15]. This results in great variation in management and increases the risk for both underdiagnosis and overtreatment.

Despite the importance of removing precancerous lesions with the potential for malignant transformation being beyond dispute, management decisions need to be balanced against the consequences of excising cervical tissue. To aid the process, individual circumstances such as general health (e.g., immunosuppression), lesion grade and size, age, parity, family planning, and the patient's wishes need to be considered. This personalised assessment and decision-making requires a fine balance of diagnostic procedures followed by adequate discussion and counselling of the patient. The use of technology, to not only improve but also standardize diagnostic abilities by adding objective measurements and improving documentation, may optimize this process.

The Dynamic Spectral Imaging (DSI) colposcope (DYSIS by DYSIS Medical Ltd, Edinburgh, UK) is a digital video colposcope that integrates the adjunctive DSI cervical mapping with standard colposcopy. DSI helps standardize the way colposcopy is performed (with respect to distance, illumination, field of view, and timing), quantifies the acetowhitening by measuring its intensity and persistence, and has been shown to increase sensitivity [16–18].

Presuming colposcopy is satisfactory and no obvious high-grade lesion is identified, a reassuring DSI map can enhance the colposcopic impression, thus assisting in reducing overtreatment. In addition, the standardization of practice as well as the introduction of an objective measure and documentation of the full acetowhitening process could facilitate follow-up of younger women with high-grade lesions, who opt to minimize risks for poor future obstetric outcomes, rather than treating them.

2. Case Presentation

A 27-year-old female was referred with cytology showing high-grade changes (moderate dyskaryosis). She was a non-smoker with no significant past medical history, nulliparous, and currently under the treatment of a fertility centre for male factor infertility, awaiting intracytoplasmic sperm injection.

During the consultation, different management options were discussed. Pending colposcopic assessment, possibly the traditional approach would be "see and treat", that is, a large loop excision of the transformation zone (LLETZ) of the cervix at the time of colposcopy, assuming colposcopy was considered to show high-grade changes. In view of her nulliparous status, age, and the wish to preserve fertility and reduce any potential risk factors for future pregnancies, the patient was alternatively offered a colposcopy with directed biopsies. Should the histology show high-grade cervical precancerous changes (CIN2+), an excision with a view to remove these changes could be performed at a second visit (select and treat).

The colposcopy was performed by an experienced colposcopist, consultant gynaecological oncologist, using the DSI colposcope.

The colposcopic impression was of low-grade changes (Figures 1(a) and 1(b)), whilst the DSI mapping suggested that the acetowhitening changes potentially corresponded to high-grade CIN (Figure 1(c)).

In view of clinical and standard colposcopic appearances consistent with bacterial vaginosis and low-grade changes only, treatment was not offered on the day. Three directed punch biopsies were taken, a high vaginal swab was obtained, and a course of topical Clindamycin cream as empiric treatment of bacterial vaginosis was prescribed.

One of the biopsy sites was selected based on clinical judgement prior to reviewing the DSI map, and two further were directed by the DSI map (Figure 1(c)). The biopsy which was based on colposcopic impression showed koilocytic changes and CIN1 only, whereas the two biopsies based on the DSI evaluation showed CIN1 and CIN2 (Figure 2). There was no evidence of CIN3, cervical glandular intraepithelial neoplasia, or invasive malignancy.

Following these results, a further clinic appointment was arranged and the patient was reexamined with the DSI colposcope. The colposcopic images and DSI map from the first visit were reviewed prior to examination to provide a reference standard. This time, neither the colposcopic impression nor the DSI map suggested any areas suspicious of high-grade disease (Figures 1(d), 1(e), and 1(f)). Notably, none of the sites biopsied at the first visit demonstrated any features in keeping with high-grade lesion neither did the DSI map, suggesting that punch biopsies likely removed all high-grade disease initially present. Therefore, the patient was offered the option of conservative management by cytology and colposcopy at 6 months versus the standard LLETZ treatment and was fully counselled, in the presence of her partner, regarding available evidence and potential risks. Pending the infertility treatment, risks such as cervical stenosis and the possibility of requiring a test run prior to embryo implantation were stressed out in particular. However, in order not to delay commencement of fertility treatment, immediate cervical excision was opted for.

A LLETZ was performed with written consent, using the DSI colposcope, under local anaesthetic. Haemostasis was achieved by ball diathermy on the cervical crater as per standard practice. The specimen measured 20 × 18 × 11 mm and weighed 1.9 grams. Final histology showed HPV-related features and CIN1 clear from all margins (endocervical, ectocervical, and deep lateral). There was no evidence of high-grade CIN or invasive cancer.

The patient was discharged back to her family doctor, with a plan for cytology and high-risk HPV cotesting in six months as a test of cure, according to the National Health Service Cervical Screening Programme guidelines.

3. Discussion

Despite organised cervical screening programmes having proven their significant value in preventing cervical cancer, there is scope for further improvement in diagnostic accuracy. Excisional treatment for CIN2 and CIN3 is at present the gold standard and is of considerable value in prevention of transformation of these lesions into cancer. However, in view of the low colposcopic accuracy, there is a risk of overtreatment and increase in unnecessary

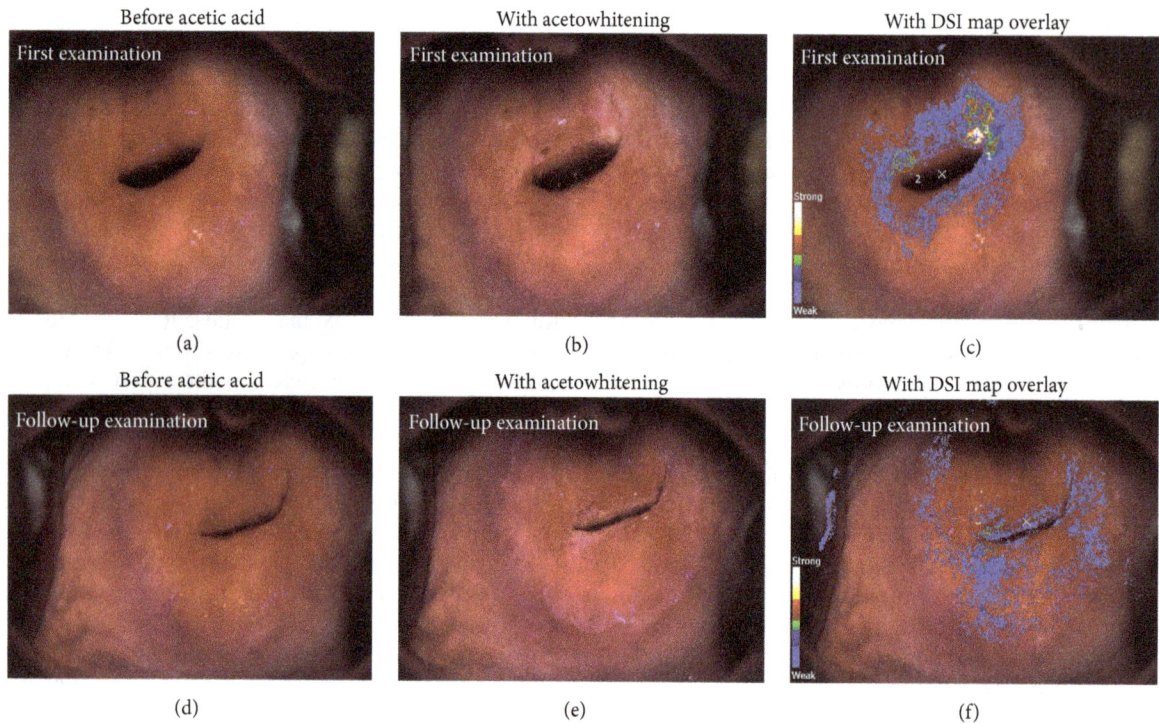

FIGURE 1: (a, b, and c) First examination. (a) Cervical appearance prior to application of acetic acid. (b) Cervical appearance after application of acetic acid. (c) DSI map overlaid on the cervix. Strong acetowhitening signal suggested potential high-grade lesion as identified by the DSI technology (colour legend on the left). The circular annotations are the biopsy sites selected and indicated during the examination; number 1 was identified by the colposcopist; numbers 2 and 3 were marked using the DSI map. (d, e, and f) Follow-up examination. (d) Cervical appearance prior to application of acetic acid. (e) Cervical colposcopic appearances after application of acetic acid. No significant acetowhitening effect is observed. (f) DSI map overlaid on the cervix, confirming the absence of significant changes. Notably, the area that yielded CIN2 at the first visit, now appears normal.

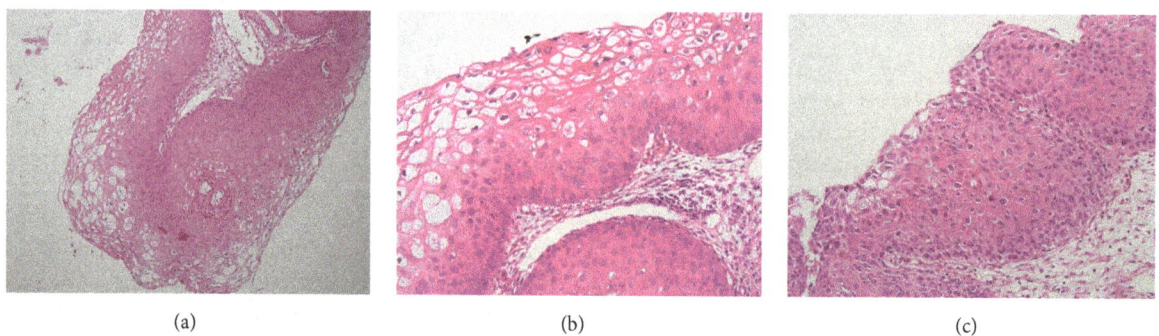

FIGURE 2: Histopathology images from the punch biopsies. (a) Mild atypia (CIN1) in lower third of cervix squamous epithelium with viral cytopathic effect in upper two-thirds (HE ×100). (b) Higher magnification (HE ×200) of CIN1 showing viral cytopathic effect in upper layers of squamous epithelium and mild atypia in lower third. (c) CIN2, showing almost full thickness epithelial atypia (HE ×200).

morbidity. There is evidence that CIN2, if left untreated, regresses spontaneously in roughly half of the cases within two years [7–9]. Hence a more conservative approach might be suitable for some women, especially those with fertility wish.

Novel technology can support the clinical diagnosis and subsequent management. Several methods, such as Dynamic Spectral Imaging, optical spectroscopy, or optical coherence tomography, have been developed aiming to aid colposcopic assessment and evaluated in regard to their clinical and

economic impact [19]. The DSI technology was shown to increase the sensitivity of colposcopy to 88% when used adjunctively to standard colposcopy [17], whilst also being cost-effective [19].

The case presented above demonstrates that the sensitivity of colposcopy when combined with DSI was indeed higher than colposcopy alone, both in terms of forming the right impression and identifying the sites to biopsy. The DSI-guided biopsy led to detection of high-grade CIN, whereas the colposcopic impression of low-grade would have otherwise been confirmed by the colposcopically directed biopsy which indeed showed CIN1.

The ability to review images and the DSI map from the first visit, performed under identical circumstances with those in the second, enabled the colposcopist to confidently advice the patient towards conservative management. The LLETZ was performed due to patient's wish and in accordance with standard guidelines following high-grade CIN on directed biopsies. The fact that the histological assessment of the treatment specimen showed no high-grade CIN illustrates that this case could have indeed been managed more conservatively, decreasing any risks associated with the excision.

This case highlights that the opportunity to compare images and DSI maps side by side, and potentially quantify cervical changes, which can be particularly valuable when patients are not seen by the same colposcopist over time, may prove invaluable in optimizing care for the selected group that will prefer conservative management to excision, and the development of appropriate guidance.

It also underlines the offered advantage to be more reassured when both colposcopic impression and the DSI map are negative for high-grade CIN, as the high negative predictive value with the use of DSI suggests [17, 18], and thus reduce unnecessary treatments.

Disclosure

This work was presented at the 2017 meeting of the International Federation of Colposcopy and Cervical Pathology (IFCPC).

Acknowledgments

The authors thank Dr. Angela Ralte (Queen Elizabeth Hospital, Sheriff Hill, Gateshead NE9 6SX, United Kingdom) for preparing and providing the histopathology images.

References

[1] J. Tidy, "NHSCSP publication number 20: NHS cervical screening programme," in *Colposcopy and Programme Management*, Public Health England, London, UK, 3rd edition, 2016, https://www.bsccp.org.uk/assets/file/uploads/resources/NHS_Cervical_Screeing_Programme._Publication_Number_20_-_Third_Edition.pdf.

[2] D. Saslow, D. Solomon, H. W. Lawson et al., "American cancer society, american society for colposcopy and cervical pathology, and american society for clinical pathology screening guidelines for the prevention and early detection of cervical cancer,"

Journal of Lower Genital Tract Disease, vol. 16, no. 3, pp. 175–204, 2012.

[3] W. P. Soutter, S. Wisdom, A. K. Brough, and J. M. Monaghan, "Should patients with mild atypia in a cervical smear be referred for colposcopy?" *BJOG: An International Journal of Obstetrics & Gynaecology*, vol. 93, no. 1, pp. 70–74, 1986.

[4] D. J. Anderson, G. M. Flannelly, H. C. Kitchener et al., "Mild and moderate dyskaryosis: can women be selected for colposcopy on the basis of social criteria?" *British Medical Journal*, vol. 305, no. 6845, pp. 84–87, 1992.

[5] M. Kyrgiou, G. Koliopoulos, P. Martin-Hirsch, M. Arbyn, W. Prendiville, and E. Paraskevaidis, "Obstetric outcomes after conservative treatment for intraepithelial or early invasive cervical lesions: systematic review and meta-analysis," *Lancet*, vol. 367, no. 9509, pp. 489–498, 2006.

[6] A. Castanon, R. Landy, P. Brocklehurst et al., "Risk of preterm delivery with increasing depth of excision for cervical intraepithelial neoplasia in England: nested case-control study," *British Medical Journal*, vol. 349, no. nov05 3, pp. g6223–g6223, 2014.

[7] P. Holowaty, A. B. Miller, T. Rohan, and T. To, "Natural history of dysplasia of the uterine cervix," *Journal of the National Cancer Institute*, vol. 91, no. 3, pp. 252–258, 1999.

[8] P. E. Castle, M. Schiffman, C. M. Wheeler, and D. Solomon, "Evidence for frequent regression of cervical intraepithelial neoplasia—grade 2," *Obstetrics & Gynecology*, vol. 113, no. 1, pp. 18–25, 2009.

[9] A.-B. Moscicki, Y. Ma, C. Wibbelsman et al., "Rate of and risks for regression of cervical intraepithelial neoplasia 2 in adolescents and young women," *Obstetrics and Gynecology*, vol. 116, no. 6, pp. 1373–1380, 2010.

[10] L. S. Massad, M. H. Einstein, W. K. Huh et al., "2012 Updated consensus guidelines for the management of abnormal cervical cancer screening tests and cancer precursors," *Journal of Lower Genital Tract Disease*, vol. 17, pp. S1–S27, 2013.

[11] L. S. Massad and Y. C. Collins, "Strength of correlations between colposcopic impression and biopsy histology," *Gynecologic Oncology*, vol. 89, no. 3, pp. 424–428, 2003.

[12] J. Jeronimo and M. Schiffman, "Colposcopy at a crossroads," *American Journal of Obstetrics & Gynecology*, vol. 195, no. 2, pp. 349–353, 2006.

[13] R. L. Bekkers, H. P. V. D. Nieuwenhof, D. E. Neesham, J. H. Hendriks, J. Tan, and M. A. Quinn, "Does experience in colposcopy improve identification of high grade abnormalities?" *European Journal of Obstetrics & Gynecology and Reproductive Biology*, vol. 141, no. 1, pp. 75–78, 2008.

[14] M. H. Stoler, M. D. Vichnin, A. Ferenczy et al., "The accuracy of colposcopic biopsy: analyses from the placebo arm of the Gardasil clinical trials," *International Journal of Cancer*, vol. 128, no. 6, pp. 1354–1362, 2011.

[15] E. H. Hopman, F. J. Voorhorst, P. Kenemans, C. J. L. M. Meyer, and T. J. M. Helmerhorst, "Observer agreement on interpreting colposcopic images of CIN," *Gynecologic Oncology*, vol. 58, no. 2, pp. 206–209, 1995.

[16] W. P. Soutter, E. Diakomanolis, D. Lyons et al., "Dynamic spectral imaging: improving colposcopy," *Clinical Cancer Research*, vol. 15, no. 5, pp. 1814–1820, 2009.

[17] J. A. Louwers, A. Zaal, M. Kocken et al., "Dynamic spectral imaging colposcopy: higher sensitivity for detection of premalignant cervical lesions," *BJOG: An International Journal of Obstetrics & Gynaecology*, vol. 118, pp. 309–318, 2011.

[18] P. J. Coronado and M. Fasero, "Colposcopy combined with dynamic spectral imaging. A prospective clinical study," *European Journal of Obstetrics & Gynecology and Reproductive Biology*, vol. 196, pp. 11–16, 2016.

[19] R. Wade, E. Spackman, M. Corbett et al., "Adjunctive colposcopy technologies for examination of the uterine cervix—DySIS, LuViva Advanced Cervical Scan and Niris Imaging System: a systematic review and economic evaluation," *Health Technology Assessment*, vol. 17, no. 8, pp. 1–240, 2013.

31

Ruptured Spinal Arteriovenous Malformation: A Rare Cause of Paraplegia in Pregnancy

Clare E. Thiele (ID)

Royal Brisbane and Women's Hospital, Cnr Butterfield St. and Bowen Bridge Rd, Herston QLD 4029, Australia

Correspondence should be addressed to Clare E. Thiele; clare.thiele@health.qld.gov.au

Academic Editor: Cem Ficicioglu

Background. Ruptured spinal arteriovenous malformation (AVM) is a rare cause of paraplegia in pregnancy, with only a few case reports describing complications from spinal AVMs during pregnancy in the literature. *Case.* A 32-year-old woman presented at 37 weeks gestation with back pain and rapidly progressive lower limb neurological symptoms. MRI showed a previously undiagnosed spinal AVM at T8. A healthy girl was delivered by caesarean under general anaesthesia to facilitate further investigation. After spinal angiography, it was concluded the most likely aetiology was acute rupture of an intra- and perimedullary AVM with associated haemorrhage at T8 secondary to venous compression from the enlarged uterus at L5 causing high pressure within the AVM and subsequent rupture. The neurosurgical and interventional radiology teams felt the lesion was not amenable to surgical or endovascular intervention. The patient remained paraplegic with no sign of neurological recovery six months after delivery. *Conclusion.* While new onset paraplegia during pregnancy secondary to ruptured spinal AVM is very rare, it is important to discuss these cases to inform future practice. In contrast to previous case reports, our patient did not spontaneously recover after delivery and was not amenable to surgical or endovascular treatment.

1. Introduction

Spinal vascular malformations, including arteriovenous malformations (AVMs), are rare. Prompt diagnosis and treatment may prevent long-term neurological disability [1–3]. Patients with spinal AVMs usually present with back pain and progressive myelopathy with gait disturbance, sensory changes, and bladder or bowel symptoms [1–3]. Proposed mechanisms for neurological deterioration include haemorrhage, redistribution of blood supply ("steal phenomena"), mass effect, or venous congestion [1, 4]. Treatment options include embolisation, surgery, combined embolisation and surgery, or conservative management depending on the specific lesion [1, 3, 4].

Ruptured spinal AVM is a rare cause of paraplegia in pregnancy, with only a few case reports describing complications from spinal vascular malformations during pregnancy in the literature [5–7]. The physiological changes of pregnancy as well as compression of venous outflow by the gravid uterus make pregnant women particularly susceptible to complications of spinal vascular malformations, precipitating venous congestion or rupture and subsequent neurological symptoms. This case describes a pregnant woman with rapidly progressive paraplegia secondary to a previously undiagnosed spinal AVM at the eighth thoracic (T8) level that ruptured during late pregnancy.

2. Case Presentation

A 32-year-old woman in her first pregnancy presented at 37 weeks gestation to the obstetric review centre in the late evening with a two-hour history of new onset right-sided leg pain and numbness. She was able to mobilise short distances and was otherwise well. Initially her symptoms were most suggestive of sciatica, a common complaint during pregnancy.

Her symptoms progressed rapidly over the next two hours and she reported bilateral lower limb numbness and severe shooting midthoracic back pain and was unable to move her legs. Initially she had no urinary retention or faecal incontinence. She also reported no history of trauma or any similar symptoms in the past.

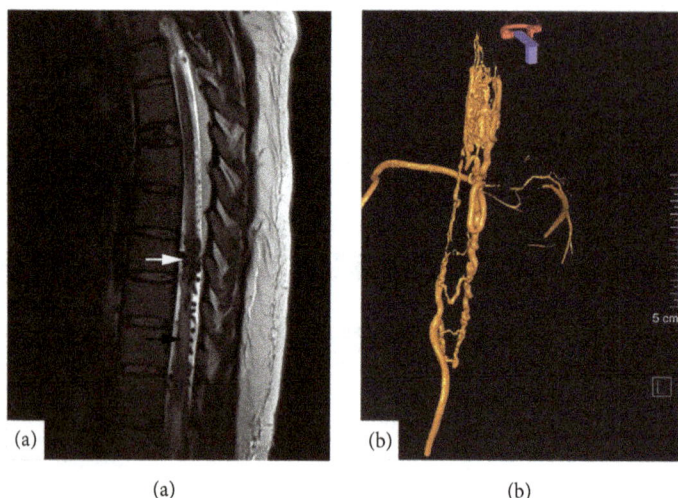

FIGURE 1: (a) Lateral T2-weighted MRI thoracic spine showing peri- and intramedullary spinal AVM at T8 (white arrow) with surrounding spinal cord oedema T6-T11 (black arrow). (b) Left lateral three-dimensional rotational spinal angiography (3D-RSA) from right T9 intercostal artery showing spinal cord AVM.

She had an otherwise low risk pregnancy and there were no signs of fetal distress on arrival. Her past medical history included asthma, allergic rhinoconjunctivitis, and depression. She was a smoker and migrated to Australia from England several years earlier.

On initial examination, vital signs were normal. She was afebrile. Cardiotocograph revealed no concerns for fetal wellbeing. Her neurological examination was inconsistent but nevertheless concerning. She was found to have patchy bilateral sensory loss up to a sensory level of T10. Lower limb examination revealed reduced power bilaterally (1-2/5) across all myotomes with hyperreflexia, clonus, and upgoing plantar reflexes. Upper limb neurological examination was normal. There was no bony tenderness on palpation of her spine. Insertion of a urinary catheter five hours after presentation drained 700 ml of urine. This was suggestive of urinary retention, particularly in the context of her advanced gestation. However, she reported normal perineal sensation on catheter insertion, again inconsistent with her other symptoms and examination findings.

Due to her pregnant state, an urgent CT was not performed. An after hours MRI was not considered necessary as it was felt an acute surgical cause for the presenting signs and symptoms was unlikely. A kidney ultrasound ruled out renal stones as a cause for severe back pain.

The next morning an MRI spine was performed. This revealed a previously undiagnosed mixed intra- and perimedullary spinal cord AVM at T8 with surrounding spinal cord oedema from T6-T11 (see Figure 1(a)). Her case was discussed with the neurosurgical team who felt she was not amenable to urgent surgical decompression or intervention based on MRI findings. A decision was made for urgent delivery to facilitate further investigation. A healthy baby girl was delivered that afternoon via caesarean under general anaesthetic. This was performed without complications.

Subsequent angiography showed a predominantly perimedullary slow flow spinal cord AVM with intramedullary extension at T8 to a compact nidus (see Figure 1(b)). The AVM received arterial supply from the radicular branches of the right T9 intercostal artery with a branch to the anterior spinal artery from the same level. The venous drainage of the AVM was via a single caudal draining vein that extended to the left internal iliac vein with attenuation at L5/S1.

In discussion between the radiology and neurosurgical teams, it was concluded the most likely aetiology for the patient's presentation was acute rupture of the AVM at T8 secondary to venous outflow compression from the enlarged uterus onto the draining vein at the level of L5 causing high pressure within the AVM and subsequent rupture. Given the lesion was partially within the spinal cord, treatment with surgical resection would risk potential permanent paraplegia. Additionally, she was considered not a good candidate for embolisation. As such, the patient was managed conservatively in the hope that she might have at least partial recovery of her neurological function. An inferior vena cava (IVC) filter was inserted at the time of initial angiography to prevent pulmonary emboli given the relative risk of anticoagulation in the setting of recent caesarean section and recent AVM rupture.

One month after admission, the patient developed left leg swelling and was diagnosed with a left leg extensive occlusive deep vein thrombosis extending to left external and common iliac vein as far as the IVC filter. There was concern about potential obstruction of venous outflow from the AVM precipitating further rupture as well as potential clot propagation above the IVC filter, so a decision was made for mechanical thrombectomy and removal of IVC filter. She was therapeutically anticoagulated on warfarin with clexane bridging and clot progression was monitored on weekly ultrasound scans.

Given the difficulties in finding a suitable discharge destination with a newborn baby, the patient's first few months of rehabilitation were as an inpatient in a private room on the neurosurgery ward. At the time of writing this article (six months after delivery), the patient remains paraplegic to the level of T8 with urinary and bowel incontinence. At this stage, she has a guarded prognosis for recovery.

3. Discussion

Cases reported in the literature of complications from spinal AVMs in pregnancy are summarised below as well as a discussion of the unique challenges of investigating and managing a pregnant woman with new onset paraplegia secondary to a spinal AVM.

Demir and colleagues published a case in *Spine* (2012) describing acute onset T8 paraplegia at 30 weeks gestation secondary to vascular congestion without rupture of a spinal vascular malformation in the setting of known Klippel-Trenaunay syndrome [5]. The patient was delivered by caesarean and her neurological symptoms improved within days of delivery without any neurosurgical intervention.

A Japanese study by Kinoshita and colleagues published in 2009 described a young woman with a known spinal vascular tumour at T2-T3 diagnosed at age 10 years [6]. She presented at 29 weeks gestation unable to walk, with progressive symptoms over the next five weeks prompting delivery via caesarean at 34 weeks gestation. Spinal angiography identified a large extradural arteriovenous fistula compressing the spinal cord at T3-T4. She was planned for endovascular embolisation but her neurological symptoms improved after delivery. She was managed conservatively and was able to walk six months after delivery.

An older study published in 1976 by Manabe and colleagues described a woman presenting at term with sudden chest pain, paraplegia, sensory level at T5, and urinary incontinence [7]. She had her delivery by caesarean and subsequently diagnosed with a typical AVM at T2-T6 on spinal angiography. Six weeks after delivery, her AVM was surgically removed and her neurological symptoms resolved.

The aforementioned studies from the literature and the one presented in this study highlight the challenges when investigating and managing paraplegia secondary to spinal vascular malformations in pregnancy.

Diagnosing spinal cord pathology in pregnancy has unique challenges. If a nonpregnant patient presented to emergency with rapidly progressive weakness and numbness suggestive of a spinal cord lesion, they would receive an urgent CT spine to rule out compressive lesions that require surgical intervention. However, radiation, especially to the abdomen, is generally avoided in pregnancy. While conventional MRI is often the first imaging performed for suspected spinal vascular malformations, it is not always readily available and is not the gold standard test. Despite advanced imaging techniques, such as time-resolved contrast-enhanced MR angiography, invasive spinal angiography is still the definitive test [1, 8]. In our patient as well as other cases in the literature, delivery of the pregnancy was necessitated to allow invasive angiography to be performed to define the lesion and determine management.

The safest choice of anaesthetic for caesarean in pregnant patients with a spinal vascular malformation requires careful consideration. A study published in 1996 by Ong et al. discussed the relative risks of different anaesthetic choices for caesarean for a patient with a known cervical (C3) AVM that was stable throughout pregnancy [9]. They commented that using general anaesthetic might be particularly dangerous in the setting of a spinal AVM, as the patient may become hypertensive with increased intrathoracic and venous pressure on waking from the anaesthetic. This has potential to precipitate rupture of the AVM. Alternatively, perfusion of the spinal cord might be compromised by epidural anaesthesia as a result of hypotension and increased epidural pressure. They elected for spinal anaesthesia and delivered her baby via caesarean without complications. However, it would not be appropriate to use their study to inform anaesthetic choice for our patient because her AVM was much lower and had associated haemorrhage and as such, general anaesthetic was considered the safest option.

Treatment of spinal AVMs generally involves surgery, endovascular embolisation, or both [1, 2]. In two of the aforementioned cases, delivery alone facilitated neurological recovery as symptoms were caused by compression of vessels by the gravid uterus that was relieved after delivery [5, 6]. Unfortunately, our patient has shown no signs of neurological recovery following delivery, likely because her symptoms are as a result of an intramedullary lesion with associated haemorrhage.

Our patient's AVM had both intra- and extramedullary components. These lesions have complex angioarchitecture and as such are particularly difficult to treat [1]. Patsalides et al. proposed that a palliative approach to patients with such complex lesions is reasonable given that curative treatment would be "extremely difficult and likely associated with increased morbidity" [1].

A recent article published in 2017 by Rashad and colleagues in *Neurosurgical Review* described a novel method for treating intramedullary AVMs using stereotactic radiosurgery [10]. Of note, this technique was used in two patients who had suffered haemorrhages and were not suitable for surgery or embolisation. As such, they performed radiosurgery using CyberKnife™, a technique that uses targeted doses of radiation. For the two patients who had evidence of haemorrhage, one had improvement of their symptoms and one remained stable with no further haemorrhagic episodes.

Rehabilitation is an important aspect of treatment for patients with paraplegia. When a mother becomes paraplegic during pregnancy, it is essential to consider the newborn baby as well as the mother's ability to care for the baby after delivery. In our patient's case, she required a special exemption from the hospital executive to be considered for spinal rehabilitation with a newborn baby. Notably, her main concern when discussing discharge destinations was her desire to remain with her daughter.

While new onset paraplegia during pregnancy secondary to ruptured spinal AVM is very rare, it is important to discuss these cases to inform future practice. Timely recognition and appropriate management of these women might help prevent permanent disability.

Consent

The patient has provided written consent for her story to be used in preparation of this case report and reviewed the manuscript prior to submission.

Disclosure

The study was conducted at Royal Brisbane and Women's Hospital, Brisbane, QLD, Australia. This case was presented as a poster at the Royal College of Obstetricians & Gynaecologists (RCOG) World Congress in Singapore March 2018.

Acknowledgments

Thanks are due to Dr. Lee Minuzzo, MBBS, FRANZCOG, an obstetrician and gynaecologist at Royal Brisbane and Women's Hospital, Brisbane, QLD, Australia.

References

[1] A. Patsalides, J. Knopman, A. Santillan, A. J. Tsiouris, H. Riina, and Y. P. Gobin, "Endovascular treatment of spinal arteriovenous lesions: beyond the dural fistula," *American Journal of Neuroradiology*, vol. 32, no. 5, pp. 798–808, 2011.

[2] J. E. Park, H.-W. Koo, H. Liu, S. C. Jung, D. Park, and D. C. Suh, "Clinical characteristics and treatment outcomes of spinal arteriovenous malformations," *Clinical Neuroradiology*, vol. 28, pp. 39–46, 2018.

[3] Y.-J. Lee, K. G. Terbrugge, G. Saliou, and T. Krings, "Clinical features and outcomes of spinal cord arteriovenous malformations: comparison between nidus and fistulous types," *Stroke*, vol. 45, no. 9, pp. 2606–2612, 2014.

[4] B. Singh, S. Behari, A. Jaiswal et al., "Spinal arteriovenous malformations: is surgery indicated?" *Asian Journal of Neurosurgery*, vol. 11, no. 2, pp. 134–142, 2016.

[5] C. F. Demir, M. Yildiz, H. Özdemir et al., "Paraplegia in pregnancy: a case of spinal vascular malformation with klippel-trenaunay syndrome," *The Spine Journal*, vol. 37, no. 19, pp. E1218–E1220, 2012.

[6] M. Kinoshita, A. Asai, S. Komeda et al., "Spontaneous regression of a spinal extradural arteriovenous fistula after delivery by cesarean sectio—case report," *Neurologia Medico-Chirurgica*, vol. 49, no. 7, pp. 313–315, 2009.

[7] T. Manabe, H. Kikuchi, S. Furuse, J. Karasawa, and T. Sakaki, "Spinal cord arteriovenous malformation during pregnancy (author's transl)," *Neurological Surgery*, vol. 4, pp. 271–276, 1976.

[8] M. Amarouche, J. L. Hart, A. Siddiqui, T. Hampton, and D. C. Walsh, "Time-resolved contrast-enhanced MR angiography of spinal vascular malformations," *American Journal of Neuroradiology*, vol. 36, no. 2, pp. 417–422, 2015.

[9] B. Y. Ong, J. Littleford, R. Segstro, D. Paetkau, and I. Sutton, "Spinal anaesthesia for Caesarean section in a patient with a cervical arteriovenous malformation," *Canadian Journal of Anesthesia*, vol. 43, no. 10, pp. 1052–1058, 1996.

[10] S. Rashad, T. Endo, Y. Ogawa et al., "Stereotactic radiosurgery as a feasible treatment for intramedullary spinal arteriovenous malformations: a single-center observation," *Neurosurgical Review*, vol. 40, no. 2, pp. 259–266, 2017.

32

Ogilvie's Syndrome after Cesarean Section: Case Report in Saudi Arabia and Management Approach

Lamiaa Elsebay[1,2,3] **and Mariam Ahmed Galal**[1,2]

[1]*Specialized Medical Center Hospital, Riyadh, Saudi Arabia*
[2]*Alfaisal University, Riyadh, Saudi Arabia*
[3]*SCFHS, Riyadh, Saudi Arabia*

Correspondence should be addressed to Mariam Ahmed Galal; melsyed@alfaisal.edu

Academic Editor: Yoshio Yoshida

Background. Acute colonic pseudoobstruction or Ogilvie's syndrome is a rare entity that is characterized by acute dilatation of the colon without any mechanical obstruction. It is usually associated with medical disease or surgery and rarely occurs spontaneously. If not diagnosed early, Ogilvie's syndrome may cause bowel ischemia and perforation. *Case.* A G7P4+2, 40-year-old woman, who is a known case of gestational diabetes mellitus during her current pregnancy, four previous cesarean sections, two early pregnancy losses at six-week gestation, and hypothyroidism, underwent uncomplicated elective cesarean section, after which she complained of abdominal distention. *Conclusion.* Ogilvie's syndrome is a rare condition yet of interest to obstetricians, midwifery staff, and general surgeons because its early diagnosis and prompt treatment are the keystones to avoid any subsequent fatal complications. This case report reviews the clinical characteristics, diagnostic methods, and management of Ogilvie's syndrome. Moreover, we suggest a management approach to help in early diagnosis and prompt management to improve the outcome of this potentially serious condition.

1. Introduction

The acute colonic pseudoobstruction (ACPO), nonobstructive colonic dilatation, or Ogilvie's syndrome is a rare entity that is characterized by acute dilatation of the colon, usually involving caecum and right hemicolon in the absence of any mechanical obstruction (80–90%), abdominal pain (80%), abdominal tenderness (62%), nausea and/or vomiting (60%), constipation (40%), and fever (37%). It is usually associated with an underlying illness, infection, or surgery and rarely occurs spontaneously. Identification of this condition is important due to the increased risk of subsequent bowel ischemia and perforation, particularly with caecal diameter >9 cm, with high mortality rate up to 50%. Here, we report a case of right colon necrosis and perforation after cesarean section that leads to urgent laparotomy and highlights early and appropriate diagnosis from an obstetric point of view.

2. Case Presentation

A 40-year-old female, G7P4+2, was admitted for elective cesarean section at 38 weeks. Her medical history included gestational diabetes mellitus (GDM) during her current pregnancy that was controlled on metformin (500 mg, three times daily), four previous cesarean sections, two early pregnancy losses at six-week gestation, hypothyroidism, and previous eye surgery at childhood for eye squint. Her family history was positive for diabetes and hypertension.

The patient had an elective cesarean section under spinal anesthesia and gave birth to a living female. It was noticed that she has been omental to the anterior abdominal wall adhesions and omental to the anterior uterine wall adhesions. There were no intraoperative complications and estimated blood loss was about 500 cc.

On the first postoperative day [POD1], the patient looked well with stable vital signs. System review was within normal,

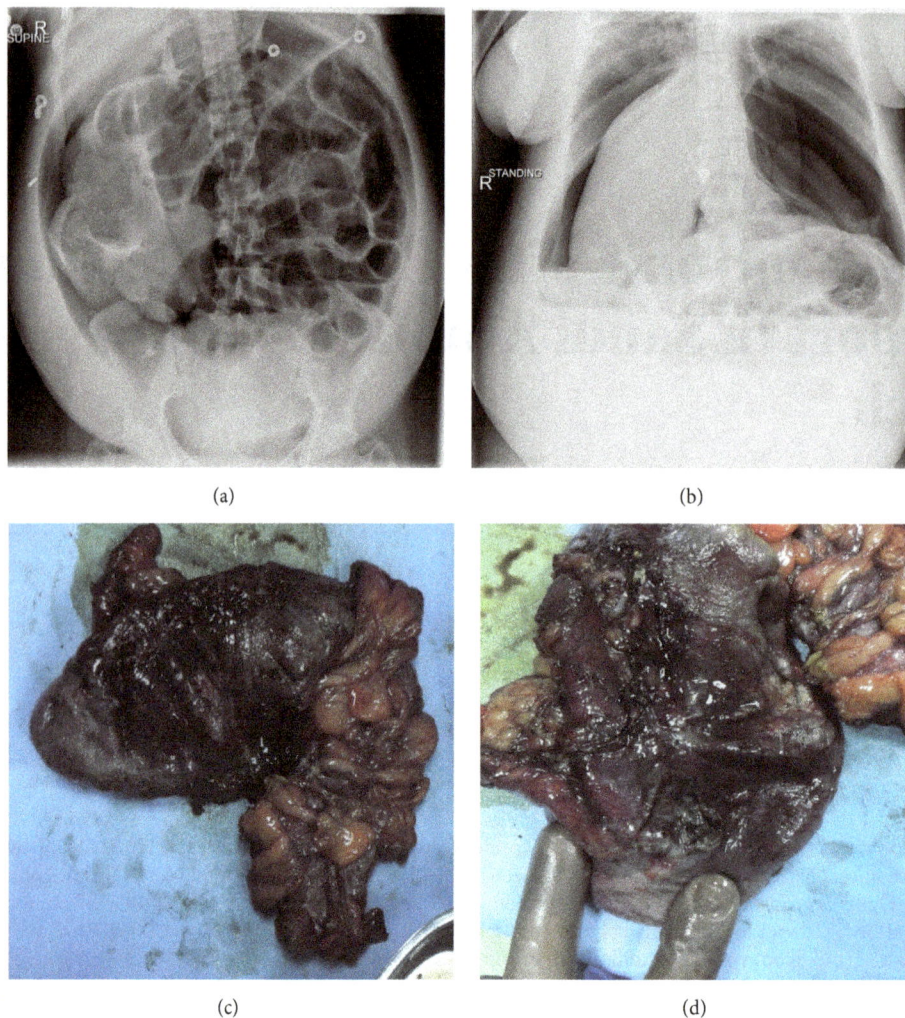

(a)

(b)

(c)

(d)

Figure 1

and physical examination showed soft and lax abdomen with audible bowel sounds. The patient was started on the liquid diet. The patient passed flatus and was started on the soft diet. The same day at night, she developed mild abdominal distension, bowel sounds still audible with stable vital signs, and the patient was advised to mobilize. The patient mentioned she used to have more abdominal distension after each caesarian delivery.

On POD2, the patient started to have more abdominal distension despite passing stool, and bowel sounds become sluggish then nonaudible. Patient was kept NPO; serum electrolytes were requested and showed mild hypokalemia 3.29 mmol/L. Patient was encouraged to mobilize and was started on potassium chloride infusion and NGT was inserted. She initially was diagnosed to have paralytic ileus, but her general condition eventually deteriorated dramatically, and she developed tachycardia and shortness of breath.

The patient was transferred to the Intensive Care Unit (ICU), reviewed by ICU and surgical team. Abdominal X-ray was performed and showed distended abdomen with pneumoperitoneum (see Figures 1(a) and 1(b)). CT scan was requested and showed small amount of free fluid collection

in the subphrenic area with subhepatic longitudinal mass and large pneumoperitoneum suggesting possible bowel perforation and dilated proximal small bowel loops without obvious transitional zone. The patient was transferred to OR for exploration laparotomy.

Exploration laparotomy performed through longitudinal abdominal incision. There was gangrenous changes of the caecum and right colon with its anterior wall showing multiple ischemic areas and necrosis; some of them are perforated with gross picture of ischemic changes, others thinned out and were about to perforate in subhepatic area; right hemicolectomy and iliostomy were performed till the area of normal color of the colon was reached (see Figures 1(c) and 1(d)). Peritoneal lavage was performed afterwards, 2 abdominal drains were inserted, and the incision site was closed with staples. The patient was properly hydrated all through the surgery, fluid input/output were properly calculated, and urine output was adequate and clear. The uterus and both adnexa were normal.

The patient was transferred back to ICU. The patient received broad-spectrum antimicrobial agents; she was under close monitoring, multidisciplinary team management and

TABLE 1: Compares between Ogilvie's syndrome and paralytic ileus.

	Ogilvie's syndrome	Paralytic ileus
Impaired area	Limited to colon	Throughout the gut
Bowel sounds	Hyperactive/high-pitched/absent	Always absent
Nausea & vomiting	Mild and inconstantly present	More common
Passing flatus	Present	Always ceased
Passing stool	Present/diarrhea/obstipation	Always ceased

discharged to regular room 6 days postoperatively. The postoperative course passed otherwise uneventful. The multidisciplinary team shared in plan of care were surgeons, pulmonologists, ICU intensivists, obstetricians, and cardiologist. Thrombophilia screening was suggested and hyperhomocysteinemia was found; homocysteine level was 14.26 Umol/L. She was discharged in a good general condition 12 days postoperatively.

3. Discussion

Ogilvie's syndrome or ACPO was first reported by Sir Ogilvie in 1948 [1]. It is described as acute dilatation of the colon usually involving caecum and right hemicolon without any existing mechanical obstruction [2, 3]. It is a rare condition yet it can result in dangerous complications with subsequent high mortality rate beyond 50% [4]. It can occur at any age with higher frequency in the sixth decade of life [5]. Its incidence in males is higher than that in females (1.5 : 1) [5].

It has been reported after pregnancy or cesarean section [6]. The condition has been also associated with trauma, severe burns, drugs (narcotic analgesics, antidepressants, corticosteroids, antipsychotic, calcium channel blockers, narcoleptics, and syntocinon), spinal anesthesia, opioid use, alcohol, cardiac failure, respiratory failure, neurological problems (Parkinson's, Multiple Sclerosis, and Alzheimer's), electrolyte imbalance, stress that causes central secretion of corticotrophin-releasing factor (which, in turn, inhibits gut motility), and hormones affecting the smooth muscles and, in rare occasions, may occur spontaneously [6–9]. The etiological factors in our case were as follows: (1) a multiparous patient; (2) previous repeated cesarean sections; (3) hormonal effect of pregnancy, GDM, and hypothyroidism; (4) receiving spinal anesthesia; and (5) age (40 years old).

The exact pathophysiology of the disease is still unclear but it was hypothesized that either the increase in the sympathetic tone or the decrease in the sacral parasympathetic innervations to the colon results in decreased colon motility with subsequent proximal colon dilation which will eventually increase the intraluminal pressure in the proximal colon and cecum, obstructing the caecal capillary circulation and causing subsequent ischemia, gangrene, and perforation [2, 8, 10]. This explanation is widely accepted due to the proximity between autonomic nerves and the structures at risk during cesarean section, including the cervix, the vagina, and the broad ligaments [6]. Regardless, the true pathogenesis of the syndrome is thought to be multifactorial.

As the ACPOs have serious complications, timely diagnosis and treatment are critical. Clinical and radiological findings are both needed to confirm the diagnosis of the syndrome [10]. Typically, it presents within 48 h and up to 12 days postoperatively and can be confused with mechanical obstruction of bowel-like paralytic ileus (see Table 1) [5, 11, 12]. Clinical features include abdominal distension with mild-to-moderate abdominal discomfort, constipation, nausea, and vomiting along with low grade fever [8, 13, 14]. Clinical examination may show mild-to-moderate tenderness with bowel sounds noted in 90% of patients [8, 10]. Abnormal bowel sounds reported were either hyperactive, high-pitched, or sometimes absent [12]. In our reported case, the clinical features included abdominal pain, distension, and vomiting.

Plain abdominal X-ray is the most useful diagnostic modality that reveals gaseous distention in colon, mostly involving the caecum and ascending colon, with or without fluid levels seen in small bowel [10, 11]. Caecal diameter of 9–12 cm warrants ischemia and subsequent perforation if not managed urgently [5]. Though X-ray is a fundamental diagnostic modality, other modalities like CT scans and water soluble contrast enema are used to confirm the diagnosis and to exclude mechanical obstruction [10]. When X-ray is indeterminate and the correct diagnosis cannot be made, gastrografin enema is desirable to detect bowel distention. However, an exploratory laparotomy in some patients will remain the final option to reach a conclusive diagnosis [13]. In our case, the initial diagnosis made was paralytic ileus and bowel perforation, yet the final diagnosis of Ogilvie's syndrome was reached only after laparotomy, when several areas of necrosis and perforation were seen.

In ACPO, laboratory findings are nondiagnostic. Some electrolyte imbalances like hyponatremia, hypomagnesemia, and hypokalemia can be seen in ACPO, but they represent a consequence of the pathological condition rather than its etiologic factor. Similarly, leukocytosis can be present, especially with perforation or bowel ischemia. Hypokalemia and leukocytosis were present in our case.

Management for uncomplicated patients is initially conservative with limiting oral intake, active mobilization, cessation of opioids, and correction of electrolytes, and underlying comorbidities should be treated [14]. Intravenous hydration, nasogastric decompression, rectal tube decompression, close clinical monitoring with serial physical examinations, laboratory studies, and abdominal radiological modalities should be done [5].

The most effective pharmacological agent is neostigmine, given intravenously at a dose of 2 mg over 3–5 min and

TABLE 2: Pre- and intraoperative measures taken in pregnant women to avoid adynamic ileus.

Preoperative measure	Intraoperative measure
Correct poor bowel habits during pregnancy Perform enema before CS	Reduce blood loss Early blood transfusion Maintain stable hemodynamic status Minimize operation time Avoid intestinal protrusion out of the abdominal cavity due to vomiting

repeated once if required in 2-3 hours [11]. Neostigmine is a reversible anticholinesterase inhibitor that potentiates the effects of the parasympathetic system and improves colonic motility, causing effective colonic decompression up to 88%. Ganglionic blockade with guanethidine followed by cholinergic stimulation with neostigmine can be effective. Neostigmine should not be used in overly distended caecum and, due to its bradycardiac hypotensive effects, it should be given to vitally stable patient with monitored setting [13]. An alternative to neostigmine is erythromycin, a motilin receptor agonist [13]. Other pharmacological agents are naloxone and cisapride [5].

If conservative and medical management, including the second dose of neostigmine, failed, colonoscopic decompression is recommended. It is successful in 68–95% of cases and prevents any ischemia and bowel perforation, yet recurrence is common. Colonoscopic decompression is contraindicated if perforation or peritonitis exists [6].

Surgery is recommended if colonoscopic decompression failed, or progressive clinical deterioration or signs of ischemia and perforation are present, or if caecal diameter is >12 cm. Surgical treatment can be either caecostomy or, in case of ischemic bowel, hemicolectomy with or without primary anastomosis or total abdominal colectomy. The surgical treatment has mortality rate ranging from 30% to 60%.

For pregnant woman with severe constipation and undergoing C-section, certain measures can be done preop and intra-op to prevent or reduce the occurrence of adynamic ileus (see Table 2) [7]. For postoperative pain control, nonsteroidal anti-inflammatory drugs may be considered in place of opioids for high-risk patients. Having similar pain relieving effect as systemic opiates, thoracolumbar epidural anesthesia can be used to reduce the duration of postoperative ileus.

After review of cases, we suggest the management algorithm (see Figure 2). Once the case is suspected (severe abdominal distention, abdominal pain, nausea, and constipations), it is required to obtain initial proper assessment including history (surgeries, caesarian section, infection, and spinal injuries, keeping in mind the previously discussed etiological factors), clinical examination, and laboratory investigations (absence of mechanical obstruction favor the diagnosis of Ogilvie's syndrome or ACPO). Conservative management should be established for 24–48 hours in the

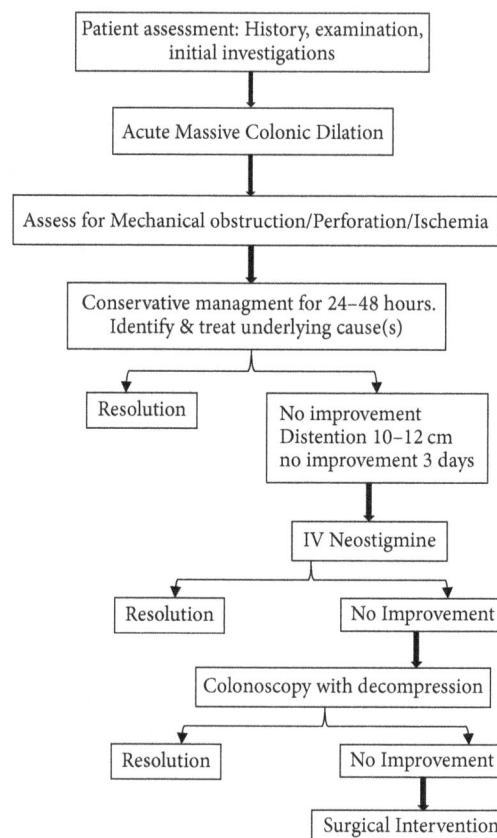

FIGURE 2: Stepwise approach to Ogilvie's syndrome.

form of close observation, hydration and correction of electrolyte imbalance, insertion of the nasogastric tube, keeping the patient fasting without using rectal enema or laxatives, cessation of all narcotic medications, and treating underlying etiological factors if any. Assess to rule out the presence of mechanical obstruction and to evaluate for perforation as this will terminate conservative management. In the case of no improvement, when abdominal X-ray shows caecal dilation, colonic distention 10–12 cm, likely normal small bowel, and no mechanical obstruction or no improvement for 3 days, pharmacological decompression with intravenous neostigmine could be started with caution if cecum is significantly dilated and if there is no response, endoscopic colonic decompression can be considered. If pharmacological/endoscopic decompression failed or signs suggestive of perforation exist, then surgical intervention should be considered in the form of caecostomy, hemicolectomy, and resection of the ischemic or perforated segment of the bowel to be performed.

To conclude, Ogilvie's syndrome is rare yet very important to obstetricians, midwifery staff, and general surgeons to diagnose and manage it as early as possible in patients who underwent C-section to avoid any subsequent fatal complications. The authors recommend precise assessment and close monitoring with conservative management in any suspected case. Reassessment is important to assess whether the disease progresses or regresses. With progression, medical, interventional, and surgical management can be considered as described in the context.

References

[1] H. Ogilvie, "Large-intestine colic due to sympathetic deprivation; A new clinical syndrome," *British Medical Journal*, vol. 2, no. 4579, pp. 671–673, 1948.

[2] M. Camilleri, "Acute Colonic Pseudo-Obstruction (Ogilvie's Syndrome)," http://www.uptodate.com.

[3] M. Cebola, E. Eddy, S. Davis, and L. Chin-Lenn, "Acute colonic pseudo-obstruction (Ogilvie's syndrome) following total laparoscopic hysterectomy," *Journal of Minimally Invasive Gynecology*, vol. 22, no. 7, pp. 1307–1310, 2015.

[4] C. Ponzano, S. Nardi, P. Carrieri, and G. Basili, "Diagnostic problems, pathogenetic hypothesis and therapeutic proposals in Ogilvie's syndrome," *Minerva Chirurgica*, vol. 11, pp. 1311–1320, 1997.

[5] A. J. Shakir, M. S. Sajid, B. Kianifard, and M. K. Baig, "Ogilvie's syndrome-related right colon perforation after cesarean section: A case series," *Kaohsiung Journal of Medical Sciences*, vol. 27, no. 6, pp. 234–238, 2011.

[6] A. K. Saha, E. Newman, M. Giles, and K. Horgan, "Ogilvie's syndrome with caecal perforation after Caesarean section: A case report," *Journal of Medical Case Reports*, vol. 3, article no. 6177, 2009.

[7] F.-N. Cho, C.-B. Liu, J.-Y. Li, S.-N. Chen, and K.-J. Yu, "Adynamic Ileus and Acute Colonic Pseudo-obstruction Occurring After Cesarean Section in Patients With Massive Peripartum Hemorrhage," *Journal of the Chinese Medical Association*, vol. 72, no. 12, pp. 657–662, 2009.

[8] V. W. Vanek and M. Al-Salti, "Acute pseudo-obstruction of the colon (Ogilvie's syndrome). An analysis of 400 cases," *Diseases of the Colon & Rectum*, vol. 29, no. 3, pp. 203–210, 1986.

[9] M. A. S. Dickson and J. H. McClure, "Acute colonic pseudo-obstruction after caesarean section," *International Journal of Obstetric Anesthesia*, vol. 3, no. 4, pp. 234–236, 1994.

[10] R. Y. Alshareef, "Pediatric acute colonic pseudo-obstruction post complicated appendicitis," *International Journal of Case Reports and Images (IJRCI)*, vol. 7, no. 1, pp. 7–10, 2016.

[11] A. O. Latunde-Dada, D. I. Alleemudder, and D. P. Webster, "Ogilvie's syndrome following caesarean section," *BMJ Case Reports*, 2013.

[12] E. Kalu, A. Fakokunde, M. Jesudason, and B. Whitlow, "Acute colonic pseudo-obstruction (Ogilvie's Syndrome) following caesarean section for triplets," *Journal of Obstetrics & Gynaecology*, vol. 25, no. 3, pp. 299-300, 2005.

[13] A. B. Bhatti, F. Khan, and A. Ahmed, "Acute colonic pseudo-obstruction (ACPO) after normal vaginal delivery," *J Pak Med Assoc*, vol. 60, no. 2, pp. 138-139, 2010.

[14] M. Khajehnoori and S. Nagra, "Acute colonic pseudo-obstruction (Ogilvie's syndrome) with caecal perforation after caesarean section," *Journal of Surgical Case Reports*, vol. 8, 2016.

33

Management of Pregnancy with Klippel-Trenaunay-Weber Syndrome: A Case Report and Review

Rati Chadha (ID)

*Department of Obstetrics and Gynecology; Division of Maternal Fetal Medicine, Foothills Medical Center,
University of Calgary, Calgary, AB, Canada*

Correspondence should be addressed to Rati Chadha; ratichadhamd@yahoo.com

Academic Editor: Erich Cosmi

Background. Klippel-Trenaunay-Weber syndrome is a rare neurocutaneous syndrome with vascular involvement. Given the rarity of the syndrome, its management in pregnancy is based on the outcome of a few case reports and expert opinion. *Case Summary.* The management of a complicated case with its antepartum, intrapartum, and postpartum concerns has been addressed in this review. *Conclusions.* Prenatal consults with anesthesia, general surgery, intervention radiology, and internal medicine should be arranged, prior to delivery in anticipation of all the possible complications. Apart from the pregnancy management, preconceptional counselling including the genetics, prognosis, and contraception has an important role in patient management.

1. Introduction

Klippel-Trenaunay Type Syndrome (KTTS) was first described in 1900 by Klippel and Trenaunay, who described it as a syndrome of osteohypertrophic varicose nevus [1]. In 1918, Weber added arteriovenous fistulae to the syndrome. It is therefore interchangeably used as KTS (Klippel-Trenaunay Syndrome) or KTW (Klippel-Trenaunay-Weber) syndrome.

KTW is a rare congenital abnormality with a variable expression [1] and an unknown etiology. The reported incidence is approximately at 1: 27500 newborns [2]. The triad that characterizes the syndrome consists of vascular skin nevus, varicose veins or venous malformations, and asymmetric hypertrophy of soft tissue and bone [2, 3]. Varicose veins or venous malformations are the most characteristic features. At least two of the three main symptoms should be present to accept the diagnosis [4]. Other features that may be seen are hyperhidrosis, scoliosis and gait abnormalities, and neuroaxial venous malformations [5].

KTS is a neurocutaneous syndrome with vascular involvement [3]. There are many theories regarding the etiology of this syndrome. It is most likely the result of a somatic mosaicism: a postzygotic mutation that only affects a subset of the cells within the body [2].

A large lateral varice is so common that it is commonly referred to the Klippel-Trenaunay vein or the Vein of Serville [6]. This vein invariably begins at the foot; tunnels laterally past the knee and then courses medially at the level of the groin. Internal iliac vein abnormalities can lead to varicosities around the colon, rectum, uterus, and bladder. The diagnosis of this disease is usually initiated by the clinical appearance in childhood [1]. During pregnancy the venous malformations increase with pelvic and intra-abdominal involvement [1]. The complications, therefore, seen are venous insufficiency, cellulitis, ulcers, thrombophlebitis, thromboembolism, lymphangiectasia [7], consumptive coagulopathy with severe thrombocytopenia (Kasabach-Merritt syndrome), and increased bleeding in the intrapartum period [8–11].

We have discussed a case of KTW syndrome below with multiple antepartum complications and their management.

2. Case Report

Our patient is a 19 yo G1P0 with an unplanned pregnancy, who was seen for the 1st time at 20+4 weeks, with syncope and right sided chest pain. Pulmonary embolism was confirmed on a spiral CT scan.

Prior to the current pregnancy, she had an extensive history of emergency room (ER) visits and pediatric intensive care unit admissions for recurrent cellulitis and septic shock secondary to lymphedema. She had been noncompliant with oral suppressive antibiotics. She had also developed toxic shock syndrome secondary to Group A streptococcal cellulitis and had multiple debridements with skin grafts as a result of necrotising fasciitis. Compounding her risk of infections was her picking behavior secondary to anxiety.

She had required ECMO (extracorporeal membrane oxygenation) for severe biventricular dysfunction from presumed septic cardiomyopathy; peritoneal hemodialysis for acute renal failure and multiple episodes of mechanical ventilation and aggressive vasopressor inotropic support.

Seven months prior to her pregnancy diagnosis, she had a bladder rupture and peritonitis after self-insertion of a pen into her urethra, requiring laparotomy. Numerous large venous bleeders were encountered in the subcutaneous tissue related to her known KTW syndrome.

She was also smoking about half to one pack of cigarettes and multiple joints of marijuana since the age of 13 years. Her overall social situation was tenuous with limited resources for food, housing, family support, and a borderline personality disorder.

At the time of presentation, her resting heart rate was 110/min and increased to 160/min on standing. On examination, she had an extremely large port wine stain extending from the right flank to midthigh with superficial excoriations (Figure 1(a)). Bilateral significant lymphedema to the lower extremities was noted. The toes were enlarged to about 5 cm in width and were overlapping with each other (Figure 1(b)). Over her abdomen she had a midline laparotomy scar that had healed along with multiple other scars from the debridements (Figure 1(c)). Her gait was abnormal, secondary to the severe scoliosis.

She was started on therapeutic enoxaparin, with the dose being adjusted on the basis of the antifactor Xa levels (goal of 0.5-1.0). Her syncope was attributed to the significant lymphedema and venous varicosities in the lower extremities, along with the consumption of very high-glucose containing fluids (juice and pop) resulting in osmotic diuresis. She also had an ECHO done which demonstrated low left ventricular function. Her compliance as an outpatient for taking heparin and antibiotics was poor. The decision was made, therefore, to keep her as an inpatient until delivery from about 24 weeks, which greatly improved her nutrition and compliance, as all medications were given under nursing supervision.

She was seen by psychiatry and social work while in the hospital. She was counselled by prenatal genetics but declined testing for herself or on her newborn.

An MRI of the abdomen and pelvis performed revealed marked hemihypertrophy of the subcutaneous soft tissues on the right side at the level of the lower abdomen (Figure 2(a)); pelvis and buttock and thigh region (Figure 2(b)), which contain innumerable venous vascular malformations and varicosities. No increase in vascularity was noted in perineal or uterine area. These changes were consistent with KTW syndrome.

The MRI of the spine revealed marked levoconvex scoliosis with a marked leftward pelvic tilt. A developmentally narrow spinal canal was noted. Numerous venous channels were noted to cross at the potential epidural injection sites from L1 to L5. The thickness from the skin to the thecal space was 9.4 cm (Figure 2(c)). No intracranial or intraspinal vascular malformations were noted. Once the MRI was completed, anesthesiology was consulted. Their recommendation was for extreme caution for neuroaxial anesthesia and if to be given to be performed above the level of L1. Given the increased risk of disseminated intravascular coagulation (DIC), several units of blood were to be cross-matched with two large bore intravenous access. Consideration for the use of cell-saver and the availability of a Trauma Pak if bleeding was a concern was proposed.

Serial scans on the fetus demonstrated as decrease in growth and along with a persistent breech presentation. A decision was made for an elective caesarian section at 37+3 weeks, given the intrauterine growth restriction with abnormal Doppler in a breech presentation. A multidisciplinary discussion between general surgery, neonatology, anesthesia, internal medicine, and nursing was arranged.

Enoxaparin was discontinued 24 hours prior to the elected time of the C-section. Four units of packed red blood cells had been placed in the OR in the event that there was a need to transfuse the patient. General anesthesia under fiber optic visualization was administrated. A midline vertical incision was made. Extensive varicosities were then found in the subcutaneous tissues closer to the level of the pelvis, which were ligated. The incision was extended superiorly to be away from the varicosities. The uterus was found to be bicornuate, which explained the breech presentation of the fetus. The neonate was at the 10th %ile for growth. No obvious stigmata of KTW syndrome were noted at the time of birth.

The patient had been counselled regarding the placement of a MIRENA IUD in the uterus at the end of the C-section for a reliable form of contraception. However, she declined contraception. She was discharged on Day# 3 with transition on to warfarin for six months. Unfortunately, given the limited compliance, she had another pulmonary embolism four months after delivery.

3. Discussion

Given the paucity of literature on this unique condition, in this case report, we have attempted to discuss the antenatal, intrapartum and postpartum management under specific areas as mentioned below, with the aim of guiding management for other healthcare professionals when such a case presents.

3.1. Genetics. Most cases are sporadic in origin. On review of literature there are a handful of familial cases of KTW syndrome. A case of reciprocal translocation [46, XX, t(5;11)(q13.3;p15.1)], suggesting that potential aetiology could be a single gene disorder [12]. However, Aelvoet [13] described a multifactorial genetic form. A somatic mutation of a factor required for vasculogenesis and angiogenesis in embryonic development has been thought to cause hypertrophy of the soft tissue and bone.

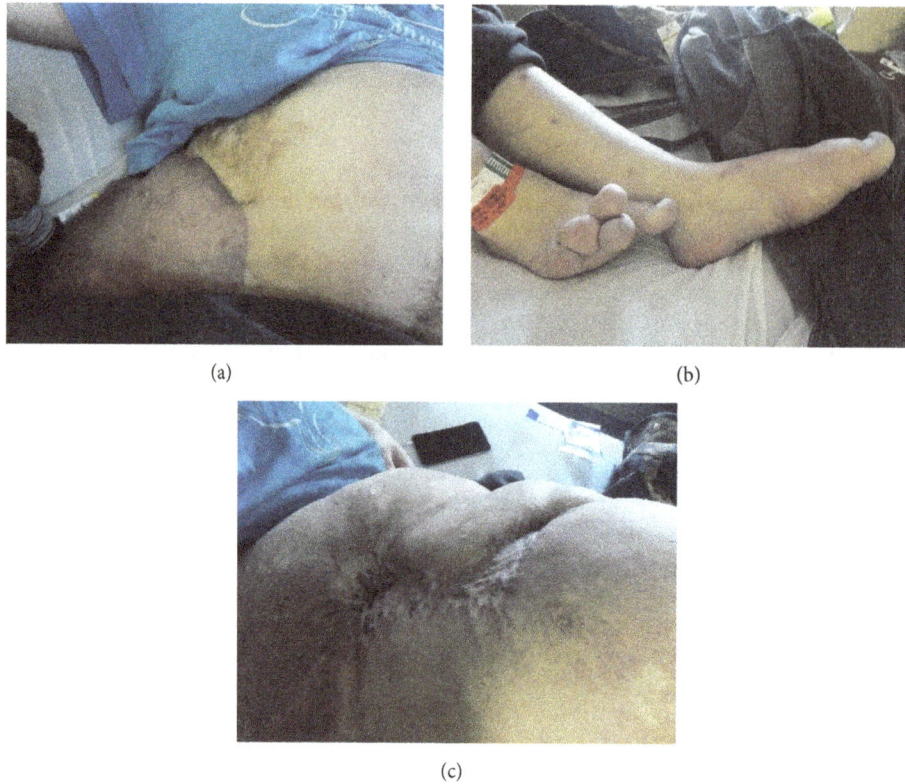

FIGURE 1: (a) Extremely large port wine stain/hemangioma extending from the right flank to midthigh with superficial excoriations. (b) Toes enlarged to about 5 cm in width and overlapping with each other. (c) Midline laparotomy scar along with multiple other scars from the debridements.

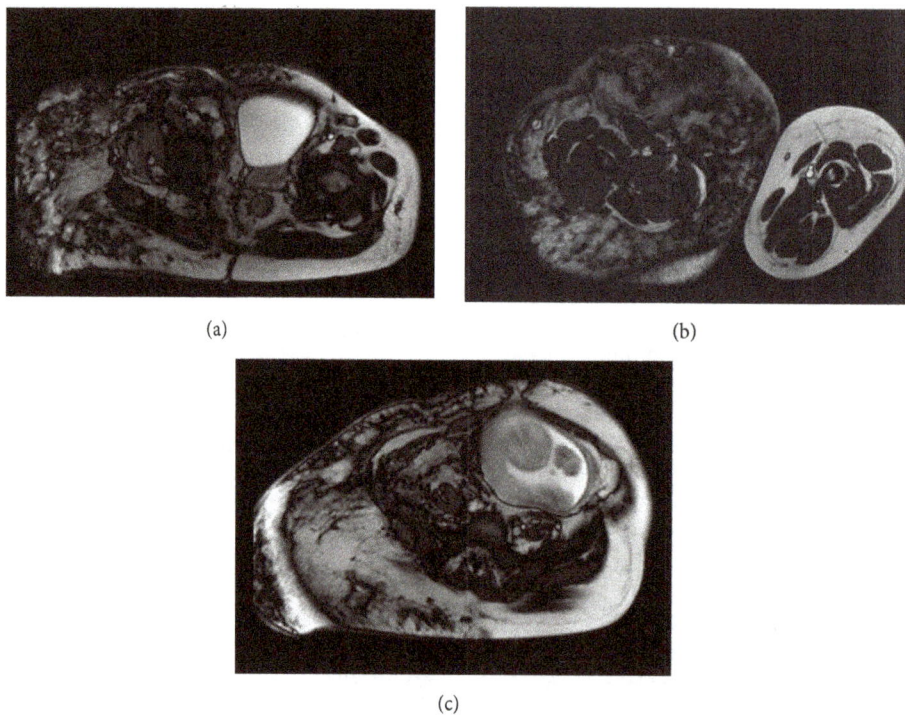

FIGURE 2: **MRI images depicting**. (a) Marked hemihypertrophy of the subcutaneous soft tissues on the right side at the level of the lower abdomen. (b) Marked hemihypertrophy of the subcutaneous soft tissues on the right thigh as compared to the left (normal). (c) Numerous venous channels were noted to cross at the potential epidural injection sites from L1 to L5. The thickness from the skin to the thecal space was 9.4 cm.

The other etiology is that there is overexpression of insulin-like growth factor-2 which causes tissue hypertrophy in different overgrowth disorders, including KTW syndrome. This was elucidated by Speradeo [14] when he described a family in which there was a case of KTW syndrome and a first cousin with Beckwith-Wiedemann syndrome.

For our patient there was no available family history and she declined genetic testing for herself.

3.2. Prenatal Diagnosis. There have been multiple case reports of prenatal diagnosis of this condition. The presentation may be in the form of multiple echo lucent areas suggestive of cutaneous vascular malformations [15] and/or hemihypertrophy of a lower extremity [16]. Roberts [17] described a case where by serial sonography was used to follow the in utero progression of the case and helped to decide the mode of delivery as a C-section, given the risk of labour dystocia and excessive fetal bleeding. In the second trimester the dominant abnormality was the cutaneous vascular lesions, while in the third trimester limb hypertrophy was the predominant finding. Other case reports have described findings of nonimmune hydrops [18] and cardiomegaly [19], secondary to the vascular malformations.

Differential diagnosis for this presentation on ultrasound is multiple congenital teratoma and cystic hygroma.

In addition, it has been suggested that fetuses in patients with KTW may be at increased risk of developing intrauterine growth restriction [20].

MRI has been extensively used in the management of KTW syndrome in children and adults. There is a case report of the prenatal use of MRI to confirm the diagnosis [21].

Our patient had multiple ultrasounds to assess fetal growth and to determine if there were any signs of a similar disorder in the fetus. No obvious cutaneous or bony anomalies were noted.

3.3. Prognosis. The main cause of complications is the presence of vascular anomalies which can cause cellulitis and resulting ulcers, sepsis, necrotising fasciitis requiring skin debridement, and vascular malformations in abdomen and pelvis. The main complications associated in pregnancy and postpartum period are thromboembolism and hemorrhage. The use of thromboembolic prophylaxis with low molecular weight heparin is generally recommended in the antepartum and the postpartum period [8]. Consideration should be given to the placement of a temporary inferior vena cava (IVC) filter to decrease the risk of pulmonary embolism.

In a cross-sectional study, KTS-related symptoms were aggravated during pregnancy in 43% of patients. Deep vein thrombosis was present in 5.8% and pulmonary embolism was present in 2.3% of pregnancies, which was extremely high compared with the reference population ($P < 0.0001$) [11].

Preterm labour has also been reported more often in patients with KTS [9]. However, in a cross-sectional study [11], this was not found.

Multiple complications such as pulmonary embolism, cellulitis, and necrotising fasciitis had occurred in our patient. However, the antepartum course after presentation to the hospital was uneventful.

3.4. Anesthesia. A MRI of the spine is recommended in the 3rd trimester to determine if neuroaxial anesthesia can be administered. In many cases such as in ours, due to the associated scoliosis or if there is a concern that a vascular malformation in the peridural space that may have been overlooked, general anesthesia is resorted to. However, general anesthesia is not without concern. In case of difficult airway secondary to vascular malformations, consideration for the use of awake fiber-optic intubation techniques to secure the airway [22] or the use of a laryngeal mask airway with continuous cricoid pressure, in an effort to minimize airway trauma and hemorrhage is recommended [23].

Additionally, given the risk of hemorrhage, arrangements for packed red blood cell and clotting factors transfusion or cell-saver technology should be made. The coagulation status of the patient should also be checked prior to delivery along with serial complete blood counts.

Getting an anesthesia consult helped the team be prepared for any complications. Fortunately, in our case no hemorrhage or another anesthetic or surgical complication was noted.

3.5. Mode of Delivery. The mode of delivery needs to be individualized per case. This will depend upon the imaging findings for the presence of vascular abnormalities in the pelvis and abdomen. The presence of varicosities/vascular malformations in the cervical, vaginal, or vulvar area will make vaginal delivery difficult because of the risk of rupture and hemorrhage. The vascular malformations are also associated with an increased risk of cerebrovascular accidents [24] in patients with intracranial anomalies. In such cases, operative vaginal delivery is recommended. If a caesarian section is the decided mode of delivery, intra-abdominal varicosities may require a midline vertical incision, such as in our patient. Disruption of the superficial draining veins of a leg during a Caesarean delivery may result in eventual amputation due to unrelieved venous engorgement [22].

3.6. Birth Control. Given the risk of thromboembolism even in the nonpregnant state, estrogen based contraception should be avoided. Depo-Provera or intrauterine device (progesterone or the copper) is good options.

Our patient received extensive counselling for contraception; however she declined to use any reliable method.

3.7. Preconceptional Counselling. Even though a few cases of familial occurrences have been described, the risk of transmission from an affected mother to her infant is unknown. There is evidence of an increased prevalence of vascular malformations in family members of these patients. Adequate counselling regarding antepartum and intrapartum complications as described above is recommended.

4. Conclusions

Less than hundred cases of pregnancies with KTW syndrome have been reported [11]. Pregnancy has historically been discouraged in women with KTW syndrome given the increased risk of complications. Prenatal consults with anesthesia, general surgery, intervention radiology, and internal medicine should be arranged prior to delivery in anticipation of all the possible complications. Therefore, an individualized multidisciplinary plan will help mitigate the complications associated with this condition for optimal results.

Abbreviations

KTTS: Klippel-Trenaunay Type Syndrome
KTS: Klippel-Trenaunay Syndrome
KTW: Klippel-Trenaunay-Weber
G1P0:   Gravida 1 para 0
CT: Computerized tomography
ECMO: Extracorporeal membrane oxygenation
ECHO: Echocardiography
MRI: Magnetic resonance imaging
DIC: Disseminated intravascular coagulation
IUD: Intrauterine device
IVC: Inferior vena cava.

Consent

Written consent was obtained from the patient as per the Alberta Health Services Guidelines.

Disclosure

The submitted manuscript is an original contribution that has not been previously published and is not under consideration for publication elsewhere.

References

[1] M. Klippel and P. D. Trenaunay, "Noevus variquex osteohypertrophique," *Archives of General Medicine*, vol. 185, pp. 641–672, 1900.

[2] C. E. U. Oduber, C. M. A. M. van der Horst, and R. C. M. Hennekam, "Klippel-Trenaunay syndrome: diagnostic criteria and hypothesis on etiology," *Annals of Plastic Surgery*, vol. 60, no. 2, pp. 217–223, 2008.

[3] S. M. Lindenauer, "The klippel-trenaunay syndrome: varicosity, hypertrophy and hemangioma with no arteriovenous fistula," *Annals of Surgery*, vol. 162, pp. 303–314, 1965.

[4] L. M. Reyes Puentes, M. J. Fuentes Camargo, and C. Perez Martinez, "Diagnostico prenatal ecografico del Sindrome Klippel-Trenaunay-Weber: a proposito de un caso," *Rev Ciencias Medicas*, vol. 14, pp. 656–661, 2010.

[5] I. W. Christie, P. A. Ahkine, and R. L. Holland, "Central regional anaesthesia in a patient with Klippel-Trenaunay Syndrome," *Anaesthesia and Intensive Care*, vol. 26, no. 3, pp. 319–321, 1998.

[6] J. G. Meine, R. A. Schwartz, and C. K. Janniger, "Klippel-Trenaunay-Weber Syndrome," *Cutis; Cutaneous Medicine for the Practitioner*, vol. 60, no. 3, pp. 127–132, 1997.

[7] M. A. Zoppi, R. M. Ibba, M. Floris, M. Putzolu, G. Crisponi, and G. Monni, "Prenatal sonographic diagnosis of Klippel-Trénaunay-Weber syndrome with cardiac failure," *Journal of Clinical Ultrasound*, vol. 29, no. 7, pp. 422–426, 2001.

[8] T. Güngor Gündoğan and Y. Jacquemyn, "Klippel-Trenaunay Syndrome and Pregnancy," *Obstetrics and Gynecology International*, vol. 2010, pp. 1–3, 2010.

[9] S. R. Stein, J. H. Perlow, and S. K. Sawai, "Klippel-Trenaunay-Type Syndrome in pregnancy," *Obstetrical & Gynecological Survey*, vol. 61, no. 3, pp. 194–206, 2006.

[10] A. George Neubert, M. A. Golden, and N. C. Rose, "Kasabach-Merritt coagulopathy complicating Klippel-Trenaunay-Weber syndrome in pregnancy," *Obstetrics & Gynecology*, vol. 85, no. 5, pp. 831–833, 1995.

[11] S. E. Horbach, M. M. Lokhorst, C. E. Oduber, S. Middeldorp, J. A. van der Post, and C. M. van der Horst, "Complications of pregnancy and labour in women with Klippel–Trénaunay syndrome: a nationwide cross-sectional study," *BJOG: An International Journal of Obstetrics & Gynaecology*, vol. 124, no. 11, pp. 1780–1788, 2017.

[12] A. J. Whelan, M. S. Watson, F. D. Porter, and R. D. Steiner, "Klippel-Trenaunay-Weber syndrome associated with a 5:11 balanced translocation," *American Journal of Medical Genetics*, vol. 59, no. 4, pp. 492–494, 1995.

[13] G. E. Aelvoet, P. G. Jorens, and L. M. Roelen, "Genetic aspects of the Klippel-Trenaunay syndrome," *Annals of Surgery*, vol. 202, pp. 624–627, 1985.

[14] M. P. Sperandeo, P. Ungaro, M. Vernucci et al., "Relaxation of insulin-like growth factor 2 imprinting and discordant methylation at KvDMR1 in two first cousins affected by Beckwith-Wiedemann and Klippel-Trenaunay-Weber syndromes," *American Journal of Human Genetics*, vol. 66, no. 3, pp. 841–847, 2000.

[15] C. G. Hatjis, A. G. Philip, G. G. Anderson, and L. I. Mann, "The in utero ultrasonographic appearance of Klippel-Trenaunay-Weber syndrome," *American Journal of Obstetrics & Gynecology*, vol. 139, no. 8, pp. 972–974, 1981.

[16] J. M. Warhit, M. A. Goldman, L. Sachs, L. M. Weiss, and H. Pek, "Klippel-Trenaunay-Weber syndrome: Appearance in utero," *Journal of Ultrasound in Medicine*, vol. 2, no. 11, pp. 515–518, 1983.

[17] R. V. Roberts, J. E. Dickinson, P. J. Hugo, and A. Barker, "Prenatal sonographic appearances of Klippel-Trenaunay-Weber syndrome," *Prenatal Diagnosis*, vol. 19, no. 4, pp. 369–371, 1999.

[18] Z. Mor, P. Schreyer, Z. Wainraub, E. Hayman, and E. Caspi, "Non-immune hydrops fetalis associated with angioosteohypertrophy (Klippel-Trenaunay) syndrome," *American Journal of Obstetrics & Gynecology*, vol. 159, no. 5, pp. 1185–1186, 1988.

[19] J. A. Drose, D. Thickman, J. Wiggins, and A. B. Haverkamp, "Fetal echocardiographic findings in the Klippel-Trenaunay-Weber syndrome," *Journal of Ultrasound in Medicine*, vol. 10, no. 9, pp. 525–527, 1991.

[20] G. Fait, Y. Daniel, M. Kupfenninc, I. Gull, M. Peyser, and J. Lessing, "Case report: Klippel-Trenaunay-Weber syndrome associated with fetal growth restriction," *Human Reproduction*, vol. 11, no. 11, pp. 2544–2545, 1996.

[21] W. L. Martin, K. M. Ismail, V. Brace, L. McPherson, S. Chapman, and M. D. Kilby, "Klippel-Trenaunay-Weber (KTW) syndrome: the use ofin utero magnetic resonance imaging (MRI) in

a prospective diagnosis," *Prenatal Diagnosis*, vol. 21, no. 4, pp. 311–313, 2001.

[22] M. J. Sivaprakasam and J. A. Dolak, "Anesthetic and obstetric considerations in a parturient with Klippel-Trenaunay syndrome," *Canadian Journal of Anesthesia*, vol. 53, no. 5, pp. 487–491, 2006.

[23] T.-H. Han, J. Brimacombe, E.-J. Lee, and H.-S. Yang, "The laryngeal mask airway is effective (and probably safe) in selected healthy parturients for elective Cesarean section: a prospective study of 1067 cases," *Canadian Journal of Anesthesia*, vol. 48, no. 11, pp. 1117–1121, 2001.

[24] R. N. Pollack, D. R. Quance, and R. M. Shatz, "Pregnancy complicated by the Klippel-Trenaunay syndrome. A case report," *The Journal of Reproductive Medicine*, vol. 40, no. 3, pp. 240–242, 1995.

34

Oncogenic Potential and Clinical Implications of Giant Endometrial Polyps: A Case Report and Literature Review

Brittany van Staalduinen,[1,2] **Andrew Stahler,**[1,2] **Catherine Abied,**[1,2]
Rita Shats,[1] **and Nisha A. Lakhi**[1,2]

[1]*Department of Obstetrics and Gynecology, Richmond University Medical Center, 355 Bard Avenue, Staten Island, NY 10310, USA*
[2]*Department of Obstetrics and Gynecology, New York Medical College, Valhalla, New York, USA*

Correspondence should be addressed to Nisha A. Lakhi; nlakhi@yahoo.com

Academic Editor: Julio Rosa-e-Silva

Endometrial polyps exceeding 4 centimeters in length are exceedingly rare and are termed "giant polyps." We describe two patients that presented to our hospital with giant endometrial polyps. Clinical implications and oncologic potential of giant endometrial polyps are discussed. Risk factors of oncologic transformation include advanced age, menopausal status, obesity, diabetes, arterial hypertension, use of tamoxifen, and size greater than 1.0 centimeter. A literature review of all documented cases of giant endometrial polyps is presented and management strategies for counseling and polypectomy are reviewed.

1. Introduction

Endometrial polyps are localized overgrowths of the endometrial lining of the uterus. Microscopically, they are composed of varying amounts of glandular tissue, stroma, and blood vessels covered by an epithelium. Their size can range from a few millimeters to beyond 5 centimeters in length. Endometrial polyps larger than 1 cm are termed "large polyps," and those that are greater than 4 cm, which are exceedingly rare, are called "giant polyps" [1].

The exact incidence of endometrial polyps is unknown; however, in women with dysfunctional uterine bleeding, the prevalence of endometrial polyps ranges from 10% to 24% [2]. 10% to 25% of symptomatic polyps may contain hyperplastic foci and malignant transformation has been observed in about 0 to 12.9% [2]. Although evidence in the literature defining factors linked to malignant transformation is contradictory, advanced age, menopausal status, obesity, diabetes, arterial hypertension, and use of tamoxifen have reached statistical significance in varying reports [3–5]. Additionally, polyp size has been found to be a predictive factor. B. P. Lasmar and R. B. Lasmar [6] found that endometrial polyps larger than 1.5 cm were associated with hyperplasia, while a separate report by Wang et al. [3] identified that

polyps measuring more than 1.0 cm were associated with malignancy.

We describe two patients that presented to our hospital with giant endometrial polyps and present a literature review of other similar cases. The oncogenic potential of large polyps is evaluated and evidence-based management strategies are discussed.

2. Case Series

2.1. Case #1. FM is a 70-year-old postmenopausal black female who presented with a chief complaint of intermittent vaginal spotting since the age of 50. She had not sought gynecologic care for several years. FM reported two episodes of vaginal spotting over the previous year, each lasting approximately one week in duration. Otherwise, she was asymptomatic and denied any recent intercourse or trauma to the vaginal area. Her past medical history was significant for poorly controlled hypertension, poorly controlled type 2 diabetes mellitus, osteoarthritis, angina, vitamin D deficiency, and glaucoma. She reported a long history of normal Pap smears over the course of her life and had one full-term normal spontaneous vaginal delivery. Family history

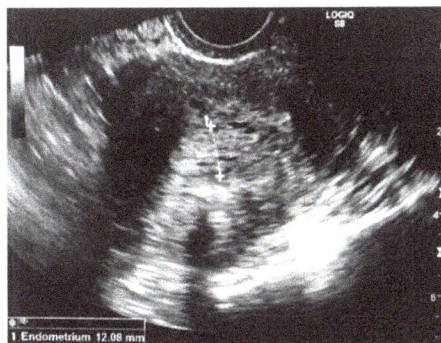

FIGURE 1: Ultrasound imaging of uterus demonstrating a 12.1 mm endometrial stripe.

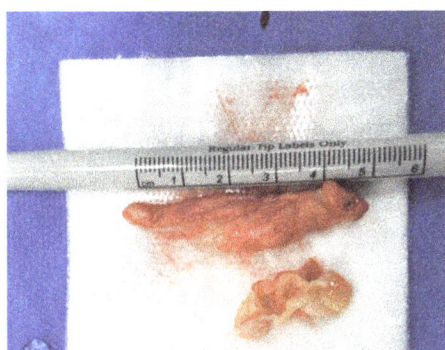

FIGURE 2: Gross specimen of polyp from case #1.

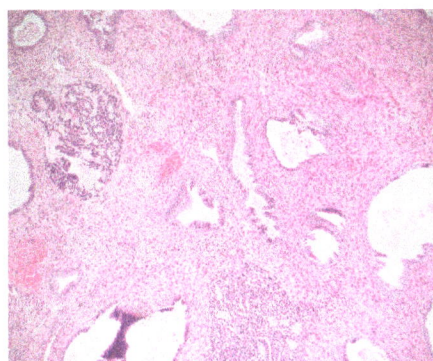

FIGURE 3: Microscopic section of polyp from case #1. H&E stain, demonstrating inactive endometrium, few glands, fibrotic stroma, and dilated, thick-walled blood vessels.

was significant for breast cancer in her mother at the age of 60 years. She denied any family history of uterine cancer, colon cancer, or ovarian cancer.

On initial evaluation, FM was alert and oriented and well nourished, with a body mass index (BMI) of $28 \, \text{kg/m}^2$. On physical examination, her vaginal mucosa was atrophic. A 1 cm polyp that originated from the endometrial cavity was found to be protruding from the cervical os and was friable to the touch. On bimanual exam, the uterus was anteverted, smooth, and mobile without palpable adnexal masses. Transvaginal ultrasound confirmed an anteverted uterus measuring 9.1×5.2×7.1 cm with a thickened, heterogeneous endometrial echo measuring 12.1 mm with multiple cystic small spaces (Figure 1). A vascular signal was seen throughout the thickened endometrium and a partially calcified leiomyoma in the left uterine body was also noted. An endometrial biopsy was obtained and showed rare superficial fragments of inactive endometrial tissue. Due to postmenopausal bleeding, the patient was booked for operative hysteroscopy, dilation and curettage, and polypectomy. On hysteroscopy, a large polyp was seen arising from the anterior uterine wall. Using operative hysteroscopy and hysteroscopic scissors, this polyp, measuring 5.3 cm in greatest dimension, was removed in its entirety (Figure 2). Endometrial curettage was performed after complete removal of the polyp. Final pathology showed inactive endometrium without evidence of hyperplasia (Figure 3). At the two-week postoperative visit, FM reported complete resolution of her symptoms.

2.2. Case #2. HA is a 66-year-old obese postmenopausal Hispanic female who presented with a chief complaint of intermittent vaginal spotting of a duration of eight months. Past medical history was significant for poorly controlled hypertension, aortic stenosis, hypercholesterolemia, and glaucoma. She reported a history of normal Pap smears throughout her life, the last one being one month prior to presentation. She had two full-term vaginal deliveries and one cesarean delivery. HA denied any significant family history of malignancy. On initial examination, she was noted to be alert and oriented and was obese with a BMI of $39.5 \, \text{kg/m}^2$. The external genitalia appeared normal and without lesions. A polyp was seen protruding 2 cm from the cervical os. On bimanual exam, the uterus was noted to be mobile, anteverted, and smooth, with no palpable adnexal masses. Transvaginal ultrasound revealed a 9.6 × 5.9 × 5.7 cm uterus with endometrial lining measuring 20 mm with small cystic appearing areas (Figure 4). Due to the large polyp protruding from the cervical os, the patient was booked for operative hysteroscopy, dilation and curettage, and polypectomy. The polyp was grasped with forceps and removed from its base prior to the hysteroscope being introduced to the uterine cavity. The polyp measured 8 cm in its greatest dimension. Hysteroscopy revealed areas of polypoid tissue which were removed under direct visualization (Figure 5). Endometrial

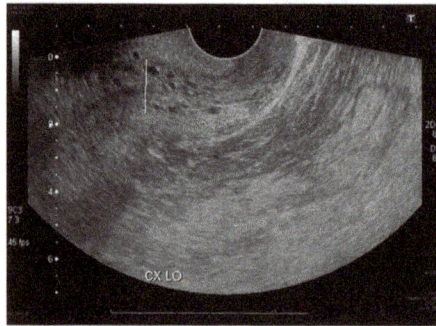

FIGURE 4: Ultrasound imaging of uterus demonstrating endometrial lining measuring 20 mm containing small cystic appearing areas.

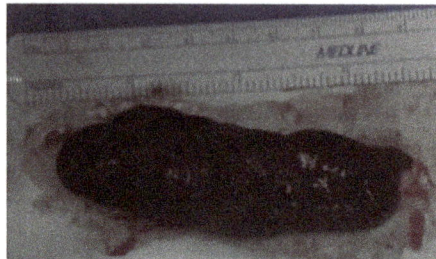

FIGURE 5: Gross specimen of polyp from case #2.

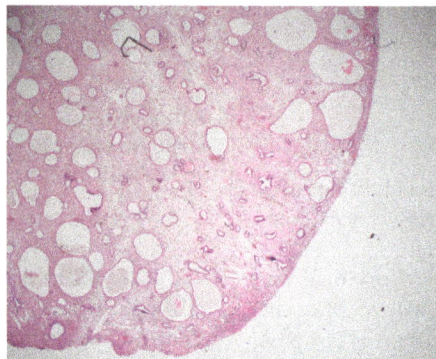

FIGURE 6: Microscopic section of polyp from case #2. H&E stain, low-power photomicrographs showing intact polypoid tissue cystic dilated glands without evidence of hyperplasia, fibrotic stroma, and dilated thick-walled vessels.

curettage was then performed. Final pathology revealed inactive endometrium with no hyperplasia or atypia (Figure 6). At her two-week postoperative visit, she reported a resolution of her symptoms.

3. Discussion

Endometrial polyps are found in both premenopausal and postmenopausal women. Patients may either be asymptomatic at the time of diagnosis or present with abnormal bleeding patterns, including intermenstrual bleeding, menorrhagia, or postmenopausal bleeding [1]. The exact cause of endometrial polyps is unknown, but estrogenic activity appears to play a crucial role in their pathogenesis and growth [2]. Several molecular mechanisms have been proposed to play a role in the development of endometrial

polyps. These include overexpression of endometrial aromatase, unbalanced activity between estrogen and progestin, inhibition of apoptosis, certain gene mutations that favor endometrial proliferation, and cellular mechanisms linked with inflammation [3, 4].

Previous case series indicate that malignancy occurs within 0% to 12.9% of endometrial polyps [4]. Although there is no consensus in the literature on the exact risk factors that are associated with malignant transformation of polyps, most authors agree that the risk of malignancy is increased with age and menopausal status and with the presence of symptomatic bleeding [1, 2]. Larger endometrial polyps also have been shown to be a risk factor for premalignant or malignant pathology, with authors advocating a cut-off point of 1.0 to 1.8 cm diameter as a risk factor [3–6].

Wang et al. retrospectively reviewed consecutive cases of patients that underwent hysteroscopic removal of an endometrial polyp and correlated malignant and premalignant lesions to clinical risk factors [3]. Of the 766 patients, polyps were histologically benign (no atypia) in 96.21% of patients, hyperplasia with atypia was identified in 3.26% of cases, and invasive endometrial carcinoma was present in only 0.52% of patients. Independent variables that were significantly related to premalignant and malignant polyps included polyp diameter greater than 1.0 cm, menopausal status, and abnormal uterine bleeding. In this report, hypertension, diabetes mellitus, body mass index, and use of tamoxifen were not found to be associated with the malignant transformation of polyps [3].

Ferrazzi et al. compared the prevalence of hyperplasia and malignancy in endometrial polyps among a cohort of 1,552 asymptomatic postmenopausal patients in comparison to a similar cohort of 770 postmenopausal patients that presented with abnormal uterine bleeding [15]. The prevalence of atypical hyperplastic polyps was 1.2% in asymptomatic versus 2.2% in symptomatic patients ($P < .005$). One single case of stage 1 grade 1 endometrial carcinoma was recorded within a polyp with a mean diameter 4 cm in an asymptomatic patient. After multivariate analysis, diameter of the polyps was the only variable significantly associated with an abnormal histology (malignancy and atypical hyperplasia) in asymptomatic women with an odds ratio of 6.9 (confidence interval: 2.2–21.4) for polyps with mean diameter > 1.8 cm [15].

Similarly, another retrospective review of 1,136 asymptomatic women that underwent hysteroscopic resection of an endometrial polyp found that polyps with diameters greater than 1.5 cm had hyperplasia rates of 14.8% compared with 7.7% in the group with smaller polyps ($P < 0.5$) [6]. Comparable to the above findings, Ben-Aire et al. assessed 430 women with endometrial polyps undergoing hysteroscopic resection and found hyperplasia without atypia in 11.4% of cases, hyperplasia with atypia in 3.3% of cases, and malignant conditions in 3.0% of cases [5]. Older age, menopause status, and polyps larger than 1.5 cm were associated with significant premalignant or malignant changes [8]. Interestingly, the presence of postmenopausal or irregular vaginal bleeding was not a predictor of malignancy in this study [8].

Giant endometrial polyps larger than 4 cm in diameter are exceedingly rare. Table 1 summarizes the management and outcomes of reported cases of giant endometrial polyps in the literature. The mean age of patients with giant endometrial polyps was 66.6 years (range: 55–70). All of the reported patients were postmenopausal. The most common presenting symptom was vaginal bleeding. Of the reported cases, 58% (7/12) were in association with use of a phytoestrogen or selective estrogen receptor modulators such as tamoxifen or raloxifene. In the report by Unal et al., the authors state that the patient consumed a large amount of thyme, a known phytoestrogen [13]. The six highest estrogen binding herbs are soy, licorice, red clover, thyme, turmeric hops, and *Verbena* [13].

Although not on exogenous drugs, the patient described by Narin et al. had several risk factors similar to our patients, including obesity, older age, and hypertension [10]. The

patient described by Meena et al. did not present with postmenopausal bleeding and did not use hormones. However, she had several risk factors including postmenopausal status, obesity, diabetes mellitus, and hypertension. Similarly, the patient in the case by Unal et al. did not report vaginal bleeding; her polyp was discovered by an incidental CT scan for complaints of lower back pain. Demographic details were not provided in the report by Çil et al.; however, the patient was of older age [1]. In addition to their menopausal status, both of our patients have medical comorbidities that may be risk factors for malignant transformation of polyps including hypertension, obesity, and type 2 diabetes mellitus. It is interesting to note that 8 of the 12 patients described were of Turkish or Mediterranean origin. It is possible that there are genetic, dietary, or ethnic factors related to the development of large polyps; however, with such a small incidence and limited reporting, no conclusions can be inferred.

The rationale for removing polyps is to exclude malignancy and to relieve symptomatic vaginal bleeding. Management of small asymptomatic polyps may be conservative with follow-up. However, conservative management should be undertaken with caution in postmenopausal patients, patients with any risk factors, or those with polyps measuring greater than 1.0–1.5 cm in size, as there is increased risk for atypical hyperplasia or malignancy [7, 15]. Risk factors for malignancy differ among reports and populations; however, larger size, advanced age, menopausal status, obesity, diabetes, arterial hypertension, and tamoxifen use have been associated with malignancy.

Hysteroscopic polypectomy remains the mainstay of evaluation and operative management of endometrial polyps as the associated morbidity is minimal when compared to a hysterectomy. Operative hysteroscopy allows for visualization of the entire uterine cavity. There are a variety of methods practiced to remove polyps at hysteroscopy (sharp scissors, electrosurgical techniques); however, there are no comparative studies for these methods with regard to efficacy. Therefore, the method of choice should be one that is most familiar to the surgeon. Regardless of which method is employed, removal of the entire polyp, including complete excision of the polyp stalk, should be achieved. Studies have indicated that removal of endometrial polyps by blind curettage is unsuccessful in more than 50% of attempts, and, in many cases, the removal is incomplete [4]. Therefore, blind curettage should not be used as a diagnostic or therapeutic intervention [4]. If malignancy is found within the polyp, the patient should be referred to a gynecological oncology specialist for further staging and management.

It should be emphasized that the clinical implications and oncogenic potential of large and giant endometrial polyps are still unclear in the literature. Information is currently derived from small studies, case series, and case reports. The pathogenesis of endometrial polyps as well as factors leading to oncogenesis is still being elucidated. Therefore, with these limitations in knowledge, caution should be taken when counseling patients that present with large or giant endometrial polyps.

TABLE 1: Summary of reported cases of giant endometrial polyps.

Report	Patient age	Polyp size (cm)	Associated drugs	Management	Pathology
Çil et al. [1] Malatya, Turkey	73	$8 \times 4 \times 3$	No	Hysteroscopic polypectomy	No hyperplasia, atypia, or malignancy
Moon et al. Busan, Republic of Korea [7]	58	$7.5 \times 5.5 \times 2.6$	Tamoxifen	Total abdominal hysterectomy	No hyperplasia, atypia, or malignancy
Nomikos et al. [8] Piraeus, Greece	74	Diameter 8 cm	Tamoxifen	Total abdominal hysterectomy	Complex hyperplasia with atypia
Kutuk and Goksedef [9] Amasya, Turkey	63	$4.5 \times 4 \times 5.2$	Raloxifene	Polypectomy under ultrasound guidance	No hyperplasia, atypia, or malignancy
Narin et al. [10] Adana, Turkey	66	$12 \times 6 \times 5$	No	Total abdominal hysterectomy, BSO	No hyperplasia, atypia, or malignancy
Erdemoglu et al. [11] Isparta, Turkey	55	$10 \times 6 \times 3$	Tamoxifen	Extraction of mass under general anesthesia	No hyperplasia, atypia, or malignancy
Caschetto et al. [12] Catania, Italy	64	$9 \times 7 \times 4.5$	Tamoxifen	Total abdominal hysterectomy, BSO	Complex hyperplasia with atypia
	67	$8 \times 6 \times 3$	Tamoxifen	Total abdominal hysterectomy, BSO	Simple hyperplasia, no atypia
Ünal et al. [13] Antalya, Turkey	78	10×9	Phytoestrogens	Total abdominal hysterectomy	No hyperplasia, atypia, or malignancy
Meena et al. [14] Delhi, India	65	8.5×1.5	No	Hysteroscopic polypectomy	Cystic hyperplasia without atypia
van Staalduinen et al. New York, USA (index cases)	70	$9.1 \times 5.2 \times 7.1$	No	Hysteroscopic polypectomy	No hyperplasia, atypia, or malignancy
	66	$8 \times 6 \times 5$	No	Polypectomy/hysteroscopy	No hyperplasia, atypia, or malignancy

Consent

Consent was obtained for publication of case and images from both patients and can be provided on request.

References

[1] A. S. Çil, M. Bozkurt, D. Kara, and B. Guler, "Giant endometrial polyp protruding from the external cervical os in a postmenopausal woman: magnetic resonance imaging and hysteroscopic findings," *Proceedings in Obstetrics and Gynecology*, vol. 3, no. 3, p. 2, 2013.

[2] S. C. Lee, A. M. Kaunitz, L. Sanchez-Ramos, and R. M. Rhatigan, "The oncogenic potential of endometrial polyps: a systematic review and meta-analysis," *Obstetrics & Gynecology*, vol. 116, no. 5, pp. 1197–1205, 2010.

[3] J. Wang, J. Zhao, and J. Lin, "Opportunities and risk factors for premalignant and malignant transformation of endometrial polyps: management strategies," *Journal of Minimally Invasive Gynecology*, vol. 17, no. 1, pp. 53–58, 2010.

[4] A. Papadia, D. Gerbaldo, E. Fulcheri et al., "The risk of premalignant and malignant pathology in endometrial polyps: should every polyp be resected?" *Minerva Ginecologica*, vol. 59, no. 2, pp. 117–124, 2007.

[5] A. Ben-Arie, C. Goldchmit, Y. Laviv et al., "The malignant potential of endometrial polyps," *European Journal of Obstetrics & Gynecology and Reproductive Biology*, vol. 115, no. 2, pp. 206–210, 2004.

[6] B. P. Lasmar and R. B. Lasmar, "Endometrial polyp size and polyp hyperplasia," *International Journal of Gynecology and Obstetrics*, vol. 123, no. 3, pp. 236–239, 2013.

[7] S. H. Moon, S. E. Lee, I. K. Jung et al., "A giant endometrial polyp with tamoxifen therapy in postmenopausal woman," *Korean Journal of Obstetrics & Gynecology*, vol. 54, no. 12, pp. 836–840, 2011.

[8] I. N. Nomikos, J. Elemenoglou, and J. Papatheophanis, "Tamoxifen-induced endometrial polyp. A case report and review of the literature," *European Journal of Gynaecological Oncology*, vol. 19, no. 5, pp. 476–478, 1998.

[9] M. S. Kutuk and B. P. C. Goksedef, "A postmenopausal woman developed a giant endometrial polyp during Raloxifene treatment," *Journal of Obstetrics & Gynaecology*, vol. 31, no. 7, pp. 672-673, 2011.

[10] R. Narin, H. Nazik, H. Aytan, M. Api, H. Toyganözü, and F. Adamhasan, "A Giant Endometrial Polyp in a Postmenopausal Woman," *Journal of Obstetrics and Gynaecology Canada*, vol. 35, no. 2, p. 105, 2013.

[11] E. Erdemoglu, M. Güney, G. Take, S. G. Giray, and T. Mungan, "Tamoxifen and giant endometrial polyp," *European Journal of Gynaecological Oncology*, vol. 29, no. 2, pp. 375–379, 2008.

[12] S. Caschetto, N. Cassaro, P. Consalvo, and L. Caragliano, "Tamoxifen and Endometrial Megapolyps," *Minerva Ginecologica*, vol. 52, no. 11, pp. 459–463, 2000.

[13] B. Unal, S. Dogan, F. Ş. Karaveli, T. Simşek, G. Erdoğan, and I. Candaner, "Giant endometrial polyp in a postmenopausal woman without hormone/drug use and vaginal bleeding," *Case Reports in Obstetrics and Gynecology*, vol. 2014, Article ID 518398, 2014.

[14] J. Meena, R. Manchanda, S. Kulkarni, N. Bhargava, and P. Mahawar, "Story of a giant endometrial polyp in asymptomatic postmenopausal female," *Journal of Clinical and Diagnostic Research*, vol. 11, no. 3, pp. QD06–QD07, 2017.

[15] E. Ferrazzi, E. Zupi, F. P. Leone et al., "How often are endometrial polyps malignant in asymptomatic postmenopausal women? A multicenter study," *American Journal of Obstetrics & Gynecology*, vol. 200, no. 3, pp. 235.e1–235.e6, 2009.

35

Conservative Management of Abnormally Invasive Placenta Previa after Midtrimester Foetal Demise

A. MacGibbon ⓘ and Y. M. Ius

Department of Obstetrics and Gynaecology, John Hunter Hospital, Newcastle, New South Wales, Australia

Correspondence should be addressed to A. MacGibbon; andrew@macgibbons.co.nz

Academic Editor: Mehmet A. Osmanağaoğlu

We present the case of a midtrimester intrauterine foetal demise (IUFD) in the context of abnormally invasive placentation. This was a grade 4 placenta previa with placenta increta in a patient requesting fertility conservation and was managed conservatively without immediate surgical intervention. The patient spontaneously delivered the fetus after 33 days, followed by a large obstetric haemorrhage requiring immediate laparotomy and hysterotomy. Her uterus was preserved and she went on to recover without further significant complication. While conservative management of morbidly adherent placentas has been well documented, there are no published cases of this strategy in the context of IUFD and fertility preservation.

1. Introduction

A morbidly adherent placenta poses a significant morbidity and mortality risk to pregnant women, primarily due to major haemorrhage at time of delivery. This includes placenta accreta where the placenta attaches to the myometrium, increta where it penetrates through the myometrium, and percreta where it invades surrounding structures such as bladder or bowel. Generally, these cases are managed by elective caesarean hysterectomy due to the risks associated with attempted removal of the placenta alone. This comes with the unfortunate consequence of loss of fertility for the patient. Of particular interest, therefore, are any strategies that can safely and effectively manage both the major praevia and the morbidly adherent placenta while providing the opportunity to preserve the uterus.

Nonsurgical strategies have effectively preserved fertility in many cases [1–3]; however no studies have yet examined the safety and efficacy of this management strategy in the complicated context of foetal demise. We present the case of a midtrimester intrauterine foetal demise in a patient with a morbidly adherent placenta and grade 4 praevia.

2. Case Description

A 31-year-old gravida 3 para 1 patient presented to antenatal clinic at 19 weeks and 3 days' gestation to discuss the results of her morphology scan which had demonstrated a grade 4 placenta previa covering the cervical os. She had a medical history significant for Arnold Chiari malformation requiring craniotomy in 2006 as well as correction of a Syringomyelia in 2005. She also suffers from irritable bowel syndrome but was taking no regular medications and had a BMI of 23. Her first pregnancy resulted in a spontaneous miscarriage that did not require dilatation and curettage. Her second pregnancy resulted in a planned elective caesarean due to concerns about raised intracranial pressure during labour, as recommended by her neurologist. She had routine antenatal care this pregnancy which had been unremarkable to date.

The morphology scan demonstrated a small omphalocele but otherwise no significant structural defects and estimated foetal weight was noted to be within the normal range. During the clinic review, the fetus was found to have a heart rate well below 100 bpm. Repeat ultrasound the following day confirmed IUFD. This ultrasound also demonstrated evidence of an abnormally invasive placenta with the appearance of dysplastic vascular hypertrophy. An obstetric MRI was performed which supported the diagnosis of morbidly adherent placenta. This showed a low lying inhomogeneous placenta, dysplastic vascular hypertrophy, ill-defined placental bands, and an overall impression of some areas of increta with no overt evidence of percreta.

Options were discussed with the patient who decided for conservative management in order to optimise her chance of preserving her fertility. This was balanced against potential complications of prolonged conservative management of an IUFD, including sepsis and coagulopathy. A plan was made for serial ultrasounds as an outpatient, to be followed by induction of labour when placental blood flow was no longer detectable. Twenty-seven days following IUFD confirmation, the patient was admitted to hospital with abdominal cramping and associated small antepartum haemorrhage (APH).

Ultrasound scan at 31 days showed a minimal reduction in blood flow through the anterior placenta and to the cervix. At day 33 she suffered a further 300mL APH. Given her increasing blood loss and minimal changes to placental blood flow on ultrasound, she was administered a dose of 80mg methotrexate intramuscularly with the hope of accelerating devitalisation of the placenta. A repeat dose of methotrexate was planned for five days' time. During the subsequent two days after the administration of methotrexate, the patient continued to suffer moderate bleeds and increasingly significant contractions. 35 days following IUFD she spontaneously delivered a male fetus with only minimal bleeding during delivery.

A brisk 2 L postpartum haemorrhage (PPH) followed delivery and the patient was immediately taken to the operating theatre for examination under anaesthesia and attempted manual removal. A urinary indwelling catheter was inserted and remained in situ for the entirety of the operation. Due to only partial removal (approximately 80%) of the placenta being achieved manually, the case quickly progressed to laparotomy. Intraoperative findings revealed a full thickness increta at the previous caesarean incision just above the level of the bladder. Hysterotomy was performed with a transverse incision made above the prior caesarean incision, and the remaining placenta was removed manually, creating a 3x3cm plug-like defect anteriorly. This defect was closed with a primary closure separate to the hysterotomy incision. In addition, the placental bed was oversewn to establish haemostasis. A Foley's catheter was inserted vaginally and inflated with 60mL normal saline. Total blood loss was 4 litres (L): 2L immediately postpartum, 1L while attempting per vaginal manual removal of the placenta, and 1L intraoperatively. Massive transfusion protocol was activated with the patient receiving 10 units of packed red cells, 6 units of fresh frozen plasma and 5 units of cryoprecipitate. The patient remained stable throughout the process. A further 3 units of packed cells was given over the next two days for persistent anaemia. The fetus was found to weigh 170g. No cause for foetal demise was identified and the family decided against an autopsy. Pathological examination of the placenta was performed. This was noted to be difficult due to extensive haemorrhage and areas of necrosis commensurate

with intrauterine foetal death and prolonged intrauterine retention. There was no evidence of funisitis or umbilical cord vasculitis to support a diagnosis of chorioamnionitis nor were any pathogens observed. The degree of decidual haemorrhage and necrosis made a histological diagnosis of placenta accreta impossible.

The patient recovered without significant complication over the following days and was discharged 1 week later on oral antibiotics and aperients. Six weeks after discharge the patient was seen in a postnatal follow-up clinic. She experienced minimal lochia in the postpartum period and was feeling generally well.

3. Discussion

Generally foetal loss in the second or third trimester is managed by either dilatation and curettage or induction of labour depending on the gestation. However, in the case of a morbidly adherent placenta, this presents a large risk of uncontrollable haemorrhage. Furthermore placenta previa increases the risk of complications as a vaginal delivery requires the placenta to deliver prior to, or simultaneously with the fetus. In this uncommon and difficult clinical scenario, the morbidly adherent placenta previa blocks the delivery of the fetus through the cervical canal. The generally accepted management strategy for abnormally adherent placentation is caesarean hysterectomy [4, 5]. However, since the 1950s, conservative treatments have been described for accreta and increta with the aim of preserving the uterus and thereby the fertility of these women [6]. This often involves leaving the placenta in situ and waiting for devascularisation of the placental bed so that remaining placental tissue may either be more safely removed or resorb itself. While there is a high rate of recurrence of placenta accreta (17-29%), several studies have reported excellent fertility rates following conservative treatment [2, 3].

Treating an abnormally adherent placenta conservatively must be weighed against the risk of several associated complications. The most significant of these is ongoing bleeding or secondary postpartum haemorrhage. A third of women being treated conservatively are likely to suffer ongoing vaginal bleeding—in the study by Timmermans et al., 15% of such patients went on to require delayed hysterectomy [1]. In a study by Sentilhes et al., 42% of women required a blood transfusion while being managed conservatively and 15% required more than 5 units [7]. Infection is another concern, however it may be difficult to diagnose clinically due to fever being a result of tissue necrosis alone in some cases [1]. Endometritis was diagnosed in 18% of patients in the Timmermans study, 18% of whom required hysterectomy as a result [1]. It must be noted however that infection rates amongst women with an IUFD and no rupture of membranes may well be lower. A further well-documented concern amongst patients conservatively managing IUFD is that of disseminated intravascular coagulopathy (DIC). While waiting for an abnormally adherent placenta to devascularise or resorb can take several months [1, 7]; the risk of DIC is up to 10% within 4 weeks of foetal death and continues to increase after this time [8]. Weighing the risk of these complications against the immediate loss of fertility from hysterectomy without clear guidelines presents an ongoing challenge for clinicians.

3.1. Monitoring of These Patients. In this presented case, the patient was initially diagnosed with placenta increta using ultrasound and subsequently MRI. She was then monitored with serial ultrasound looking for devascularisation of the placental bed. Ultrasound is an effective imaging modality for diagnosing and monitoring placental invasion [1]. There has been no consistently demonstrated superiority in sensitivity or specificity of MRI over serial ultrasound in the diagnosis of morbidly adherent placenta. However, the use of both techniques may be useful to evaluate the extent of placental tissue invasion [5, 9]. HCG has previously been suggested as a method of monitoring placental vascular activity [10] but there are several documented cases of persistent vascularity despite undetectable HCG levels making it an unreliable marker [1].

3.2. Methotrexate. Since the 1980s methotrexate has been suggested as an adjuvant treatment during the observation period in order to target folate metabolism in the rapidly growing tissues of the trophoblast [11]. There is currently no clear evidence as to the benefit of methotrexate in conservative management of placenta accreta after delivery [12]. This has been attributed to limited or absent trophoblastic proliferation at term [13] and as such is not recommended by UK or American guidelines [4, 5]. In the case of IUFD or midtrimester miscarriage, however, the much higher rate of proliferation could make methotrexate a more effective treatment. Consideration must also be given to the adverse effects of methotrexate which range from nausea, headache, and fevers to nephrotoxicity and rarely severe myelosuppression that can be fatal [7].

3.3. Learnings from This Case. The aim of conservative management of abnormally invasive placentation is to allow the placenta time to devitalise and hopefully make removal less difficult. While this case resulted in a 4L PPH and surgical removal of the invasive placental tissue, the uterus was ultimately preserved. If delivery and removal of the placenta had been attempted at time of diagnosis bleeding from the placental bed may well have been more difficult to control leading to a hysterectomy. Both UK and American guidelines are clear that these women must be managed in a centre capable of rapid blood transfusions, with emergency operating theatres, experienced multidisciplinary surgeons, and intensive care [4, 5]. This is well supported by the outcome of this case. Other significant risks during the observation period include infection, ongoing bleeding, and DIC along with what may be a traumatic psychological experience for the woman [1, 14]. Placental vascularity has been shown to persist for months in some cases [1] and in many women; having a retained fetus for this length of time would not be acceptable. Despite these risks, conservative management will continue to be a desirable option for women wanting to preserve their fertility, particularly in the context of IUFD. With the number of

caesarean deliveries increasing worldwide, this complex clinical scenario is likely to become more common [15]. Further investigation into the best markers for placental vascularity and possible benefits of methotrexate in midtrimester loss would be helpful to develop an appropriate management protocol for these patients.

References

[1] S. Timmermans, A. C. van Hof, and J. J. Duvekot, "Conservative management of abnormally invasive placentation," *Obstetrical & Gynecological Survey*, vol. 62, no. 8, pp. 529–539, 2007.

[2] L. Sentilhes, G. Kayem, C. Ambroselli et al., "Fertility and pregnancy outcomes following conservative treatment for placenta accreta," *Human Reproduction*, vol. 25, no. 11, pp. 2803–2810, 2010.

[3] M. Alanis, B. S. Hurst, P. B. Marshburn, and M. L. Matthews, "Conservative management of placenta increta with selective arterial embolization preserves future fertility and results in a favorable outcome in subsequent pregnancies," *Fertility and Sterility*, vol. 86, no. 5, pp. 1514–e7, 2006.

[4] Royal College of Obstetricians and Gynaecologists, *Green-top guideline 27. Placenta praevia, placenta praevia accreta and vasa praevia: diagnosis and management*, Royal College of Obstetricians and Gynaecologists, London, UK, 2011.

[5] American College of Obstetricians and Gynecologists Committee on Obstetric Practice, "Committee Opinion No. 529: Placenta Accreta," *Obstetrics and Gynaecology*, vol. 120, no. 1, pp. 207–2011, 2012.

[6] R. P. McKeough and E. D'Errico, "Placenta accreta: clinical manifestations and conservative management," *The New England Journal of Medicine*, vol. 245, no. 5, pp. 159–165, 1951.

[7] L. Sentilhes, C. Ambroselli, and G. Kayem, "Maternal outcome after conservative treatment of placenta accreta," *Obstetrics Gynaecology*, vol. 115, no. 3, pp. 526–534, 2010.

[8] H. Parasnis, B. Raje, and I. N. Hinduja, "Relevance of plasma fibrinogen estimation in obstetric complications," *Journal of Postgraduate Medicine*, vol. 38, no. 4, pp. 183–185, 1992.

[9] B. K. Dwyer, V. Belogolovkin, L. Tran et al., "Prenatal diagnosis of placenta accreta: Sonography or magnetic resonance imaging?" *Journal of Ultrasound in Medicine*, vol. 27, no. 9, pp. 1275–1281, 2008.

[10] N. Matsumura, T. Inoue, M. Fukuoka, N. Sagawa, and S. Fujii, "Changes in the serum levels of human chorionic gonadotropin and the pulsatility index of uterine arteries during conservative management of retained adherent placenta," *Journal of Obstetrics and Gynaecology Research*, vol. 26, no. 2, pp. 81–87, 2000.

[11] S. Arulkumaran, C. S. A. Ng, I. Ingemarsson, and S. S. Ratnam, "Medical Treatment of Placenta Accreta with Methotrexate," *Acta Obstetricia et Gynecologica Scandinavica*, vol. 65, no. 3, pp. 285–286, 1986.

[12] K. Lin, J. Qin, K. Xu, W. Hu, and J. Lin, "Methotrexate management for placenta accreta: a prospective study," *Archives of Gynecology and Obstetrics*, vol. 291, no. 6, pp. 1259–1264, 2015.

[13] M. Winick, A. Coscia, and A. Noble, "Cellular growth in human placenta. I. Normal placental growth," *Pediatrics*, vol. 39, no. 2, pp. 248–251, 1967.

[14] I. Radestad, G. Steineck, B. Sjogren, and C. Nordin, "Psycholog-
      ical complications after stillbirth—influence of memories and
      immediate management: Population based study," *BMJ*, vol. 312,
      no. 7045, pp. 1505–1508, 1996.

[15] D. A. Miller, J. A. Chollet, and T. M. Goodwin, "Clinical risk fac-
      tors for placenta previa-placenta accreta," *American Journal of
      Obstetrics & Gynecology*, vol. 177, no. 1, pp. 210–214, 1997.

36

Prenatal Diagnosis of a Segmental Small Bowel Volvulus with Threatened Premature Labor

Barbara Monard,[1] Nicolas Mottet,[1] Rajeev Ramanah,[1,2] and Didier Riethmuller[1,2]

[1]Obstetrics and Gynecology Department, Besancon University Medical Center,
 3 boulevard Alexandre Fleming, 25000 Besancon, France
[2]University of Franche-Comte, Hauts de Chazal, 19 rue Ambroise Paré, 25000 Besancon, France

Correspondence should be addressed to Barbara Monard; monard.barbara@gmail.com

Academic Editor: Svein Rasmussen

Fetal primary small bowel volvulus is extremely rare but represents a serious life-threatening condition needing emergency neonatal surgical management to avoid severe digestive consequences. We report a case of primary small bowel volvulus with meconium peritonitis prenatally diagnosed at 27 weeks and 4 days of gestation during threatened premature labor with reduced fetal movements. Ultrasound showed a small bowel mildly dilated with thickened and hyperechogenic intestinal wall, with a typical whirlpool configuration. Normal fetal development allowed continuation of pregnancy with ultrasound follow-up. Induction of labor was decided at 37 weeks and 2 days of gestation because of a significant aggravation of intestinal dilatation appearing more extensive with peritoneal calcifications leading to the suspicion of meconium peritonitis, associated with reduced fetal movements and reduced fetal heart rate variability, for neonatal surgical management with a good outcome.

1. Introduction

Intestinal volvulus is a serious life-threatening disease and it can cause severe digestive consequences in children. Prenatal diagnosis is very difficult because its occurrence is rare and its nonspecific clinical signs are variable. Intestinal volvulus is commonly associated with malrotation or atresia. A primary small bowel volvulus is extremely rare. Prenatal diagnosis enables appropriate surgical management immediately after birth and improves neonatal outcome. We report a case of prenatally diagnosed primary small bowel volvulus with meconium peritonitis at 27 weeks and 4 days of gestation during threatened premature labor with a good outcome.

2. Case Report

A 30-year-old primiparous woman was seen at our hospital for preterm contractions for seven days with reduced fetal movements at 27 weeks and 4 days of gestation. A threatened premature labor was diagnosed. Ultrasound showed a female fetus with normal development and amniotic fluid volume.

Small bowel appeared mildly dilated (14 mm) with thickened and hyperechogenic intestinal wall. There was a typical whirlpool configuration of the bowel (Figure 1). First and second trimester ultrasounds were unremarkable. Screening for infectious diseases was negative. A molecular genetic testing of CFTR was realized in the parents who were tested for the 32 main mutations of CFTR during a genetic counseling. This testing was negative in both of the parents. So, the fetus was not screened for cystic fibrosis. The patient received atosiban for tocolysis and steroids for fetal lung maturation. Ultrasound follow-up one week later and every two weeks showed absence of significant modification in small bowel dilatation and normal fetal development and amniotic fluid volume up to 33 weeks and 1 day of gestation when a peritoneal calcification appeared leading to the suspicion of meconium peritonitis. Fetal biometry measures including the abdominal circumference and amniotic fluid volume were normal throughout the follow-up in antepartum period. Ultrasound follow-up at 36 weeks and 4 days of gestation revealed a significant aggravation of intestinal dilatation (30 mm) appearing more extensively with persistent intestinal

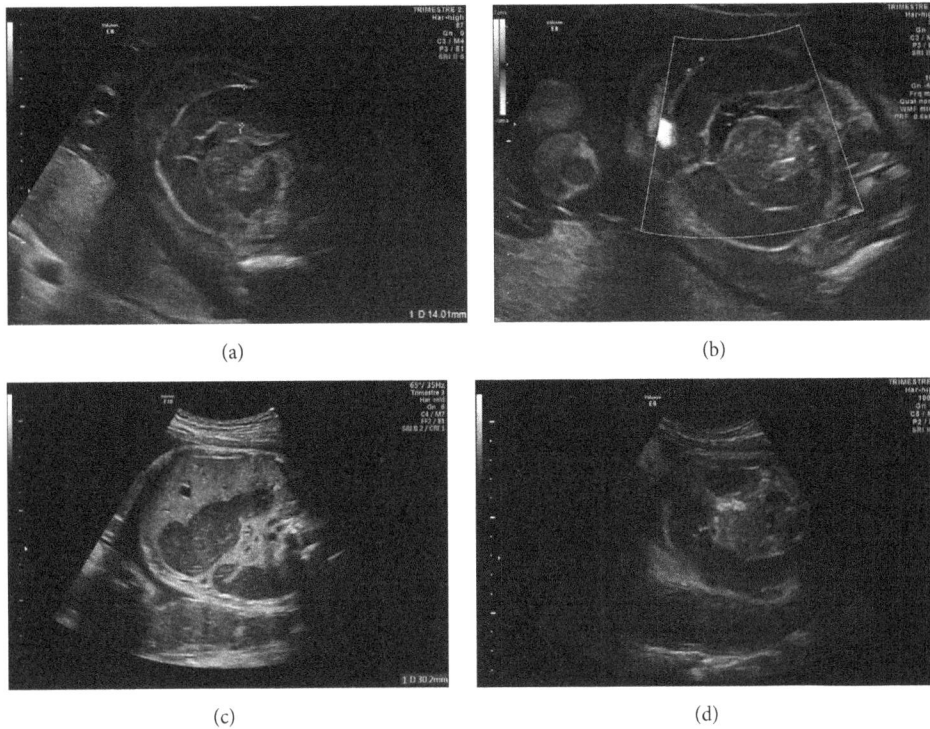

FIGURE 1: Mildly dilated small bowel with thickened and hyperechogenic intestinal wall (a) in a typical whirlpool configuration (a, b). Aggravation of intestinal dilatation (c) and peritoneal calcifications leading to the suspicion of meconium peritonitis (d).

peristalsis, and some parietal calcifications appeared with a meconium pseudocyst but there were no ascites (Figure 1). Fetal vitality was good with a satisfying Manning's score; there were neither ascites nor significant increasing in abdominal circumference nor abnormality in fetal heart rate and the amniotic fluid volume was normal. So, the patient was hospitalized for close monitoring of fetal heart rate. After consultation with members of pediatric surgery team, induction of labor was decided at 37 weeks and 2 days of gestation given the worsening ultrasound images associated with reduced fetal movements and reduced fetal heart rate variability for neonatal surgical management. Furthermore, the patient had a favorable Bishop score of 6 on clinical examination. A 2,470 g girl was born vaginally with vacuum assistance at 37 weeks and 2 days of gestation, with Apgar scores of 3, 7, and 10 at 1, 3, and 5 minutes, respectively. The neonate was ventilated for three minutes after birth with good neonatal adaptation. She received a nasogastric tube and was immediately hospitalized in pediatric intensive care unit. Her vital and biological parameters were normal except for hemoglobin. The newborn was mildly anemic with a hemoglobin level of 15 g/dl. She had neither hyperthermia nor biological inflammatory syndrome (leukocyte count = 12,0 $\times 10^9$/l, CRP < 2,9 mg/l). Clinical examination showed no abnormality with an abdomen soft and painless on palpation but slightly distended. The postnatal plain abdominal X-ray showed a voluminous dilated bowel loop (Figure 2). The water-soluble contrast enema revealed a vacuous colon in normal position, a caecum in the right iliac fossa, and an opacification of a few centimeters of the last ileal loop

(Figure 2). A right transverse laparotomy was performed the day after birth and revealed a segmental small bowel volvulus with a perforated meconium pseudocyst secondary to in utero perforation of distal ileum and a type II small bowel atresia five centimeters above ileocaecal valve (Figure 3). The residual length of small bowel was sufficient with 100 cm above atresia and 4 cm below atresia. No microbiological test has been performed during surgery because there was no sign of extensive inflammation. The meconium pseudocyst, the volvulus loop, and 16 cm of very dilated and unstressed small bowel were resected. The diameter of the loop below atresia was much smaller but ileocaecal valve was permeable. Given the significant difference in the diameter of the two loops, the distal loop was opened on its antimesenteric side to realize a termino-terminal ileoileal anastomosis more congruent without perioperative complication (Figure 3). Immediate postoperative care was simple. Recovery of bowel movements occurred two days after surgery and a normal diet with breast milk was started three days after surgery. The Guthrie (neonatal heel prick) test was negative. The anatomopathological examination revealed peritonitis signs on the serosa and the mesentery of the surgical specimens in the form of more or less voluminous calcifications. Moreover, there was panparietal ischemic necrosis of the mucosa and all other layers of the intestinal wall. Finally, there was diffuse vascular congestion and stigma of intraparietal hemorrhage. A satisfying weight curve permitted her return home thirteen days after surgery. One year after surgery, feeding and bowel movements were normal with a good growth. She did not suffer from short bowel syndrome.

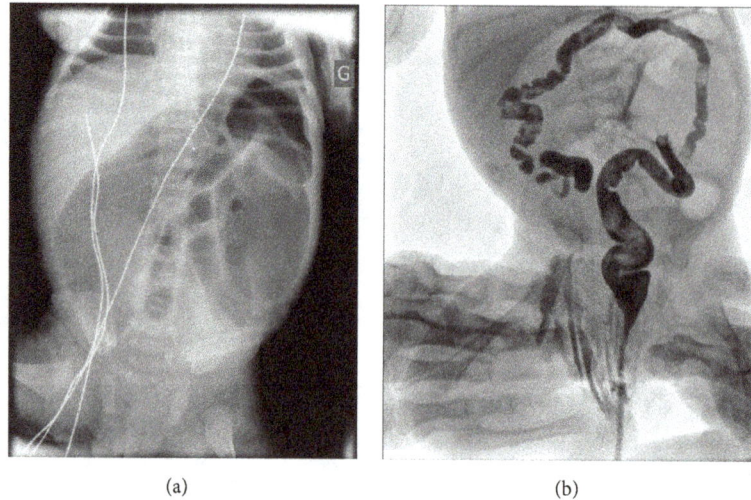

FIGURE 2: Postnatal plain abdominal X-ray showing a voluminous dilated bowel loop (a). Water-soluble contrast enema with opacification of a few centimeters of the last ileal loop (b).

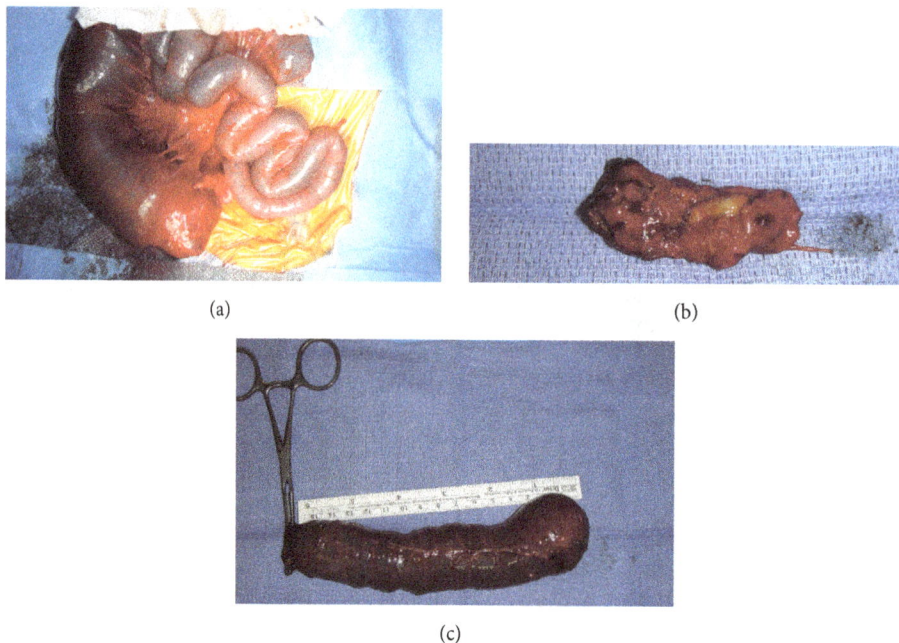

FIGURE 3: Small bowel atresia with dilated small bowel five centimeters above ileocaecal valve (a). Volvulus loop resected (b) and 16 cm of dilated small bowel resected (c).

3. Discussion

Fetal intestinal volvulus is rare and several modes of diagnosis are described in the literature. It can be diagnosed during a routine ultrasound [1] or if the patient presents clinical signs. The most common signs are reduced fetal movements and fetal heart rate abnormalities [2–7]. Another symptom frequently described in the literature is the presence of uterine contractions with or without associated threatened premature labor [8, 9]. De Felice et al. proposed an explanation of relationship between intrauterine midgut volvulus and preterm delivery. Acute fetal stress would activate both the fetal-placental adrenal and hypothalamic stress hormones, leading to premature uterine activity and preterm delivery [10]. Many of these symptoms led to prenatal diagnosis in our case report.

Prenatal ultrasound signs commonly described in the literature are polyhydramnios, hyperechogenic and dilated bowel loop, typical whirlpool sign, fetal ascites, peritoneal calcifications, and meconium peritonitis with stopped, persistent, or intensive intestinal peristalsis [1–9, 11–13]. In our case, we showed small bowel dilatation with thickened and hyperechogenic intestinal wall and there was a typical whirlpool configuration of the bowel at diagnosis. During the ultrasound follow-up, peritoneal calcifications appeared and led to suspect a meconium peritonitis. Amniotic fluid volume was normal and intestinal peristalsis was persistent.

Despite a significant aggravation of intestinal dilatation at 36 weeks and 4 days of gestation, we decided to continue pregnancy. Indeed, recurrence of intestinal dilatation if isolated was not a sufficient argument to justify premature birth. There was no other ultrasound sign of poor prognosis; fetal vitality was good with a satisfying Manning's score; there were neither ascites nor significant increasing in abdominal circumference nor abnormality in fetal heart rate. Moreover, the gestational age of birth in these children is determinant in postnatal evolution. In our team, planned vaginal delivery is considered in fetuses with gastrointestinal malformations if there is no major abnormality in fetal heart rate.

In all the cases of intestinal volvulus described in the literature, an early neonatal laparotomy was performed with intestinal resection and either termino-terminal anastomosis at the same time [1, 3, 14–17] or temporary enterostomy with secondary restoration of intestinal continuity [4, 6, 11, 18–20]. According to Raherison et al., ileostomy seems to be the best option in case of intestinal perforation or necrosis, or if there is atresia associated with peritonitis, because of a high risk of anastomotic leaks in an inflammatory or septic context. A resection with anastomosis at the same time can be performed if necrosis is restricted without peritonitis [14]. However, if there is a complete ischemic damage, simple detorsion and closing without pressure followed by a secondary reevaluation seem to be the best choice to limit intestinal resection in case of partial recovery seen during reevaluation [3, 13]. In our case, we performed an intestinal resection with termino-terminal anastomosis at the same time because there was no sign of extensive inflammation, without postoperative complication.

Intestinal volvulus and atresia often coexist [7, 14, 15]. When intestinal volvulus occurs in utero and is complicated with ischemic necrosis, secondary intestinal atresia can appear [7, 13, 14]. Primary intestinal atresia can be complicated with volvulus because of an increased peristalsis within dilated bowel close to atresia [14, 15]. According to Raherison et al., volvulus would be secondary when there is a 180- or 360-degree torsion of a dilated bowel loop above atresia, and volvulus would be primary leading to ischemia and atresia below the volvulus intestinal loop when a necrotic intestinal portion is located in the aplomb of atresia [3, 14]. This latter explanation seems to be the most probable hypothesis in our case report.

Despite a few cases of neonates with postoperative short bowel syndrome [11, 13], long-term prognosis was good overall with normal growth and feeding [1, 4, 6, 11, 13–16, 18, 20].

4. Conclusion

Prenatal small bowel volvulus should be suspected in case of reduced fetal movements associated with small bowel dilatation with or without polyhydramnios, especially if there are abnormalities in fetal heart rate or in a context of threatened premature labor. It is a life-threatening condition

requiring an emergency neonatal surgical management with a good prognosis and a survival rate greater than 95% in case of isolated abnormality. Therefore, its early detection is important to provide for ultrasound follow-up and to reduce its morbidity and mortality. The outcome depends on the amount of residual bowel and the gestational age at the time of the event. It is a third trimester condition, when fetal lung maturity is sufficient. However, there is no prenatal imaging for assessing the risk of short bowel syndrome.

References

[1] S.-J. Yoo, K. W. Park, S. Y. Cho, J. S. Sim, and K. S. Hhan, "Definitive diagnosis of intestinal volvulus in utero," *Ultrasound in Obstetrics & Gynecology*, vol. 13, no. 3, pp. 200–203, 1999.

[2] J. J. Terzibachian, J. D. Shu, G. Levy, O. Destuynder, G. Agnani, and J. Daucourt, "Prenatal diagnosis of a small intestinal volvulus," *J Gynécologie Obstétrique Biol Reprod*, vol. 24, no. 8, Article ID 83942, 1995.

[3] K. Miyakoshi, M. Tanaka, T. Miyazaki, and Y. Yoshimura, "Prenatal ultrasound diagnosis of small-bowel torsion," *Obstet Gynecol*, vol. 91, no. 5, part 2, article 8023, 1998.

[4] K. Miyakoshi, H. Ishimoto, S. Tanigaki et al., "Prenatal diagnosis of midgut volvulus by sonography and magnetic resonance imaging," *American Journal of Perinatology*, vol. 18, no. 8, pp. 447–450, 2001.

[5] B. Uerpairojkit, D. Charoenvidhya, S. Tanawattanacharoen, S. Manotaya, T. Wacharaprechanont, and Y. Tannirandorn, "Fetal intestinal volvulus: A clinico-sonographic finding," *Ultrasound in Obstetrics & Gynecology*, vol. 18, no. 2, pp. 186-187, 2001.

[6] R. N. Sammour, Z. Leibovitz, S. Degani, I. Shapiro, and G. Ohel, "Prenatal diagnosis of small-bowel volvulus using 3-dimensional Doppler sonography," *Journal of Ultrasound in Medicine*, vol. 27, no. 11, pp. 1655–1661, 2008.

[7] J. H. Chung, G.-Y. Lim, and J. S. We, "Fetal primary small bowel volvulus in a child without intestinal malrotation," *Journal of Pediatric Surgery*, vol. 48, no. 7, pp. e1–e5, 2013.

[8] Y. Yilmaz, G. Demirel, H. O. Ulu, I. H. Celik, O. Erdeve, S. S. Oguz et al., "Urgent surgical management of a prenatally diagnosed midgut volvulus with malrotation," *European Review for Medical and Pharmacological Sciences*, vol. 16, supplement 4, article 524, 2012.

[9] Z. F. Takacs, C. M. Meier, E.-F. Solomayer, L. Gortner, and G. Meyberg-Solomayer, "Prenatal diagnosis and management of an intestinal volvulus with meconium ileus and peritonitis," *Archives of Gynecology and Obstetrics*, vol. 290, no. 2, pp. 385–387, 2014.

[10] C. De Felice, C. Massafra, G. Centini, G. Di Maggio, G. Tota, and R. Bracci, "Relationship between intrauterine midgut volvulus without malrotation and preterm delivery [1]," *Acta Obstetricia et Gynecologica Scandinavica*, vol. 76, no. 4, p. 386, 1997.

[11] R. Has and S. Gunay, "'Whirlpool' sign in the prenatal diagnosis of intestinal volvulus [4]," *Ultrasound in Obstetrics & Gynecology*, vol. 20, no. 3, pp. 307-308, 2002.

[12] M. G. Mercado, D. I. Bulas, and R. Chandra, "Prenatal diagnosis and management of congenital volvulus," *Pediatric Radiology*, vol. 23, no. 8, pp. 601-602, 1993.

[13] N. Samuel, D. Dicker, D. Feldberg, and J. A. Goldman, "Ultrasound diagnosis and management of fetal intestinal obstruction and volvulus in utero," *J Perinat Med*, vol. 12, article 3337, no. 6, 1984.

[14] R. Raherison, C. Grosos, J. Lemale et al., "Prenatal intestinal volvulus: a life-threatening event with good long-term outcome," *Archives de Pédiatrie*, vol. 19, no. 4, pp. 361–367, 2012.

[15] L. V. Baxi, M. N. Yeh, W. A. Blanc, and J. N. Schullinger, "Antepartum diagnosis and management of in utero intestinal volvulus with perforation," *The New England Journal of Medicine*, vol. 308, no. 25, pp. 1519–1521, 1983.

[16] S. Jéquier, S. Hanquinet, P. Bugmann, and M. Pfizenmaier, "Antenatal small-bowell volvulus without malrotation: Ultrasound demonstration and discussion of pathogenesis," *Pediatric Radiology*, vol. 33, no. 4, pp. 263–265, 2003.

[17] A. Weissman and I. Goldstein, "Prenatal sonographic diagnosis and clinical management of small bowel obstruction," *American Journal of Perinatology*, vol. 10, no. 3, pp. 215-216, 1993.

[18] R. Heydanus, M. C. Spaargaren, and J. W. Wladimiroff, "Prenatal ultrasonic diagnosis of obstructive bowel disease: A retrospective analysis," *Prenatal Diagnosis*, vol. 14, no. 11, pp. 1035–1041, 1994.

[19] F. Bargy and S. Beaudoin, "Urgences chirurgicales du nouveauné et du nourrisson," *Pédiatrie - Maladies Infectieuses*, 2006, http://www.em-consulte.com/article/38685/urgences-chirurgicales-du-nouveau-né-et-du-.

[20] A. Pierro and E. Ong, "Malrotation," in *Pediatric surgery*, P. Puri and M. E. Höllwarth, Eds., Springer, Berlin, Germany, 2006.

37

Facilitation of Vaginal Delivery in an Infant with Complete Heart Block Secondary to Maternal Anti-Ro Antibodies

E. Thornton,[1] L. Tripathi,[2] S. Shebani,[3] I. Bruce,[4] and L. Byrd[5]

[1]ST1 Obstetrics and Gynaecology, Royal Bolton Hospital, Bolton, UK
[2]North Manchester General Hospital, Manchester, UK
[3]Glenfield Hospital, Leicester, UK
[4]Department of Rheumatology, Manchester Royal Infirmary, Manchester, UK
[5]St Mary's Hospital, Manchester, UK

Correspondence should be addressed to E. Thornton; emmathornton@doctors.org.uk

Academic Editor: Irene Hoesli

Congenital heart block (CHB) is a rare disorder that may be associated with a high morbidity and even mortality, with a risk of death both in utero and during infancy. Women with serum titres of anti-Ro and/or anti-La antibodies carry a risk of CHB of 1–5% in their offspring, with a recurrence risk of approximately 20%. We present a case of a 36-year-old female with a pregnancy complicated by congenital heart block. Autoimmune profiling at booking showed she was positive for lupus anticoagulant and anti-Ro antibodies. A fetal echocardiogram at 21 + 3 showed complete heart block. She was monitored throughout the remainder of her pregnancy with serial growth scans, cardiovascular profiling, and BPP scoring. She had a normal vaginal delivery at term to a female infant.

1. Background

Congenital heart block (CHB) is a rare disorder with an incidence of 1 in 22,000 live births [1]. It may be associated with high morbidity and even mortality (15–30%) with a risk of death both in utero and during infancy, particularly if the heart is structurally abnormal. As many as 67% of survivors require permanent cardiac pacing. Women with serum titres of anti-Ro and/or anti-La antibodies carry a risk of CHB of 1–5% in their offspring, with a recurrence risk of approximately 20%. The condition carries not only neonatal risks but a burden of maternal risk with approximately 50% of mothers developing obstetric complications [2].

2. Case Report

Mrs. N is a 36-year-old with G 4 P3 booked at 7-week gestation and viability and EDD of 10/3/10 confirmed by ultrasound scan. She had a history of Sjogren's Syndrome and postpartum DVT and was positive for lupus anticoagulant and anti-Ro antibodies. This pregnancy was managed in the multidisciplinary joint Obstetric and Haematology Clinic and Low Molecular Weight Heparin (LMWH) was commenced at presentation.

An anomaly scan at 20 weeks was unremarkable and a fetal echocardiogram confirmed a structurally normal heart with a normal PR interval (see Figures 1 and 2). Unfortunately 10 days later a repeat scan confirmed complete heart block, with a ventricular rate of 65 bpm (see Figure 3). There were no fetal hydrops or any evidence of heart failure. The couple was counselled regarding the potentially poor outcome and possible risk of fetal death in utero. A plan was agreed to assess fetal cardiac function every week throughout the remainder of the pregnancy. Dexamethasone was given (4 mg daily) the following week as the scan suggested incomplete 2:1 block. However, two weeks later complete heart block was reconfirmed and dexamethasone was then discontinued. Its use would however be reconsidered if cardiac failure ensued.

Mode of delivery was initially discussed at 28 weeks and agreed at 36 weeks gestation. Given her parity and history of quick labours the aim was to avoid surgery. Serial growth scans confirmed a fetal AC on the 50th centile, with good

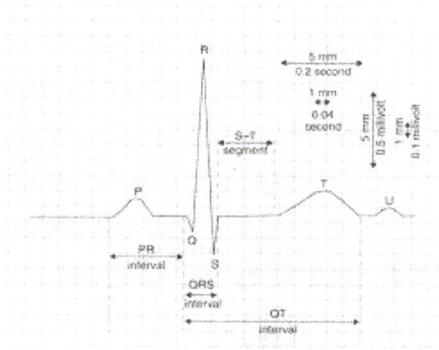

FIGURE 1: Normal electrical PR (ePR) interval on surface ECG as a guide.

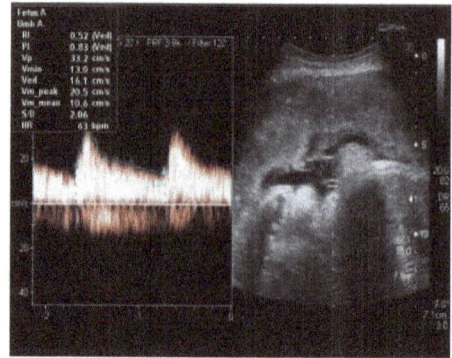

FIGURE 2: Normal mechanical PR interval (mPR) 10 days earlier in our case; fetal cardiac Doppler sampling the mitral inflow to aortic outflow.

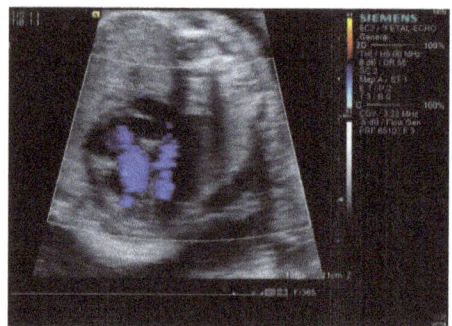

FIGURE 3: Complete heart block.

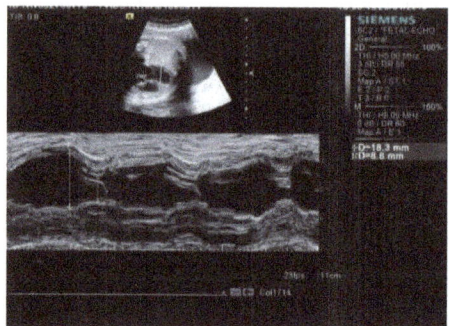

FIGURE 4: (Umbilical artery Doppler. Good EDF, PI 0.83).

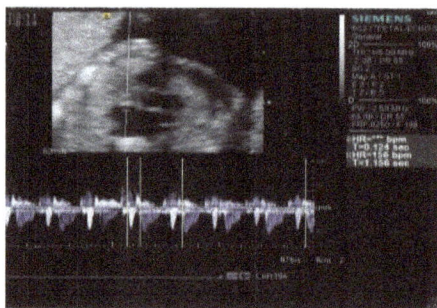

FIGURE 5: (No atrioventricular regurgitation. No cardiomegaly).

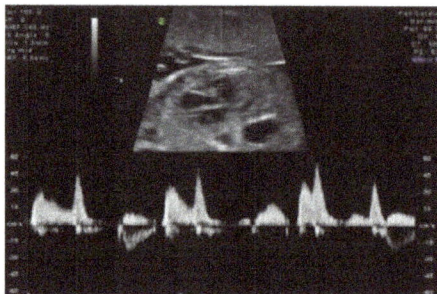

FIGURE 6: Preserved ventricular contractility (indicated by Fractional Shortening of 52%).

growth velocity. Umbilical artery Doppler showed good end diastolic flow and a pulsatility index of 0.83 (Figure 4). Cardiac function, CVP score (see discussion), was maintained throughout (Figures 5 and 6), with a ventricular rate between 65 and 75 bpm. Biophysical Profile (BPP) was assessed from 36 weeks. Good fetal movements were regularly reported by mum. Intermittent auscultation +/− FBS if required, was to be used in labour.

At term a membrane sweep was offered and Mrs. N was admitted to hospital (at her request) 24 hours later with mild tightening. A BPP during the latent phase of labour was reassuring. Labour established later the same day, progressing rapidly to a spontaneous vaginal delivery of a female infant weighing 3.02 kg with Apgars of 9 at 1 and 5 minutes. She was transferred to SCBU for assessment and observation. An ECG

confirmed complete heart block, and an echocardiogram reaffirmed good cardiac function despite a ventricular rate of 55 bpm. She established demand feeding over the next 48–72 hours without compromise and was discharged home with mum within the week. Although she remains under review, at the time of Mrs. N's postnatal review in the JOHC her daughter was thriving and had not required cardiac pacing.

3. Discussion

At approximately 12 weeks of gestation maternal IgG antibodies against Ro and La intracellular ribonuclear protein are *actively transferred* across the placenta. These are thought to bind to specific cells within the fetal conducting system, resulting in inflammation, scarring, and/or fibrosis. With this in mind Saxena et al. (2015) [3] showed an elevation in cord blood inflammatory markers including CRP and NT-ProBNP in infants who subsequently developed neonatal lupus syndrome.

Whilst CHB is the main cardiac manifestation in infants exposed to anti-Ro/La antibodies other pathologies (to include cardiomyopathy and/or valvular heart disease) also occur [4].

Mortality from heart disease unfortunately remains high with the majority of deaths occurring in utero or early infancy [5] secondary to CHB [6]. Risk factors for poor outcome include presence of structural heart disease, hydrops fetalis, low heart rate (<55 bpm), prematurity, and/or male gender.

Whilst fluorinated steroids, like dexamethasone, can cross the placenta and may treat first or second degree heart block, they have no benefit in third degree heart block which is considered complete and irreversible [7]. A secondary role in improving cardiac function in those fetuses in utero with heart failure has also been considered [8] but robust data is lacking and therefore a pragmatic approach is required as maternal use of dexamethasone is, of course, not without risks. These include the glucocorticoid associated risks of increased infection, loss of bone density, diabetes, hypertension, and cataracts. The fetal risks of maternal steroids include oligohydramnios, intrauterine growth retardation, and adrenal suppression. There is also some suggestion of a risk to the developing fetal brain when exposed to steroids [9].

Based on the assumption that treatment for identified heart block in utero may be effective if it can reduce a generalized inflammatory insult and lower the titre of maternal autoantibodies, several prenatal therapeutic protocols have been utilized. All women at risk with antibodies present should be closely followed during the pregnancy with serial echocardiograms, specifically looking for the earliest signs of conduction system disease such as PR interval prolongation by Doppler (see later discussion). If complete heart block is recently diagnosed (within three weeks of onset), a therapeutic course of dexamethasone 4 mg orally once a day may be tried.

Prenatal dexamethasone may have a role in preventing late onset cardiomyopathy, which frequently requires pacing; however, this viewpoint is far from universal [10]. By contrast a more consistent preventative approach is the use of maternal hydroxychloroquine in high risk pregnancies, though further study is required [11].

It has hitherto been suggested that all women at risk of fetal cardiac disease because of a previous history and/or high positive antibodies should be followed up with serial echocardiograms specifically looking for any prolongation in the PR interval. Nevertheless it has subsequently been established that the onset of CHB is far from predictable and measurement of the mechanical PR interval lacks sensitivity (44%) and/or specificity (88%). Whilst it may be useful in diagnosis, it has no role in prediction or prognosis. However, the electrical PR interval (whilst not available at the time of this case) is proving to be more useful (sensitivity 66%, specificity 96% [12]).

In our patient, Mrs. N, the changes in the degree of heart block was sudden and unpredictable. However, regular/frequent surveillance permitted prompt recognition which was then amenable to steroid therapy; despite this no benefit was achieved as therapy did not reverse the heart block. This agrees with outcome data from larger data sets. Prenatal dexamethasone would appear to have a role in the prevention of cardiomyopathy necessitating frequent cardiac pacing.

For those infants that survive pregnancy the main dilemma is then how to deliver. Continuous CTG is not possible and there is concern that the fetal heart in heart block does not have the capacity to withstand the demands of labour. The BPP is a 10-point fetal assessment tool first described by Manning et al. [9] in 1980. It evaluates fetal breathing, movement, tone, reactivity, and amniotic fluid volume and has been shown to correlate with fetal asphyxia, acidosis, and poor outcome. However, as the most sensitive marker of acidosis is the heart rate component which clearly cannot be assessed in cases of CHB, the BPP is then less than ideal in this situation. With this in mind Donofrio et al. [13] in 2004 utilised a Cardiovascular Profile (CVP) score, originally described by Huhta in 2001 [14] to assess cardiac function, since its introduction CVP scoring has also become valuable in evaluating the prognosis of hydrops when seen on echocardiography [15]. The score subtracts points for the presence of abnormal signs to include hydrops (late sign), venous pulsations, umbilical artery Doppler, cardiac enlargement, and atrioventricular valve regurgitation. To be used effectively the CVP score should be interpreted in consideration with the underlying disease pathology, for example, distinguishing between overload, myocardial disease, and arrhythmias [16]. A similar approach was adopted here. In CVP assessment in CHB then

(i) umbilical venous pulsation is only scored when noted to be at the atrial rate;

(ii) intermittent holosystolic tricuspid and/or mitral regurgitation is normal in CHB and therefore not scored;

(iii) diastolic AV valve regurgitation is low, common, and not scored;

(iv) small effusion can be seen secondary to inflammation and should therefore be scored.

Excellent cardiac function was maintained throughout pregnancy (CVP score 10/10) and vaginal delivery, at term, of a female infant, was achieved.

4. Conclusion

With the advances in the ultrasound technology the prenatal diagnosis of autoimmune CHB has become standard care in most institutions. Fetal echocardiogram with measurement of the mechanical PR interval would not predict but will allow earlier diagnosis of heart block and/or the possibility of very early treatment, which may be able to reverse the disease [12].

On the other hand electrical PR reproducibility, sensitivity, and specificity are superior, which, if available, would be the diagnostic tool of choice to use in any trial to investigate both the natural history and therapy of conduction abnormalities in Ro/La pregnancies.

What really made a difference is that this case was the consistently reassuring high CVP score through cardiothoracic ratio, atrioventricular valve regurgitation fraction shortening, absence of hydrops, and normal fetal umbilical Doppler.

Disclosure

An earlier version of this work was presented as a poster at Arch Dis Fetal Neonatal Ed in 2013.

References

[1] N. J. Kertesz, A. L. Fenrich, and R. A. Friedman, "Congenital complete atrioventricular block," *Texas Heart Institute Journal*, vol. 24, no. 4, pp. 301–307, 1997.

[2] I. M. Jakobsen, R. B. Helmig, and K. Stengaard-Pedersen, "Maternal and foetal outcomes in pregnant systemic lupus erythematosus patients: An incident cohort from a stable referral population followed during 1990-2010," *Scandinavian Journal of Rheumatology*, vol. 44, no. 5, pp. 377–384, 2015.

[3] A. Saxena, P. M. Izmirly, S. W. Han et al., "Serum Biomarkers of Inflammation, Fibrosis, and Cardiac Function in Facilitating Diagnosis, Prognosis, and Treatment of Anti-SSA/Ro-Associated Cardiac Neonatal Lupus," *Journal of the American College of Cardiology*, vol. 66, no. 8, Article ID 21508, pp. 930–939, 2015.

[4] P. Brito-Zerón, P. M. Izmirly, M. Ramos-Casals, J. P. Buyon, and M. A. Khamashta, "Autoimmune congenital heart block: Complex and unusual situations," *Lupus*, vol. 25, no. 2, pp. 116–128, 2016.

[5] E. T. Jaeggi, R. M. Hamilton, E. D. Silverman, S. A. Zamora, and L. K. Hornberger, "Outcome of children with fetal, neonatal or childhood diagnosis of isolated congenital atrioventricular block: A single institution's experience of 30 years," *Journal of the American College of Cardiology*, vol. 39, no. 1, pp. 130–137, 2002.

[6] M. Dey, T. Jose, A. Shrivastava, R. D. Wadhwa, R. Agarwal, and V. Nair, "Complete congenital foetal heart block: a case report," *Facts, Views & Vision in ObGyn*, vol. 6, no. 1, pp. 39–42, 2014.

[7] Carolis S. D., Salvi S., Botta A. et al., "Which Intrauterine Treatment for Autoimmune Congenital Heart Block?" *Open Autoimmunity Journal*, vol. 2, pp. 1–10, 2010.

[8] D. M. Friedman, A. Rupel, J. Glickstein, and J. P. Buyon, "Congenital heart block in neonatal lupus: The pediatric cardiologist's perspective," *The Indian Journal of Pediatrics*, vol. 69, no. 6, pp. 517–522, 2002.

[9] F. A. Manning, L. D. Platt, and L. Sipos, "Antepartum fetal evaluation: Development of a fetal biophysical profile," *American Journal of Obstetrics & Gynecology*, vol. 136, no. 6, pp. 787–795, 1980.

[10] K. Shinohara, S. Miyagawa, T. Fujita, T. Aono, and K.-I. Kldoguchi, "Neonatal lupus erythematosus: Results of maternal corticosteroid therapy," *Obstetrics & Gynecology*, vol. 93, no. 6, pp. 952–957, 1999.

[11] N. Costedoat-Chalumeau, Z. Amoura, D. Le Thi Hong et al., "Questions about dexamethasone use for the prevention of anti-SSA related congenital heart block," *Annals of the Rheumatic Diseases*, vol. 62, no. 10, pp. 1010–1012, 2003.

[12] H. M. Gardiner, C. Belmar, L. Pasquini et al., "Fetal ECG: A novel predictor of atrioventricular block in anti-Ro positive pregnancies," *Heart*, vol. 93, no. 11, pp. 1454–1460, 2007.

[13] M. T. Donofrio, S. D. Gullquist, I. D. Mehta, and W. B. Moskowitz, "Congenital complete heart block: Fetal management protocol, review of the literature, and report of the smallest succesful pacemaker implantation," *Journal of Perinatology*, vol. 24, no. 2, pp. 112–117, 2004.

[14] J. C. Huhta, "Right ventricular function in the human fetus," *Journal of Perinatal Medicine*, vol. 29, no. 5, pp. 381–389, 2001.

[15] J. C. Huhta, "Diagnosis and treatment of foetal heart failure: Foetal echocardiography and foetal hydrops," *Cardiology in the Young*, vol. 25, no. 2, pp. 100–106, 2015.

[16] V. Thakur, J. Fouron, L. Mertens, and E. T. Jaeggi, "Diagnosis and management of fetal heart failure," *Canadian Journal of Cardiology*, vol. 29, no. 7, pp. 759–767, 2013.

38

A Triple Obstetric Challenge of Thoracopagus-Type Conjoined Twins, Eclampsia, and Obstructed Labor: A Case Report from Sub-Saharan Africa

Mariatu Binta Leigh,[1,2] Valerie John-Cole,[1] Mike Kamara,[1]
Alimamy Philip Koroma,[1] Michael Momoh Koroma,[3] Edward Ejiro Emuveyan,[1,4]
Peter Bramlage,[2] and Ivo Buschmann[2]

[1]Department of Obstetrics and Gynecology, Princess Christian Maternity Hospital (PCMH), University Teaching Hospitals Complex, University of Sierra Leone, Freetown, Sierra Leone
[2]Center for Internal Medicine I, Department for Angiology, Medical School Brandenburg Theodor Fontane (MHB), Campus Brandenburg, Brandenburg, Germany
[3]Department of Anesthesia, Princess Christian Maternity Hospital (PCMH), University Teaching Hospitals Complex, University of Sierra Leone, Freetown, Sierra Leone
[4]Department of Obstetrics and Gynecology, College of Medicine, University of Lagos, Akoka, Lagos, Nigeria

Correspondence should be addressed to Mariatu Binta Leigh; leigh@esvm.eu

Academic Editor: Giovanni Monni

Conjoined twins are very rarely seen. We present a case of thoracopagus that was undiagnosed prior to delivery and combined with eclampsia and obstructed labor in a low-resource setting in sub-Saharan Africa. A 27-year-old pregnant woman was presented to the maternity emergency unit of Princess Christian Maternity Hospital (PCMH) in Freetown at term in labor. Upon admission, the patient was awake and orientated and presented a blood pressure of 180/120 mmHg and a protein value of 3+ on urine dipstick test. Clinical examination—ultrasound was not available—led to the admission diagnosis: obstructed labor with intrauterine fetal death and preeclampsia. Application of Hydralazine 5 mg (i.v.) under close blood pressure monitoring was performed. Under spontaneous progression of labor, one head of the yet unknown conjoined twin was born. The patient developed eclamptic fits. Ceasing of seizures was achieved after implementing the loading dose of the $MgSO_4$ protocol. A vaginal examination led to the unexpected diagnosis of conjoined twins. An emergency cesarean section under general anesthesia via a longitudinal midline incision was performed immediately. The born head was repositioned vaginally. The stillborn conjoined twins presented a female thoracopagus type that seemed to involve the heart. After 8 weeks, the woman was clinically fully recovered.

1. Introduction

Conjoined twins represent one of the rarest forms of twin gestation. They are always identical and occur in about 1 in every 200 sets of monozygotic twin pregnancies. The estimated overall incidence ranges from 1 in 50,000 to 1 in 250,000 live births [1–3]. However, about 40–60% of the cases are stillborn [2, 3].

Conjoined twins are suggested to result from aberrant embryogenesis in monozygotic twins. Two main theories are being proposed. In the fission theory, it is speculated that the origin of conjoined twins is an incomplete division of a single zygote at the primitive streak stage of the embryonic plate (15–17 days) [4]. In the fusion theory, it is proposed that a fertilized egg completely separates; however, stem cells lead to the fusion of both embryos [4, 5]. Importantly *high maternal and fetal risks* are present in all these conjoined twin cases, and even under the best of circumstances good outcomes for mother and both babies are rarely achieved. Considering termination of pregnancy might be the ultimate choice [6–8].

Preeclampsia is a pregnancy-associated disorder characterized by high blood pressure and significant proteinuria after 20 weeks of gestation. Eclampsia is a hypertensive disorder in pregnancy combined with convulsions [9].

Among the risk factors for hypertensive disorders are preexistent hypertension, existence of antiphospholipid syndrome or other coagulopathies, occurrence of certain biochemical markers such as the soluble fms-like tyrosine kinase-1 (sFlt-1)/placental growth factor (PLGF) ratio, status of primigravida, past obstetric history of preeclampsia, twin pregnancy, ethnicity, and low socioeconomic status.

The incidence of preeclampsia and related hypertensive disorders of pregnancy ranges from 2 to 5% for the United States, Canada, and Western Europe [10, 11], whereas in so-called developing countries, hypertensive disorders of pregnancy have the huge impact of 4–18% of all deliveries [10, 11]. The variation in incidence rates is due to the diversity of definitions, tests, and their methodologies and the differences in healthcare standards in the various African countries [10]. In fact, severe preeclampsia and eclampsia remain a significant public health threat in both developed and developing countries. They are accountable for 12% of all maternal deaths worldwide, which represent the third leading cause of maternal mortality and equal 76,000 women who die in childbirth every year [12]. 99% of all maternal deaths occur in so-called developing countries [13].

Apart from maternal mortality, hypertensive disorders in pregnancy have considerable adverse impacts on maternal, fetal, and neonatal health.

Early diagnosis, close prenatal management, and the choice of proper route of delivery will determine the best possible outcomes in both pathologies, respectively. In the present article, we are reporting a case of thoracopagus that was undiagnosed prior to delivery and combined with eclampsia and obstructed labor in Freetown, Sierra Leone, a low-resource country in sub-Saharan Africa.

2. Case Presentation

We report the case of a 27-year-old pregnant woman, gravida 3 para 2, who was presented to the maternity emergency unit of Princess Christian Maternity Hospital (PCMH) in Freetown at term in labor. The patient was referred from a health center for prolonged labor and arrest of descent at complete cervical dilatation despite being in active labor for the past 9 hours. She was an illiterate street trader. In terms of past obstetric history, there was a spontaneous vaginal delivery (SVD) at term of a healthy live born boy and a fresh stillbirth at term for an unknown reason. During this present pregnancy, she did not make any antenatal care visit. Therefore, blood pressure levels during pregnancy were undocumented and no obstetric ultrasound examination was performed. Her last menstrual date was unknown. Other relevant risk factors, such as gestational diabetes and infectious diseases, were also not known or documented.

Upon admission, the patient was awake and orientated and presented the following vital signs: blood pressure of 180/120 mmHg and a protein value of 3+ on urine dipstick

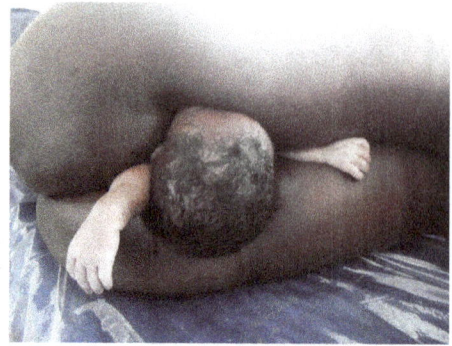

FIGURE 1: One head and two arms born.

test. Clinical examination revealed anasarca and hyperreflexia and a gravid abdomen with assumed term pregnancy and assumed singleton. The cervix was fully dilated with dystocia of labor; the presentation was cephalic. On auscultation with Pinard stethoscope, fetal heartbeat was absent. Ultrasound was not available. The findings led to the admission diagnosis of "obstructed labor with intrauterine fetal death (IUFD) and preeclampsia."

The patient was admitted to the eclamptic ward to be stabilized, and application of Hydralazine 5 mg (i.v.) every 20 minutes under close blood pressure monitoring was performed.

Under spontaneous progression of labor (no application of oxytocin), the patient was transferred to the labor ward, where one head of the yet unknown conjoined twin was born. Even though blood pressure was controlled (140/95 mmHg), the patient developed eclamptic fits. Ceasing of seizures was achieved after implementing the loading dose of the $MgSO_4$ protocol [14].

The consultant obstetrician was now involved, and a new clinical assessment revealed a somnolent patient that was now stable, reflexes were low, and the blood pressure was controlled: 140/95 mmHg. The fundal height corresponded to term; there were no adequate contractions, and the fetal heart was absent. On vaginal examination, the presentation was left occiput posterior with stuck fetal head and a turtleneck phenomenon. With regard to the unknown presence of conjoined twins, the diagnosis of obstructed labor (suspicion of shoulder dystocia) and IUFD was confirmed and eclampsia was added. In an attempt to deliver the shoulders, manual extraction of both arms was performed as follows: reaching up along the dorsal shoulder blade, sweeping the humerus down, and thereby bringing the left arm out of the vagina. The same procedure was performed at the anterior shoulder for the right arm (Figure 1). Since shoulders were still not following and due to the unordinary presentation of the fetus, a second deep vaginal examination along the fetus' back was done, and further membranes were discovered. This led to the sudden and unexpected diagnosis of conjoined twins.

An emergency cesarean section under general anesthesia via a longitudinal midline incision was performed immediately. The fetus was extracted by breech, whilst the born head was repositioned vaginally by a midwife (Figure 2). External

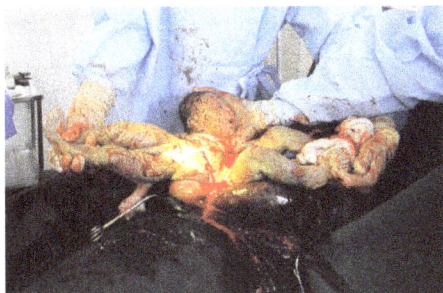

FIGURE 2: Surgery site during cesarean section.

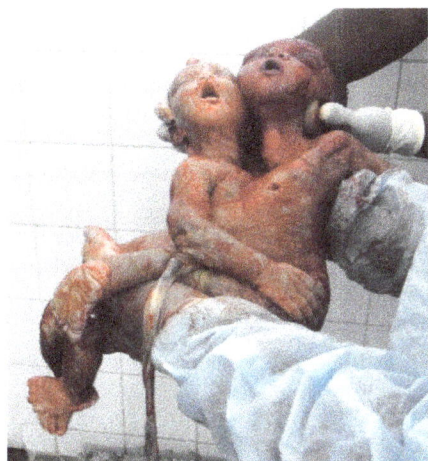

FIGURE 3: Stillborn thoracopagus-type conjoined twins.

inspection of the conjoined twins after surgery revealed a female thoracopagus type that seemed to involve the heart (Figure 3). Apgar score (Appearance, Pulse, Grimace, Activity, and Respiration) was 0/0/0, and pH was generally not available. The gestational age was estimated to be about 37–39 weeks of gestation.

The $MgSO_4$ protocol was maintained further for 48 hours, and the antihypertensive therapy was continued with Hydralazine and later changed to 3×20 mg Nifedipine orally. The patient was kept under close monitoring of blood pressure, reflexes, respiration rate, and input-output evaluation.

During the postpartum period, there was no reappearance of seizures, and the anasarca disappeared fully. In the absence of proper laboratory facilities, no parameters concerning the hepatic or renal status could be done. Oral antihypertensive therapy was maintained for 6 weeks. On the control visit after 8 weeks, the patient was clinically fully recovered.

3. Discussion

Conjoined twins represent one of the rarest forms of twin gestation.

In the present article, we present the unique, and so far undescribed, case of a triple coincidence of conjoined twins, eclampsia, and obstructed labor. This scenario is further complicated due to unavailability of obstetric ultrasound in a low-resource setting.

3.1. The Challenge of Conjoined Twins. Anatomically, conjoined twins are classified based upon the site of attachment: thorax (thoracopagus), abdomen (omphalopagus), sacrum (pygopagus), pelvis (ischiopagus), skull (cephalopagus), and back (rachipagus). The extent of organ sharing, especially of the heart, determines the possibility and prognosis of a surgical separation procedure [2]. The most common types are thoracopagus [6, 15] with fusion from the anterior thorax to the umbilicus. A common pericardial sac is present in 90% of thoracopagus twins, and conjoined hearts are seen in 75% [16].

In general, there is higher predisposition towards female than male gender with a ratio of $3:1$ [2, 3].

Early diagnosis of conjoined twins via ultrasound is reported in the first trimester but not before the 10th week of gestation [17]. Once the diagnosis is made, further characterization of the type and severity of the abnormality can be performed by three-dimensional ultrasound, computed tomography, or magnetic resonance imaging [18]. Based on these imaging techniques, the decision of carrying on with the pregnancy or its termination can be made.

Thus, early diagnosis, close prenatal management, and the choice of a proper route of delivery will assure the best possible outcome for mother and both babies [6–8, 19].

Nevertheless, the situation of conjoined twins carries high maternal and fetal risks. Even in high-resource settings, conjoined conditions present an enormous challenge of a catastrophic obstetric event. Even under optimal clinical care, a good outcome is rarely achieved [6]. Approximately 40–60% of conjoined twins arrive stillborn, and about 35% survive for only one day. The overall survival rate of conjoined twins is estimated between 5 and 25% [2, 3]. The surgical separation of conjoined twins is a delicate and risky procedure. Mortality rates for twins who undergo separation vary, depending on their type of connection and the organs they share. For example, twins joined at the sacrum, the base of the spine, have a 68% chance of successful separation, whereas in cases of twins with conjoined hearts at the left ventricular level, there are no known survivors. Although success rates have improved over the years, surgical separation is still rare. Since 1950, in about 75% of the cases, at least one twin has survived separation. After separation, most twins need intensive rehabilitation because of the malformation and position of their spines; they often have difficulties bending their backs and sitting up straight.

In West Africa between 1963 and 1978, 12 cases of conjoined twins have been reported [20]: 8 sets were live born and 4 sets were stillborn. The 8 live born sets were surgically separated either in local hospitals or abroad. Surgical separation was successful in 6 cases (in 2 cases both twins did not survive surgery). In 4 cases, one twin died during surgery or was sacrificed, whereas the other twin survived. In 2 cases, both twins initially survived surgery, but in one set both died about a month later. The most common type and the ones most likely to be live born were the omphalopagus twins [20].

In all of Africa, only two sets of nonseparated conjoined twins have ever been reported in the current literature to be alive, namely, (i) the 19-year-old female thoracopagus Maria and Consolata Mwakikuti, born and raised in Tanzania, where they graduated from high school in 2017 and aim to become teachers [21, 22], and (ii) the Ethiopian mother who delivered in May 2017 a set of live born male thoracopagus conjoined twins who seem to be sharing a common heart and lung [23].

Taking all this information into account, and with respect to the ethical controversy of pregnancy termination, it becomes clear in the case presented here that the early diagnosis via ultrasound would have been fundamentally important: a potential pregnancy termination could have avoided unnecessary but life-threatening maternal complications. The low-resource setting would not have allowed surgical separation, the overall risk for stillbirth in conjoined twins is significantly high, and even if the diagnosis had been made early and an elective cesarean section had been performed, the risk for unseparated twins to die soon after birth would have been very high. In contrast, the choice of pregnancy termination would have spared the mother undergoing unnecessary surgery and the experience of life-threatening complications of preeclampsia and eclampsia.

3.2. The Challenge of Preeclampsia and Eclampsia.
Hypertensive disorders in pregnancy are one of the major causes of maternal mortality and morbidity worldwide [11, 24–26]. 12% of all maternal deaths are due to preeclampsia/eclampsia and HELLP syndrome (hemolysis, elevated liver enzymes, low platelets, and pain), representing the third leading cause of maternal mortality worldwide [12, 13]. Thus, the impact of the disease is felt more severely especially in low-resource countries, such as sub-Saharan African countries, where severe forms of preeclampsia and eclampsia are far more common [27–31].

In our case, the patient presented with several independently known risk factors for developing a hypertensive disorder in pregnancy: (a) unfavourable obstetric history, (b) twin pregnancy, (c) no visits to the antenatal care (ANC) clinic/late referral to the clinic, (d) ethnicity, and (e) low socioeconomic status.

3.2.1. Unfavourable Obstetric History.
The stillbirth of unknown origin in our patient's past obstetric history may allude to a history of preeclampsia in the previous pregnancy, since preeclampsia can lead to complications like placental abruption and IUFD. If she has had preeclampsia in a prior pregnancy, that would be a risk factor for the current pregnancy to get preeclampsia again.

3.2.2. Twin Pregnancy.
The incidence of preeclampsia in twin pregnancies is 2-3 times higher than that in singleton pregnancies [32]. Since the pathogenesis of preeclampsia is to be found in abnormal placentation, it is supposed that the higher incidence in twin pregnancies is due to the increased placental mass compared to singleton pregnancies.

Circulating biomarkers such as PAPP-A, PlGF, and sFlt-1 have been identified to play a role in diagnosis and prediction of preeclampsia [33, 34].

Similarly in twin pregnancies, circulating sFlt-1 levels and sFlt-1/PlGF ratios can be found twice as high as those in singleton pregnancies [35].

Among twin pregnancies, monochorionic types have the highest risk of preeclampsia [36].

3.2.3. No Visits to ANC Clinic/Late Referral to the Clinic.
In developed countries, pregnant women are commonly followed up by a healthcare specialist (doctor, midwife, or nurse) with frequent antenatal evaluations, even without presenting any risk factor. The role of early diagnosis and management of pregnancy-associated conditions has been numerously published worldwide. Special emphasis is placed on the importance of the first-trimester screening via ultrasound [37, 38]. Combined with clinical examination and detection of biochemical markers, it leads to early diagnosis and treatment of pregnancy-associated conditions and permits significantly reducing complications [33, 34, 39, 40]. Preeclampsia should be detected and appropriately managed before the onset of convulsions (eclampsia) and other life-threatening complications. Administering drugs for preeclampsia, such as magnesium sulfate, can lower a woman's risk of developing eclampsia.

Being exposed during her entire pregnancy to an undiagnosed preeclampsia and even having to undergo an eclamptic fit put the mother presented here under a life-threatening maternal mortality risk [25, 26, 30]. Moreover, we cannot even estimate whether she remains with residual kidney, liver, or brain damage, since laboratory parameters could not be performed.

The impact can clearly be seen in our case, where no visits to the ANC clinic and delay in the referral lead to undetected preeclampsia with the consequence of avoidable and life-threatening complication of eclampsia. Due to unavailability of early obstetric ultrasound, the conjoined twins still might not have been detected, even if the patient had attended ANC clinic.

3.3. The Challenge of a Low-Resource Setting

3.3.1. The Presented Patient Case.
The impact of an early diagnosis of pregnancy-associated conditions may be even greater in so-called developing countries, where significant avoidable maternal and neonatal morbidity and mortality often result.

This is perfectly reflected in our presented case. There is no doubt that access to healthcare is the main complicating factor for our patient.

It is well known that in developing countries medical conditions during pregnancy commonly advance to more complicated stages of disease, and many unreported births and deaths occur at home. Also, medical interventions may be ineffective due to late presentation of the cases.

(1) Unavailability of early ultrasound led to undiagnosed conjoined twins. If known, termination could have

been offered, or at least an elective cesarean section could have been performed, and the complication of obstructed labor would have been prevented.

(2) No visits to ANC clinic led to undiagnosed preeclampsia and therefore to a more advanced stage and then finally to the unnecessary and dangerous complication of eclampsia.

(3) Delay in referral and treatment led to obstructed labor and eclampsia.

(4) Deficiency in skills leads to delay and complications of obstructed labor and eclampsia.

(5) There is no doubt that the indication for cesarean section was already given on admission for obstructed labor and severe preeclampsia, respectively. Also the situation of severe preeclampsia in labor would have indicated an immediate onset of the $MgSO_4$ protocol. The explanation can only be insufficiently skilled staff or insufficiently motivated staff.

(6) Even to prevent a cesarean section would have been beneficial for the mother: being a postcesarean case with an uterine scar, the mother runs a high risk of further complications and even maternal death in a future childbirth when being in a low-resource setting.

Inaccessibility is a major barrier resulting in morbidity and mortality, which would otherwise have been prevented.

3.3.2. The Setting of the Princess Christian Maternity Hospital (PCMH) in Sierra Leone. Sierra Leone is on the West Coast of sub-Saharan Africa. The population is about 7,09 million people and life expectancy is as low as 50,1 years for both sexes. The literacy rate is low with an average of 43%. Half of the population live on only 1,25 Dollar per day [41]. Many births occur at home, which leads to the fact that skilled health personnel are only present in 59,7% of all births in total. Furthermore, physicians density and nursing and midwifery personnel density are extremely low, 0,03/1000 and 0,8/1000, respectively, and are insufficient for the need of the population [41].

In April 2010, the government of Sierra Leone launched free healthcare services for pregnant women, lactating mothers, and children under 5. Nevertheless, maternal mortality is estimated at 1,360/100,000 live born births, and it is considered as one of the highest worldwide (also in the subregion) [42].

The Princess Christian Maternity Hospital (PCMH) is the biggest referral hospital for Obstetrics and Gynecology in this country with about 4,000 births per year.

Laboratory investigations are limited to hemoglobin (Hb), blood grouping, malaria, human immunodeficiency virus (HIV), and urine tests using dip sticks; a limited blood bank facility is available. Very often there is a lack of basic equipment and medication, such as IV lines, surgical sutures, antibiotics, antihypertensive medication, $MgSO_4$, Ringer, or N/S, due to a poor distribution system for drugs. Unstable power supply leads to inaccessibility to electronic devices,

such as perfusors or cardiotocogram (CTG). Concerning ultrasound, there is one machine with only an abdominal probe and no Doppler available. The machine is not accessible in the emergency department, labor ward, or theatre; and ultrasound skills are possessed by only one consultant obstetrician. The number of trained health professionals is unacceptably inadequate. Skills and motivation of health workers, that is, midwives, nurses, and doctors, are insufficient with regard to the medical challenges faced. This leads to a lack of implementation of mandatory guidelines and structured procedures; thus timelines are not respected, often through incapacity or even neglect.

3.3.3. The Low-Resource Setting in a Global Context. In the year 2000, the international community committed to 8 Millennium Development Goals (MDG) to be achieved by 2015 [43]. MDG number 5 commits to reducing maternal mortality by three quarters worldwide, which would have required an annual decline of 5.5% until 2015. However, between 1990 and 2013, the global maternal mortality ratio declined by only 2.6% per year.

Albeit shocking, the course of events in the case presented here is more common than unusual—seen from a global perspective and especially in the context of a low-resource setting [10, 13, 24, 25, 27, 29, 31, 43]. It is well known that in developing countries medical conditions during pregnancy commonly advance to more complicated stages of disease, and many unreported births occur at home. Also, medical interventions may be ineffective due to late presentation of the cases [25, 26]. Every year, over half a million women die globally from pregnancy and childbirth-related complications [13]. Out of these, 99% of all maternal deaths occur in so-called developing countries.

The main causes for maternal deaths accounting for 80% of the cases are severe bleeding, infections, preeclampsia and eclampsia, and unsafe abortion [12, 13].

Most maternal deaths are avoidable, since the healthcare solutions to prevent or manage complications are well known. But why do not women get the care they need?

According to World Health Organization (WHO), worldwide factors preventing women from receiving or seeking care during pregnancy and childbirth are poverty, distance, lack of information, cultural practices, and inadequate services [13].

Access to ANC clinic, facility deliveries, a skilled birth attendant at delivery, and family-planning methods are crucial in preventing these complications. Timely management and treatment can make the difference between life and death.

The higher number of maternal deaths in sub-Saharan Africa reflects inequities regarding access to health services.

"Access" in this case does not only mean rural and remote areas but also stands for

(i) the gap between rich and poor,

(ii) lower social status of women; lack of education leads to not claiming health service that is provided,

(iii) traditional health practices which are usually inadequate to detect medical conditions early,

(iv) low numbers of skilled health workers.

World Health Organization reports that only 46% of women in low-income countries benefit from skilled care during childbirth [12, 13]. This means that millions of births are not assisted by a midwife, a doctor, or a trained nurse. Many unreported births and deaths occur at home.

Moreover, women in developing countries have on average many more pregnancies than women in developed countries, and their lifetime risk of death due to pregnancy is thus significantly higher.

4. Summary

In the present article, we present the unique and so far undescribed case of a triple coincidence of conjoined twins, eclampsia, and obstructed labor which occurred in Freetown, Sierra Leone, a low-resource country in sub-Saharan Africa.

Conjoined twins represent one of the rarest forms of twin gestation. The situation of conjoined twins carries high maternal and fetal risks, thus holding the absolute challenge of preventing a catastrophic obstetric event. Even under the best of circumstances, a good outcome is rarely achieved. Therefore, termination of pregnancy may be the choice. Although success rates have improved, surgical separation of conjoined twins is a delicate and risky procedure. Cases where at least one twin has survived separation are reported to be about 75%. In Africa, there are only two sets of nonseparated thoracopagus conjoined twins reported to be alive: the 19-year-old Maria and Consolata Mwakikuti from Tanzania and the male thoracopagus set born in May 2017 in Ethiopia [21–23].

Severe preeclampsia and eclampsia have remained a significant public health threat in both developed and developing countries, as they have considerable adverse impacts on maternal, fetal, and neonatal health. However, the impact of the disease is felt more severely, especially in low-resource countries, where conditions are often complicated, since medical interventions may be ineffective due to late presentation of cases. Advances to more complicated stages of disease are common.

The role of early diagnosis for conjoined twins and preeclampsia, respectively, is crucial.

The occurrence of both conditions, conjoined twins and preeclampsia, in a developing country is demonstrated in the present article to be the main complicating factor for the fetal and maternal outcomes (fetal mortality and maternal morbidity).

Worldwide factors preventing pregnant women from seeking or receiving healthcare, such as poverty, distance, lack of information, inadequate services, and cultural practices, are discussed.

In the 21st century, it is unacceptable that mothers die from preventable conditions or go through life-threatening preventable complications.

If substantial reductions in maternal mortality are to be achieved, universal coverage of life-saving interventions needs to be matched with comprehensive emergency care and overall improvements in the quality of maternal healthcare.

To improve maternal health worldwide, barriers that limit access to quality maternal health services must be identified and addressed at all levels of the health system.

The implementation of guidelines and policies and the application of a profound quality management system would crucially improve performances at health centers and hospitals in low-resource settings and therefore lead to a better functional medical system in its entirety.

Consent

Informed consent was obtained from the patient for publication of this case report and accompanying images.

Disclosure

Mariatu Binta Leigh and Ivo Buschmann are members in the European Society for Vascular and Preventive Medicine (ESVM).

Authors' Contributions

Mariatu Binta Leigh was the consultant obstetrician in charge at the maternity unit who diagnosed and treated the patient and performed the surgery. She had the conceptional idea of the report and drafted and reviewed the manuscript for important intellectual content. Valerie John-Cole and Mike Kamara assisted with surgery; Michael Momoh Koroma was the anesthetist at surgery. Alimamy Philip Koroma and Edward Ejiro Emuveyan supported the medical team in postoperative care. Peter Bramlage and Ivo Buschmann revised the manuscript. All authors agreed on the final version submitted and take full responsibility for the work.

Acknowledgments

The authors would like to thank all the midwives and theatre nurses at Princess Christian Maternity Hospital for their tireless efforts dedicated to saving newborns' and women's lives.

References

[1] G. J. Amiel, "Conjoined entire twins: a case of thoraco-omphalopagus with discussion on nomenclature, obstetric management and anatomical note," *The British Journal of Clinical Practice*, vol. 21, no. 3, pp. 141–146, 1967.

[2] A. Mian, N. I. Gabra, T. Sharma et al., "Conjoined twins: From conception to separation, a review," *Clinical Anatomy*, vol. 30, no. 3, pp. 385–396, 2017.

[3] D. Montandon, "The unspeakable history of thoracopagus twins' separation," *ISAPS News*, p. 9, 2015.

[4] T. Abossolo, P. Dancoisne, J. Tuaillon, E. Orvain, J. C. Sommer, and J. P. Rivière, "Early prenatal diagnosis of asymmetric

cephalothoracopagus twins," *Journal de Gynécologie Obstétrique et Biologie de la Reproduction*, vol. 23, no. 1, pp. 79–84, 1994.

[5] R. Spencer, "Theoretical and analytical embryology of conjoined twins: Part I: Embryogenesis," *Clinical Anatomy*, vol. 13, no. 1, pp. 36–53, 2000.

[6] T. C. MacKenzie, T. M. Crombleholme, M. P. Johnson et al., "The natural history of prenatally diagnosed conjoined twins," *Journal of Pediatric Surgery*, vol. 37, no. 3, pp. 303–309, 2002.

[7] A. Kirbas, E. Biberoglu, S. Celen, E. Oztas, D. Uygur, and N. Danisman, "A case of thoracopagus conjoined twins," in *Proceedings of the 13th World Congress in Fetal Medicine*, Nice, France, 2014.

[8] M. A. Osmanağaoğlu, T. Aran, S. Güven, C. Kart, Ö. Özdemir, and H. Bozkaya, "Thoracopagus conjoined twins: a case report," *ISRN Obstetrics and Gynecology*, vol. 2011, Article ID 238360, 3 pages, 2011.

[9] K. Lim and G. Steinberg, "Preeclampsia," *Medscape*, 2016.

[10] R. Carine and J. G. Wendy, "Maternal mortality: who, when, where, and why," *The Lancet*, vol. 368, no. 9542, pp. 1189–1200, 2006.

[11] C. Dolea and C. AbouZahr, "Global burden of hypertensive disorders of pregnancy in the year 2000," Evidence and Information for Policy (EIP), World Health Organization, 2003.

[12] W.H.O., "The World Health report 2005: make every mother and child count," *World Health Organization*, 2005.

[13] W. H. O., "Maternal mortality— fact sheet," *World Health Organization*, 2016.

[14] J. F. Lu and C. H. Nightingale, "Magnesium sulfate in eclampsia and pre-eclampsia. Pharmacokinetic principles," *Clinical Pharmacokinetics*, vol. 38, no. 4, pp. 305–314, 2000.

[15] J. A. Noonan, "Twins, Conjoined Twins, and Cardiac Defects," *American Journal of Diseases of Children*, vol. 132, no. 1, pp. 17-18, 1978.

[16] R. Tandon, L. P. Sterns, and J. E. Edwards, "Thoracopagus twins. Report of a case," *Archives of Pathology*, vol. 98, pp. 248–251, 1974.

[17] C. Hubinont, P. Kollmann, V. Malvaux, J. Donnez, and P. Bernard, "First-trimester diagnosis of conjoined twins," *Fetal Diagnosis and Therapy*, vol. 12, no. 3, pp. 185–187, 1997.

[18] K. Kuroda, Y. Kamei, S. Kozuma et al., "Prenatal evaluation of cephalopagus conjoined twins by means of three-dimensional ultrasound at 13 weeks of pregnancy," *Ultrasound in Obstetrics & Gynecology*, vol. 16, no. 3, pp. 264–266, 2000.

[19] A. C. Wittich, "Conjoined twins: report of a case and review of the literature," *The Journal of the American Osteopathic Association*, vol. 89, no. 9, pp. 1175–1179, 1989.

[20] O. A. Mabogunje and J. H. Lawrie, "Conjoined twins in West Africa," *Archives of Disease in Childhood*, vol. 55, no. 8, pp. 626–630, 1980.

[21] B.B.C., "The conjoined twins hoping to become teachers," *BBC.com*, 2017.

[22] Bellanaija, "19-Year old Tanzanian conjoined twins aim to become teachers," *Bellanaija.com*, 2017.

[23] A. Shaban, "Ethiopian delivers conjoined twin boys in 'historic' birth," *Africanews*, 2017.

[24] E. M. McClure, S. Saleem, O. Pasha, and R. L. Goldenberg, "Stillbirth in developing countries: A review of causes, risk factors and prevention strategies," *The Journal of Maternal-Fetal and Neonatal Medicine*, vol. 22, no. 3, pp. 183–190, 2009.

[25] S. O. Onuh and A. O. Aisien, "Maternal and fetal outcome in eclamptic patients in Benin City, Nigeria," *Journal of Obstetrics & Gynaecology*, vol. 24, no. 7, pp. 765–768, 2004.

[26] J. I. Ikechebelu and C. C. Okoli, "Review of eclampsia at the Nnamdi Azikiwe University teaching hospital, Nnewi (January 1996–December 2000)," *Journal of Obstetrics & Gynaecology*, vol. 22, no. 3, pp. 287–290, 2002.

[27] G. Igberase and P. Ebeigbe, "Eclampsia: Ten-years of experience in a rural tertiary hospital in the Niger delta, Nigeria," *Journal of Obstetrics & Gynaecology*, vol. 26, no. 5, pp. 414–417, 2006.

[28] Y. M. Adamu, H. M. Salihu, N. Sathiakumar, and G. R. Alexander, "Maternal mortality in Northern Nigeria: A population-based study," *European Journal of Obstetrics & Gynecology and Reproductive Biology*, vol. 109, no. 2, pp. 153–159, 2003.

[29] A. Shah, B. Fawole, J. M. M'Imunya et al., "Cesarean delivery outcomes from the WHO global survey on maternal and perinatal health in Africa," *International Journal of Gynecology and Obstetrics*, vol. 107, no. 3, pp. 191–197, 2009.

[30] S. Ngwenya, "Severe preeclampsia and eclampsia: incidence, complications, and perinatal outcomes at a low-resource setting, Mpilo Central Hospital, Bulawayo, Zimbabwe," *International Journal of Women's Health*, vol. Volume 9, pp. 353–357, 2017.

[31] K. O. Osungbade and O. K. Ige, "Public health perspectives of preeclampsia in developing countries: implication for health system strengthening," *Journal of Pregnancy*, vol. 2011, Article ID 481095, 6 pages, 2011.

[32] C. Francisco, D. Wright, Z. Benkő, A. Syngelaki, and K. H. Nicolaides, "Hidden high rate of pre-eclampsia in twin compared with singleton pregnancy," *Ultrasound in Obstetrics & Gynecology*, vol. 50, no. 1, pp. 88–92, 2017.

[33] I. Herraiz, E. Simón, P. I. Gómez-Arriaga et al., "Angiogenesis-related biomarkers (sFlt-1/PLGF) in the prediction and diagnosis of placental dysfunction: An approach for clinical integration," *International Journal of Molecular Sciences*, vol. 16, no. 8, pp. 19009–19026, 2015.

[34] C. Francisco, D. Wright, Z. Benkő, A. Syngelaki, and K. H. Nicolaides, "ompeting-risks model in screening for pre-eclampsia in twin pregnancy according to maternal factors and biomarkers at 11–13 weeks' gestation," *Ultrasound in Obstetrics & Gynecology*, vol. 50, no. 5, pp. 589–595, 2017.

[35] Y. Bdolah, C. Lam, A. Rajakumar et al., "Twin pregnancy and the risk of preeclampsia: bigger placenta or relative ischemia?" *American Journal of Obstetrics & Gynecology*, vol. 198, no. 4, pp. 428.e1–428.e6, 2008.

[36] D. M. Campbell and I. MacGillivray, "Preeclampsia in twin pregnancies: Incidence and outcome," *Hypertension in Pregnancy*, vol. 18, no. 3, pp. 197–207, 1999.

[37] K. H. Nicolaides, "Some thoughts on the true value of ultrasound," *Ultrasound in Obstetrics & Gynecology*, vol. 30, no. 5, pp. 671–674, 2007.

[38] K. H. Nicolaides, "Turning the pyramid of prenatal care," *Fetal Diagnosis and Therapy*, vol. 29, no. 3, pp. 183–196, 2011.

[39] C. Francisco, D. Wright, Z. Benkő, A. Syngelaki, and K. H. Nicolaides, "Competing-risks model in screening for pre-eclampsia in twin pregnancy by maternal characteristics and medical history," *Ultrasound in Obstetrics & Gynecology*, vol. 50, no. 4, pp. 501–506, 2017.

[40] H. Stepan, I. Herraiz, D. Schlembach et al., "Implementation of the sFlt-1/PlGF ratio for prediction and diagnosis of preeclampsia in singleton pregnancy: Implications for clinical

practice," *Ultrasound in Obstetrics & Gynecology*, vol. 45, no. 3, pp. 241–246, 2015.

[41] W.H.O., "Country cooperation strategy—Sierra Leone," *World Health Organization*, 2017.

[42] W.H.O., "Sierra Leone statistics summary (2002—present). Global health observatory country views," *World Health Organization*, 2017.

[43] D. Chou, D. Hogan, S. Zhang et al., "Global, regional, and national levels and trends in maternal mortality between 1990 and 2015, with scenario-based projections to 2030: a systematic analysis by the UN Maternal Mortality Estimation Inter-Agency Group," *The Lancet*, vol. 387, no. 10017, pp. 462–474, 2016.

39

Bicornuate Bicollis Uterus with Obstruction of the Lower Uterine Segment and Cervical Prolapse Complicating Pregnancy

Kristen Stearns ⓘ [1] **and Antoun Al Khabbaz** ⓘ [2]

[1] *Medical College of Wisconsin and Affiliated Hospitals, Department of Obstetrics and Gynecology, 9200 W. Wisconsin Ave, Milwaukee, WI 53226, USA*

[2] *University of Illinois College of Medicine-Rockford, Department of Obstetrics and Gynecology, 1601 Parkview Ave, Rockford, IL 61101, USA*

Correspondence should be addressed to Antoun Al Khabbaz; akhabbaz@crusaderhealth.org

Academic Editor: Julio Rosa-e-Silva

Congenital Mullerian duct anomalies are conditions involving the female genital tract. Cases of complex Mullerian duct anomalies with involvement of the renal system are rare. Occasionally, these cases can be associated with obstetrical complications. Cervical prolapse infrequently complicates pregnancy, and an association between uterine malformations and cervical prolapse has not been cited in the literature. We describe the case of a primigravid patient at 38 weeks of gestation noted to have cervical prolapse during evaluation for preeclampsia and labor induction. Obstetrical ultrasound at presentation to the labor and delivery suite revealed a high suspicion for a bicornuate uterus. The patient was delivered by cesarean section due to obstruction of the lower uterine segment of the gravid uterus. Further evaluation post-partum revealed a bicornuate bicolis uterus and renal agenesis. Pregnancies in patients with bicornuate bicollis uterus can be complicated by obstruction of the gravid uterus, resulting in cervical prolapse and necessitating cesarean section.

1. Introduction

Congenital Mullerian duct anomalies are conditions involving the female genital tract. They involve abnormalities of the fallopian tubes, uterus, cervix, and/or upper vagina. The etiology of Mullerian duct anomalies is multifactorial. These abnormalities may result from agenesis or failed fusion of the paramesonephric ducts or from failed resorption of the uterine septum in utero. It is estimated that the incidence of various congenital uterine anomalies is between 0.5% and 5.0% [1]. Bicornuate uterus represents approximately one-fourth of such anomalies, whereas didelphic or "double uterus" is among the least common and represents only 8% of these anomalies [2]. Mullerian duct anomalies have been found to be associated with infertility, early pregnancy loss, preterm labor and delivery, and fetal malpresentation [3]. Other studies have found an association between congenital Mullerian duct anomalies and an increased incidence of renal and urinary tract abnormalities, often leading to more complex cases [4].

The etiology of cervical prolapse is also multifactorial and usually occurs secondary to weakening of the supportive ligaments of the uterus. Cervical prolapse occurs rarely in pregnancy and complicates between 1 in 10,000 and 1 in 15,000 pregnancies [5]. Additional factors have been cited as contributors to this phenomenon including multiparity, increased intra-abdominal pressure, genetic predispositions, collagen abnormalities, and history of pelvic floor surgery. Cervical prolapse can result in vascular congestion of the cervix, cervical edema, cervical insufficiency, and dystocia. Studies have also found an increased risk of spontaneous abortion in patients with cervical prolapse [6].

In this case report, we describe the presentation of a nulliparous patient with cervical prolapse, bicornuate bicollis uterus, and obstruction of the lower uterine segment of the gravid uterus by the nongravid uterus.

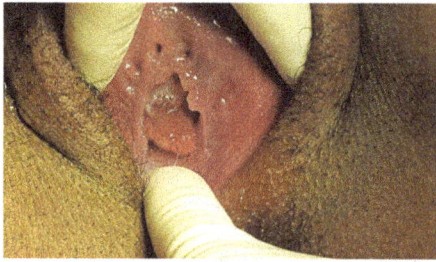

FIGURE 1: Cervical prolapse reaching the level of the introitus.

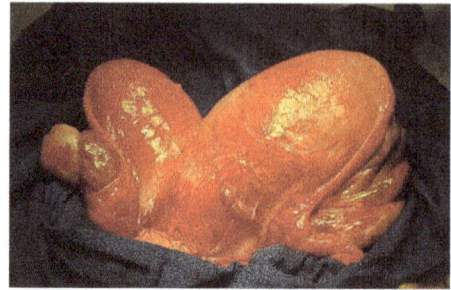

FIGURE 2: Intraoperative finding of bicornuate uterus (right hemi-uterus on the left side of image, left hemiuterus on right side of image).

2. Presentation of Case

A 17-year-old gravida 1 para 0 patient at 38 weeks of gestation was admitted to the labor and delivery suite for labor induction secondary to diagnosis of preeclampsia with severe features (hypertension, proteinuria, and a creatinine level of 1.2 mg/dL). The patient had an uncomplicated course of pregnancy prior to this diagnosis. The patient initiated prenatal care at 16 weeks of gestation and had a normal baseline pelvic examination. The fetal anatomic survey at 20 weeks of gestation was also normal.

Pelvic examination on admission to the labor suite revealed a moderate to severe cervical prolapse with the cervix noted at the introitus (Figure 1). Digital examination revealed a closed cervix, and a posterior mass was suspected in the lower uterine segment. Transvaginal ultrasound demonstrated a mass posterior to the cervix, resulting in displacement of the gravid uterus markedly anteriorly. On ultrasound, the mass appeared to be uterine in origin with normal appearing myometrium and decidualized endometrium. Initial findings were suggestive of a uterine malformation with obstruction of the lower uterine segment of the gravid and anterior left-sided uterus by its nongravid, right-sided, and posterior counterpart.

The patient was counseled about the need for delivery due to preeclampsia. Complete obstruction of the lower uterine segment of the gravid uterus prompted recommendation for primary cesarean section. A primary low-segment transverse cesarean section via Pfannenstiel skin incision was performed after obtaining patient's informed consent. The patient delivered a live female newborn from a vertex presentation with a birthweight of 2840 grams and Apgar scores of 8 and 9 at one and five minutes, respectively. Intraoperative findings included apparently noncommunicating uteri and normal fallopian tubes and ovaries (Figure 2). The patient received magnesium sulfate prophylaxis for seizures for 24 hours postpartum. During admission, renal ultrasound revealed an absent left kidney with compensatory hypertrophy of the right kidney. Her postpartum course was uncomplicated. Creatinine level normalized postpartum. The patient was discharged home on postpartum day 3. At her 6-week postpartum check-up, speculum examination revealed two cervixes, with the right cervix notably smaller and more superior than the left. There was no evidence of a vaginal septum. Cervical prolapse was noted to have resolved. At 8 weeks postpartum, pelvic MRI demonstrated bicornuate

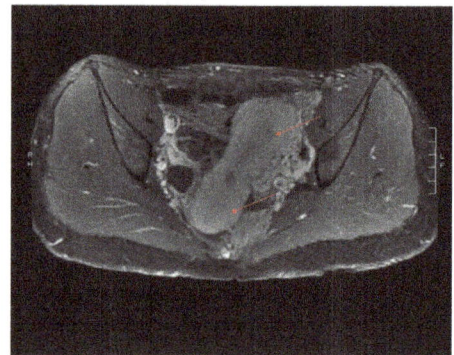

FIGURE 3: MRI demonstrating bicornuate uterus.

uterus (Figure 3) with cervical bicollis (Figure 4). There was no evidence of communication between the two uterine horns on MRI. Postpartum hysterosalpingogram was not performed secondary to patient loss to follow-up.

3. Discussion

We report the case of a primigravid patient with bicornuate bicollis uterine anatomy, cervical prolapse, preeclampsia, and unilateral renal agenesis who was delivered with cesarean section due to obstruction of the lower uterine segment of the gravid uterus. Bicornuate uterus is a common Mullerian duct anomaly and can be accompanied with a single cervix (unicollis) or a double cervix (bicollis) depending on the extent of the duplication. Differentiating bicornuate bicollis uterus from didelphic uterus can be challenging, as the anatomy of these anomalies is similar. The key difference between these anomalies is that a didelphic uterus has two widely spaced and completely separate uterine cavities. By comparison, bicornuate anatomy demonstrates some degree of fusion between the two uterine horns, although the septum can extend to the level of the cervix to yield two cervices in some cases (Figure 5). Pelvic MRI is the modality of choice for differentiating the two aforementioned abnormalities.

This case highlights numerous points of discussion including the relationship between bicornuate uterus and cervical prolapse. In this patient's case, the lower uterine segment of the left-sided, gravid uterus was obstructed by the right-sided, nongravid uterus. The cervix of the gravid uterus was

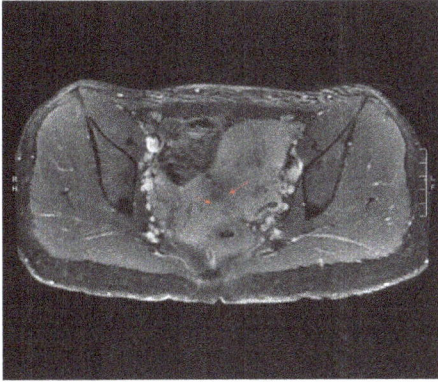

FIGURE 4: MRI demonstrating bicollis uterus.

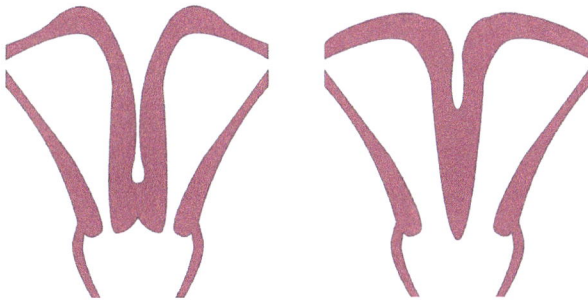

FIGURE 5: Didelphic uterus (left), bicornuate bicollis uterus (right), courtesy of Kyle Koniewicz.

displaced downward by its nongravid counterpart, resulting in cervical prolapse. Neither bicornuate bicollis uterus or cervical prolapse is an indication for cesarean section delivery in isolation, and many patients with these conditions are able to progress and deliver vaginally [7]. However, in this case, cesarean section was indicated due to obstruction of the lower uterine segment of the gravid uterus. Bicornuate bicollis uterus and cervical prolapse are relatively rare phenomena. After an extensive literature search, we could not find a case describing the combined presentation of these two conditions.

This case highlights the relationship between bicornuate uterus and preeclampsia. Mullerian duct anomalies are known to be associated with renal and urinary tract abnormalities. Studies have reported that renal anomalies are found in 20-30% of patients with Mullerian duct anomalies, and these cases represent complex mesonephric anomalies stemming from abnormal development of both renal and reproductive anatomy in utero [4]. In this case, further workup postpartum revealed left renal agenesis. The absence of the left kidney probably contributed to the development of this patient's preeclampsia. Heinonen retrospectively studied the possible connection between gestational hypertensive disease and unilateral renal agenesis in women with Mullerian duct anomalies. He concluded that women with uterine anomalies and unilateral renal agenesis have greater than three times the risk for development of preeclampsia than women with normal renal anatomy. This is thought to be a consequence of

the increased burden on the solitary kidney due to functional renal changes during pregnancy.

Abnormal uterine anatomy has been well-documented and studied, and complex distal mesonephric congenital anomalies including cases of unilateral renal agenesis and ipsilateral cervicovaginal atresia or an ipsilateral blind hemivagina have been described [8]. Similarly, there have been cases with communicating bicornuate bicollis uterine anatomy associated with atretic blind hemivagina and ipsilateral renal agenesis [8]. Thus, in patients presenting with bicornuate uterine anatomy and unilateral renal agenesis, it is reasonable to suspect anomalies of this nature. This patient did not have evidence of any of the aforementioned cervical and/or vaginal findings. Rather, the patient had apparently noncommunicating uterine horns with respective cervices; a true bicornuate bicollis anatomy with unilateral renal agenesis. This anatomy has not been documented in the literature and represents a very rare anomaly. It is possible that a communication between the uterine horns existed in this patient. It would have been difficult to diagnose at the time of cesarean section and it was not seen on subsequent pelvic MRI. Further evaluation with a hysterosalpingogram could have helped determine if a communication existed between the two uterine horns and if the patient had an atretic cervix.

The finding of cervical prolapse in a pregnant patient at term, particularly in a nulligravid patient, should prompt evaluation for a uterine malformation. In this case, the uterine anomaly was diagnosed at term after finding cervical prolapse and a pelvic mass. The diagnosis was missed at the time of the fetal anatomic survey, likely because the nongravid uterus was positioned posterior to its gravid counterpart. All patients with bicornuate uterus should be evaluated for renal agenesis or other renal and urinary tract malformations. In case of such abnormalities or malformations, these patients should be diligently monitored for hypertensive disease of pregnancy.

Additional Points

Teaching Points. (1) Patients presenting with cervical prolapse and obstruction of the lower uterine segment should be evaluated for a uterine malformation. (2) Uterine malformations can be associated with renal agenesis, which can be associated with preeclampsia.

Consent

Written permission for publication was obtained from the patient.

References

[1] P. K. Heinonen, "Clinical implications of the didelphic uterus: long-term follow-up of 49 cases," *European Journal of Obstetrics*

& *Gynecology and Reproductive Biology*, vol. 91, no. 2, pp. 183–190, 2000.

[2] G. F. Grimbizis, M. Camus, B. C. Tarlatzis, J. N. Bontis, and P. Devroey, "Clinical implications of uterine malformations and hysteroscopic treatment results," *Human Reproduction Update*, vol. 7, no. 2, pp. 161–174, 2001.

[3] M. Hua, A. O. Odibo, R. E. Longman, G. A. MacOnes, K. A. Roehl, and A. G. Cahill, "Congenital uterine anomalies and adverse pregnancy outcomes," *American Journal of Obstetrics & Gynecology*, vol. 205, no. 6, pp. 558–e5, 2011.

[4] P. K. Heinonen, "Gestational hypertension and preeclampsia associated with unilateral renal agenesis in women with uterine malformations," *European Journal of Obstetrics & Gynecology and Reproductive Biology*, vol. 114, no. 1, pp. 39–43, 2004.

[5] H. L. Brown, "Cervical prolapse complicating pregnancy," *Journal of the National Medical Association*, vol. 89, pp. 346–348, 1997.

[6] P. Tsikouras, A. Dafopoulos, N. Vrachnis et al., "Uterine prolapse in pregnancy: Risk factors, complications and management," *The Journal of Maternal-Fetal and Neonatal Medicine*, vol. 27, no. 3, pp. 297–302, 2014.

[7] P. Acién, "Reproductive performance of women with uterine malformations," *Human Reproduction*, vol. 8, no. 1, pp. 122–126, 1993.

[8] P. Acién and M. Acién, "Diagnostic imaging and cataloguing of female genital malformations," *Insights into Imaging*, vol. 7, no. 5, pp. 713–726, 2016.

40

Sertoli-Leydig Cell Tumour and *DICER1* Mutation: A Case Report and Review of the Literature

B. Wormald ⓘ,[1] **S. Elorbany,**[1] **H. Hanson,**[1] **J. W. Williams,**[1] **S. Heenan,**[1] **and D. P. J. Barton**[2]

[1]*St George's Hospital, UK*
[2]*St George's Hospital and the Royal Marsden Hospital, UK*

Correspondence should be addressed to B. Wormald; ben.wormald@nhs.net

Academic Editor: Giampiero Capobianco

Sertoli-Leydig cell tumours of the ovary (SLCT) are rare tumours predominantly caused by mutations in the *DICER1* gene. We present a patient with a unilateral SLCT who had an underlying germline *DICER1* gene mutation. We discuss the underlying pathology, risks, and screening opportunities available to those with a mutation in this gene as SLCT is only one of a multitude of other tumours encompassing *DICER1* syndrome. The condition is inherited in an autosomal dominant fashion. As such, genetic counselling is a key component of the management of women with SLCT.

1. Introduction

Sertoli-Leydig cell tumours of the ovary (SLCTs) are a rare type of sex cord-stromal tumour, constituting less than 0.5% of all ovarian cancers. SLCTs contain Sertoli and Leydig cells which are somatic cells found within the male gonad. It is likely that SLCTs derive from primitive pregranulosa cells and therefore represent a pseudo–male gonadal genesis in the ovary. Patients typically present in the 2nd or 3rd decade of life and often have features of androgen excess, such as amenorrhoea, hirsutism, deepening of the voice, and clitoral enlargement. The vast majority, more than 95% of tumours, are unilateral, FIGO Stage 1, and either moderately or poorly differentiated. It is increasingly clear that the pathogenesis of SLCT is through mutation in the *DICER1* gene [1].

2. Case Presentation

A 15-year-old girl presented with a background of erratic menstrual periods following menarche at age of 12 years. By first contact she had experienced amenorrhoea for 6 months followed by continuous daily vaginal bleeding for 3 months. She had noticed hair loss, receding hairline, and coarse dark hair on her abdomen, thighs, and bottom. Clinical examination revealed a normally developed female without virilisation of the external genitalia or a change in voice. She was pain free.

Hormone profile revealed raised testosterone (10.1 nmol/l Ref: 0.5-3.0 nmol/l), suppressed FSH (<0.1 IU/L Ref: 1-11 iu/L), and borderline SHBG (21 nmol/l Ref: 18 – 114 nmol/L). AFP was raised (137 kU/L Ref: 0-5.8 kU/L) but all other tumour markers, including Beta-HCG and Inhibin, were normal. Urine steroid profile was normal.

Ultrasound examination of the abdomen and pelvis, Figure 1, revealed a complex 7 cm left ovarian lesion with internal vascularity but otherwise normal pelvic organs and adrenal glands. MRI, Figure 2, confirmed an abnormal but well-defined 7 cm left adnexal lesion of predominant intermediate T2 signal interspersed with high signal cystic areas separated by low signal septa. The clinical picture was of a primary ovarian tumour with ectopic production of androgens, and not the more common germ cell tumour.

The case was discussed at the paediatric and gynaecologic oncology MDT. A laparoscopic left oophorectomy with preservation of the ipsilateral fallopian tube was performed with a secondary Pfannenstiel incision used to extract intact the specimen. The tumour which was more solid than cystic was 11 cm in size with no discernible normal ovarian tissue visible. A small nodule on the right ovary was excised. There were no other sites of disease. All other organs and

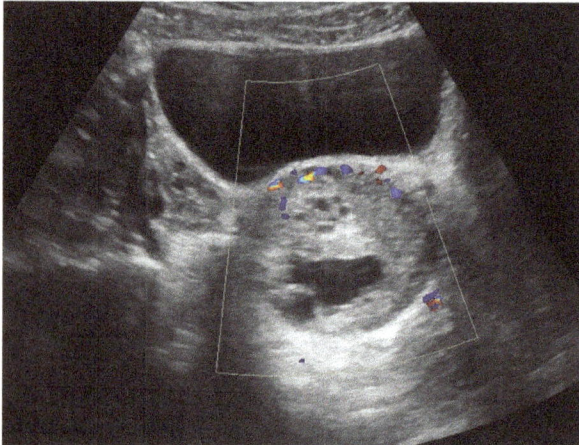

FIGURE 1: Ultrasound image of ovarian lesion.

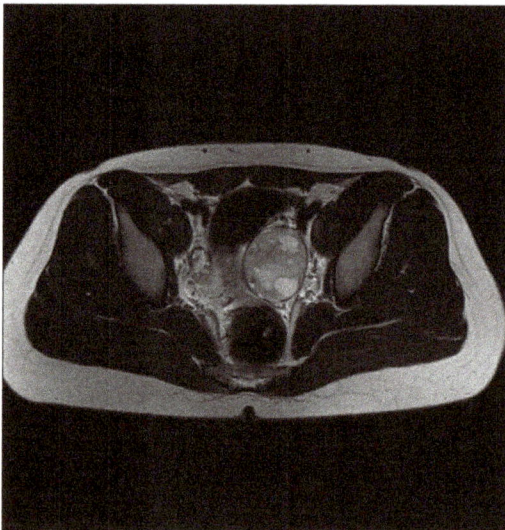

FIGURE 2: MRI image of ovarian lesion.

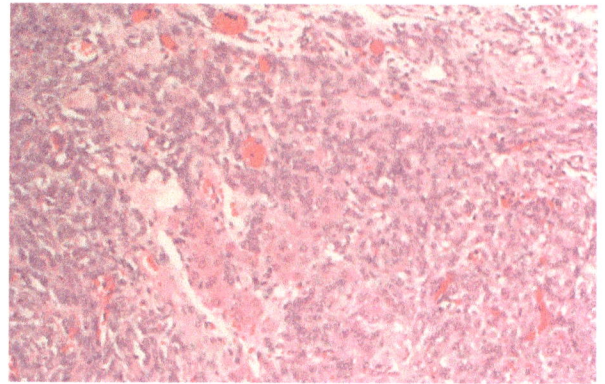

FIGURE 3: Microscopic view of specimen.

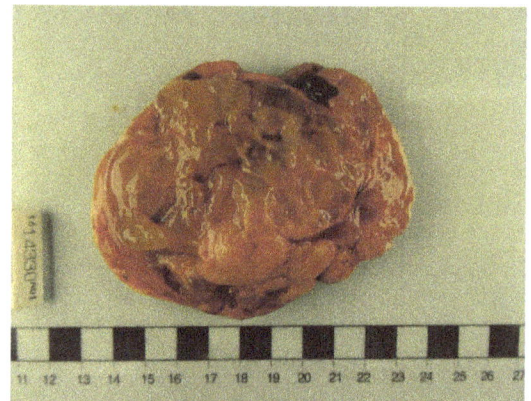

FIGURE 4: Macroscopic specimen.

peritoneal surfaces were normal. The postoperative course was uneventful.

Histological analysis, Figures 3 and 4, indicated a predominantly poorly differentiated Sertoli-Leydig cell tumour, retiform pattern, with heterologous mucinous elements. The right ovarian nodule was benign.

Following multidisciplinary team discussion and parental consent, adjuvant chemotherapy was commenced, in a monthly regime of Bleomycin 28500 IU on Day 1, Etoposide 190 mg daily on Days 1-5, and Cisplatin 38 mg daily on Days 1-5 for 3 cycles. Starting prior to chemotherapy commencement, a GNRH analogue, Leuprorelin 3.75mg per month, was administered for 4 months for ovarian protection. The patient became neutropenic following cycle 1 and received Filgrastim 300mcg for 6 days on Days 6-10 of Cycle 2. There were no further episodes of neutropenia. Following cessation of Leuprorelin, menstruation resumed on a regular monthly cycle. She completed her treatment 2 years ago and been reviewed every 3 months. She has had normal

tumour markers, including testosterone and AFP, and normal abdominopelvic ultrasound scans throughout this period. Following genetic analysis a germline *DICER1* mutation was discovered, inherited from her father and shared by her 19-year-old sister.

3. Discussion

DICER1 is located on chromosome 14q32.13 and contains 27 exons. Dicer1 is an RNase III endoribonuclease which has several functions but crucially is involved in the microRNA (miRNA) biogenesis pathway. Dicer1 processes precursor miRNA into functional mature miRNA through the cleaving of dsRNA into two RNA strands. RNA IIIa and RNA IIIb domains are responsible for 3p and 5p miRNAs, respectively. The miRNAs act as tumour suppressors in silencing mRNA expression [2].

DICER1 syndrome is a familial tumour susceptibility syndrome associated with pleuropulmonary blastoma; ovarian sex cord-stromal tumours; cystic nephroma; thyroid gland neoplasia; and other rare benign and malignant tumours. Features of *DICER1* syndrome may present in childhood, but up to 95% of *DICER1* carriers do not develop any significant clinical features by age 10 [3, 4].

DICER1 related conditions are inherited in an autosomal dominant fashion. Penetrance is currently unknown but thought to be low except patients who have thyroid neoplasia. This is supported by the most recent estimated prevalence of germline *DICER1* mutation from population databases which is 1:10600 [4].

Germline mutations are typically truncating loss of function mutations. These are mainly single-nucleotide substitutions that produce new stop codons and small insertions or deletions within exons that shift reading frame. The mutations truncate the open reading frame before the end of the RNase IIIb domain, and as such result in complete loss of Dicer protein function [5].

Typically, pathology results from a somatic mutational insult to the remaining wild type allele. This mutation predominantly occurs within exons 24 or 25 in the RNase IIIb domain at one of five hotspot sites (E1705, D1709, E1788, D1810, or E1813) located in the metal-binding site. This affects balance between 5p and 3p miRNA [6].

Previously, up to 60% of SLCT were thought to contain somatic *DICER1* mutations; however, more recently, when centrally reviewed pathology was used to discriminate SLCT pathology, nearly all SLCT contained *DICER1* somatic mutations, especially in those determined to be moderately or poorly differentiated. This is against a background of at least 60% of patients having a germline mutation. Given this, all patients diagnosed with an SLCT should be tested for germline *DICER1* mutation and referred for genetic counselling [7–9].

The effect of this mutation in ovarian tissue includes deregulation of genes that control gonadal differentiation and cell proliferation, downregulation of key ovarian development genes, upregulation of Sertoli cell differentiation genes, and suppression of CYP19A1 leading to reduced aromatase activity causing androgenic effect [10].

3.1. Screening. Once *DICER1* syndrome is identified and the initial neoplasm has been treated, surveillance for recurrence and development of additional *DICER* related tumours should be considered. Genetic counselling regarding the implications of a diagnosis of *DICER1* familial mutation is recommended.

In the case we present the most common residual risk including multinodular goitre and a recurrence or metachronous SLCT. There is also a small increased lifetime risk of other *DICER1* related tumours such as pineoblastoma or cervical embryonal rhabdomyosarcoma. A surveillance program incorporated into the usual ovarian cancer 5-year follow-up protocol would include pelvic ultrasound every 6 months until age of 18, changing to transvaginal approach for better sensitivity in ovarian imaging, and the serum tumour markers AFP and testosterone. Pelvic imaging would be recommended until age 40 to rule out metachronous SLCT, which can be found in 6% of cases up to 14 years following initial development [7]. Symptom awareness for thyroid gland problems is advised, with low threshold for TFTS and thyroid ultrasound. Typically thyroid problems present with palpable neck lumps. The cumulative risk of multinodular goitre or thyroidectomy in women affected by *DICER1* syndrome by age 40 is 75% [11].

Educating those affected to be vigilant of symptoms such as postcoital bleeding, menstrual abnormalities, thyrotoxicity, headache, and visual disturbance and seeking medical review should they occur is also key.

Descendants of those affected have a 50% chance of inheriting the germline mutation and could be offered screening from a much earlier age. This is to incorporate pleuropulmonary blastoma, cystic nephroma, and pineoblastoma and other rarer phenotypes of *DICER1* syndrome.

Screening recommendations in each country are different due to the current evidence base being inconclusive. An international consensus on surveillance guideline is not yet available. However, the following surveillance options have been suggested by teams in Canada and the USA to consider. In the UK, screening is not currently offered but guidelines will be reviewed once international consensus recommendations are published.

Current preliminary recommendations include baseline CT examination of the chest between 3 and 6 months from birth, and if normal, it is repeated when they are 2.5 to 3 years old, sandwiched by chest radiographs every 6 months to age 8 and then annually to age 12.

Abdominal/pelvic ultrasound from birth are repeated every 6 months until age 40. Thyroid palpation annually from age 8 with ultrasound is repeated every 3 years. Brain MRI annually from birth to age 25 is controversial [12, 13].

The risk of repeated ionising radiation exposure is balanced against the early detection of malignant conditions and thus likely improvement in morbidity and mortality. Units have utilised whole-body MRI to ameliorate this; however in very young patients (< 6 years old) the long sequencing time often requires sedation or anaesthesia, which, albeit very low, has its own risk of complications [14, 15].

3.2. Conclusion. A diagnosis of Sertoli-Leydig cell tumour should prompt a referral to Clinical Genetics service due to the possibility of germline mutation and familial risk of malignancy. Knowledge of a *DICER1* mutation can inform the individual regarding management of the current tumour and also potential future cancer risks.

Consent

Written informed consent was obtained from the patient and parents for publication of this case report and accompanying images. A copy of the written consent is available for review by the Editor-in-Chief of this journal on request.

Disclosure

The present address of B. Wormald is The Institute of Cancer Research.

Authors' Contributions

All authors wrote sections of the manuscript. All authors contributed to manuscript revision and read and approved the submitted version.

References

[1] T. Gui, D. Cao, K. Shen et al., "A clinicopathological analysis of 40 cases of ovarian Sertoli-Leydig cell tumors," *Gynecologic Oncology*, vol. 127, no. 2, pp. 384–389, 2012.

[2] W. D. Foulkes, J. R. Priest, and T. F. Duchaine, "DICER1: mutations, microRNAs and mechanisms," *Nature Reviews Cancer*, vol. 14, no. 10, pp. 662–672, 2014.

[3] L. Doros, K. A. Schultz, D. R. Stewart, A. J. Bauer, G. Williams, C. T. Rossi et al., "DICER1-related disorders," in *GeneReviews(R). Seattle (WA): University of Washington, Seattle University of Washington*, M. P. Adam, H. H. Ardinger, R. A. Pagon, S. E. Wallace, L. J. H. Bean, and H. C. Mefford, Eds., Seattle University of Washington, Seattle, DC, USA, 2014.

[4] J. Kim, A. Field, K. A. P. Schultz, D. A. Hill, and D. R. Stewart, "The prevalence of DICER1 pathogenic variation in population databases," *International Journal of Cancer*, vol. 141, no. 10, pp. 2030–2036, 2017.

[5] M. Brenneman, A. Field, J. Yang et al., "Temporal order of RNase IIIb and loss-of-function mutations during development determines phenotype in pleuropulmonary blastoma / DICER1 syndrome: a unique variant of the two-hit tumor suppression model," *F1000Research*, vol. 4, p. 214, 2015.

[6] M. S. Anglesio, Y. Wang, W. Yang et al., "Cancer-associated somatic DICER1 hotspot mutations cause defective miRNA processing and reverse-strand expression bias to predominantly mature 3p strands through loss of 5p strand cleavage," *The Journal of Pathology*, vol. 229, no. 3, pp. 400–409, 2013.

[7] K. A. P. Schultz, A. K. Harris, M. Finch et al., "DICER1-related Sertoli-Leydig cell tumor and gynandroblastoma: clinical and genetic findings from the international ovarian and testicular stromal tumor registry," *Gynecologic Oncology*, vol. 147, no. 3, pp. 521–527, 2017.

[8] L. De Kock, T. Terzic, W. G. McCluggage et al., "DICER1 mutations are consistently present in moderately and poorly differentiated sertoli-leydig cell tumors," *The American Journal of Surgical Pathology*, vol. 41, no. 9, pp. 1178–1187, 2017.

[9] L. Witkowski, J. Mattina, S. Schönberger et al., "DICER1 hotspot mutations in non-epithelial gonadal tumours," *British Journal of Cancer*, vol. 109, no. 10, pp. 2744–2750, 2013.

[10] Y. Wang, J. Chen, W. Yang et al., "The oncogenic roles of DICER1 RNase IIIb domain mutations in ovarian sertoli-leydig cell tumors," *Neoplasia*, vol. 17, no. 8, pp. 650–660, 2015.

[11] N. E. Khan, A. J. Bauer, K. A. P. Schultz, L. Doros, R. M. Decastro, and A. Ling, "Quantification of thyroid cancer and multinodular goiter risk in the DICER1 syndrome: a family-based cohort study," *The Journal of Clinical Endocrinology & Metabolism*, vol. 102, no. 5, pp. 1614–1622, 2017.

[12] K. A. P. Schultz, S. P. Rednam, J. Kamihara et al., "PTEN, DICER1, FH, and their associated tumor susceptibility syndromes: Clinical features, genetics, and surveillance recommendations in childhood," *Clinical Cancer Research*, vol. 23, no. 12, pp. e76–e82, 2017.

[13] K. van Engelen, A. Villani, J. D. Wasserman et al., "DICER1 syndrome: Approach to testing and management at a large pediatric tertiary care center," *Pediatric Blood & Cancer*, vol. 65, no. 1, 2018.

[14] D. G. Sabapathy, R. Paul Guillerman, R. C. Orth et al., "Radiographic screening of infants and young children with genetic predisposition for rare malignancies: DICER1 mutations and pleuropulmonary blastoma," *American Journal of Roentgenology*, vol. 204, no. 4, pp. W475–W482, 2015.

[15] M. T. Bueno, C. Martínez-Ríos, A. D. la Puente Gregorio et al., "Pediatric imaging in DICER1 syndrome," *Pediatric Radiology*, vol. 47, no. 10, pp. 1292–1301, 2017.

41

Asymptomatic Bacteriuria in Pregnancy Complicated by Pyelonephritis Requiring Nephrectomy

Sharon J. Kim ⑩,[1] Pavan Parikh,[2] Amanda N. King,[1] and Mary L. Marnach[1]

[1]*Mayo Clinic, Department of Obstetrics and Gynecology, Rochester, MN, USA*
[2]*Mayo Clinic, Department of Obstetrics and Gynecology, Division of Maternal Fetal Medicine, Rochester, MN, USA*

Correspondence should be addressed to Sharon J. Kim; kim.sharon@mayo.edu

Academic Editor: Seung-Yup Ku

Routine prenatal care in the United States includes screening for asymptomatic bacteriuria (ASB), which occurs in 2 to 7 percent of pregnant women and can cause urinary tract infection and pyelonephritis. We present the case of a pregnant woman affected by multidrug resistant Klebsiella induced ASB during her prenatal screen, which was untreated due to a repeat urine culture showing mixed flora; subsequently, the patient's postpartum course was complicated by pyelonephritis and perinephric abscess, concluding in a radical nephrectomy. Current recommendations are to treat ASB after two consecutive voided urine cultures showing the same bacterial strain in quantitative counts of =/> 10(5) colony forming units (cfu)/mL or a single-catheterized specimen with quantitative count of =/> 10(2) cfu/mL. For women with ASB in their prenatal screen or other high risk factors, consideration should be given to testing urine cultures every trimester until the completion of pregnancy to prevent the complications of persistent bacteriuria.

1. Introduction

Screening for asymptomatic bacteriuria (ASB) is part of routine prenatal care in the United States, as ASB occurs in 2 to 7 percent of pregnant women [1, 2]. Up to 40% of untreated pregnant women with ASB will develop a urinary tract infection (UTI), including pyelonephritis, with 80 percent risk reduction if bacteriuria is eradicated forming the basis for ACOG treatment recommendations [1–4].

In the absence of strong risk factors for recurrent or persistent bacteriuria such as sickle cell trait or renal transplantation, there is no guidance available to inform the care of other patients at moderately increased risk. These risk factors include a history of prior UTI, nulliparity, pre-existing diabetes mellitus, smoking, late presentation to care, and low socioeconomic status [3, 5–7]. Herein, we discuss the case of a woman affected by multidrug resistant Klebsiella induced ASB untreated in the antenatal period, leading to pyelonephritis and perinephric abscesses and concluding in radical nephrectomy in the postpartum period.

2. Case Presentation

The patient is a 30-year old now gravida 2 para 2, status post complete left nephrectomy in the setting of multidrug resistant Klebsiella urosepsis and left pyelonephritis during her immediate postpartum phase. The Anuak speaking woman immigrated from Kenya to the United States nine months prior to her second pregnancy and presented to care at 15 weeks' gestation. Her history included chronic hypertension without a previous history of UTI.

At her new obstetrical visit, a urinalysis demonstrated 4-10 white blood cells (WBC) per high power field and gram stain positivity for gram-negative bacilli and gram-positive bacilli. Urine culture yielded multidrug resistant Klebsiella pneumoniae, 10(4) to 10(5) colony forming units (cfu)/mL). The organism was susceptible to quinolones, carbapenems, and piperacillin/tazobactam. An Infectious Disease consultation recommended a repeat clean catch culture with treatment using IV ertapenem if the culture showed the same organism. The repeat urine culture showed mixed

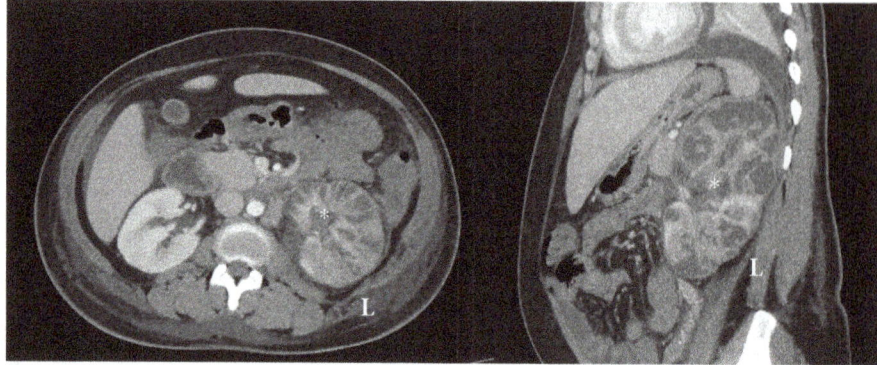

FIGURE 1: CT of abdomen, axial and sagittal views, with findings of multifocal areas of parenchymal infection and necrosis to left kidney∗.

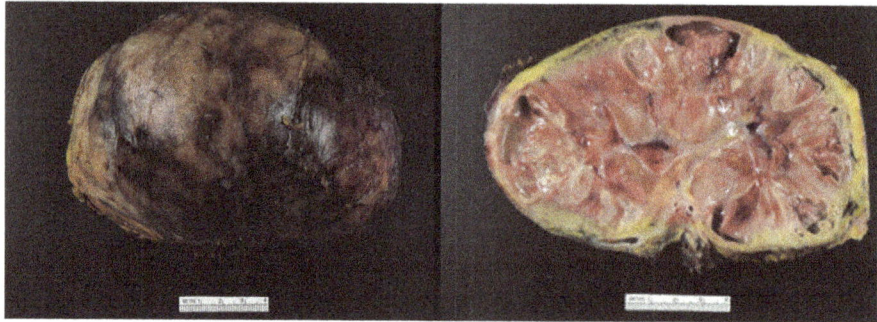

FIGURE 2: Renal parenchyma shows severe acute pyelonephritis with multifocal abscess formation and multifocal renal infarction.

flora without a specific organism identified. Because the patient remained asymptomatic, she did not have an additional gram stain or urine culture through the remainder of pregnancy.

At 37 weeks' gestation, the patient developed superimposed preeclampsia and underwent induction of labor with a normal spontaneous vaginal delivery without complications. On postpartum day (PPD) 0, she was afebrile but reported left sided abdominal and flank pain. A urine culture on PPD1 was positive for multidrug resistant Klebsiella/Raoultella species (sp) > 10(5) cfu/mL and sensitive to quinolones, gentamicin, and piperacillin/tazobactam. She began PO ciprofloxacin 500 mg twice daily with creatinine rising to 1.1. By PPD3, she continued to have abdominal and flank pain with creatinine rise to 1.5, and based on urine culture sensitivities, antibiotic was changed from ciprofloxacin to PO levofloxacin 500 mg daily. By PPD4 she developed new onset tachycardia, tachypnea, fever of 38.6 degrees celsius, and continued pain. As such, she was transferred to the intensive care unit with lactate 2.8 and WBC 18,000 and started on IV piperacillin/tazobactam 3.375 grams every 6 hours. A chest computerized tomography (CT) was negative for pulmonary embolism, showing a moderate left pleural effusion, and abdominal/pelvic CT compatible with pyelonephritis but no abscess. Blood cultures were positive for Klebsiella/Raoultella sp. On PPD5, when stable, she was transferred to the postpartum unit and switched to IV meropenem 500 mg every 6 hours due to persistent fevers. On PPD7, with ongoing fevers, tachycardia, and pain, a left kidney ultrasound confirmed a 5.1 cm left subcapsular

abscess which was aspirated 30 cc of purulent discharge. An echocardiogram for endocarditis and HIV testing were negative. By PPD9, with continued fevers to 39.3 degrees celsius, abdominal CT imaging was concerning for left renal multifocal infection and parenchymal necrosis (Figure 1). On PPD10, after Urology and Maternal Fetal Medicine consultations, the patient underwent an open left nephrectomy. Pathology confirmed severe diffuse pyelonephritis, multifocal abscesses, and diffuse parenchymal infarction (Figure 2).

The patient recovered well thereafter with symptom resolution, creatinine 1.0, and was discharged on postoperative day 3 with a 14-day course of IV ertapenem 1 gram daily.

3. Discussion

While our patient's early pregnancy urine culture demonstrated multidrug resistant Klebsiella pneumonia complex at 10(4) to 10(5) cfu/ml, she was not treated antenatally due to a repeat urine culture showing mixed flora likely related to inappropriate collection technique [8]. Through the remainder of her pregnancy, she had no urinary symptoms and no additional gram stain or urine culture was obtained until complaint of left abdominal and flank pain on the night of delivery.

The immunosuppression of pregnancy, mechanical bladder compression, and ureteral dilatation facilitates the ascent of bacteria resulting in a 20-fold increased risk of pyelonephritis in gravidas [2, 7, 9, 10]. For asymptomatic women, bacteriuria is defined as two consecutive voided urine specimens with isolation of the same bacterial strain in quantitative counts > 10(5) cfu/ml or a single-catheterized urine specimen with one bacterial species isolated in a quantitative count of =/> 10(2) cfu/mL [2]. In typical practice, however, only one voided urine specimen is usually obtained and diagnosis is made with =/> 10(5) cfu/mL without obtaining a confirmatory repeat urine culture. Asymptomatic bacteriuria > 10(5) cfu/ml is treated with an antibiotic tailored to the susceptibility of the isolated organism [4]. The threshold for diagnosis and treatment of asymptomatic bacteriuria due to group B Streptococcus, during pregnancy, is lower at =/> 10(4) cfu/mL [11].

In this patient's particular case, a repeat culture revealed mixed flora. While the general interpretation of mixed flora is one that does not need to be followed up, it should be emphasized that the more appropriate interpretation is that the culture is contaminated and must be repeated especially in the case with a prior positive test. Further, positive cultures that have been treated should be repeated to ensure appropriate clearance of the pathogen. The timing for this is as yet undetermined [2]; however 1 to 2 weeks following completion of antibiotic therapy is reasonable. In our case, empiric treatment of multidrug resistant Klebsiella would have been inappropriate as it is normal skin flora; yet, ensuring that the culture was truly negative thereafter should have been a priority to reduce the subsequent morbidity experienced by the patient and staying true to the core value of antibiotic stewardship.

Proper management of ASB during pregnancy is critical to decrease the risks of maternal and neonatal adverse events. Suspicion for renal or perinephric abscess should arise when there are prolonged fever and flank pain, despite antimicrobial therapy [12]. When renal abscesses are less than 5 cm in diameter, antimicrobial therapy alone may be adequate initial management [13, 14]. When clinical symptoms persist after several days of antimicrobial therapy, percutaneous drainage of abscesses less than 5 cm should be considered. Patients with renal abscesses greater than 5 cm should be managed with percutaneous drainage in conjunction with antimicrobial therapy [14, 15]. In the antepartum period, ultrasound imaging should be considered to evaluate for structural abnormalities. Computed tomography with contrast enhancement is the ideal imaging for assessing a perinephric abscess and the extension of suppuration; however, in the antepartum period, the risks of fetal harm should be weighed [14, 16, 17]. Early surgical consultation is recommended for abscesses not amenable to drainage, anatomic abnormalities, or failed medical treatment.

For low-risk women with a negative urine test in their initial prenatal visit, rescreening for ASB is not indicated. For women with ASB in their prenatal screen or other risk factors, consideration should be given to urine cultures performed every trimester until the completion of pregnancy.

Consent

Informed consent was obtained from the patient included in the study.

References

[1] L. E. Nicolle, "Asymptomatic bacteriuria: when to screen and when to treat," *Infectious Disease Clinics of North America*, vol. 17, no. 2, pp. 367–394, 2003.

[2] L. E. Nicolle, S. Bradley, R. Colgan, J. C. Rice, A. Schaeffer, and T. M. Hooton, "Infectious diseases society of America guidelines for the diagnosis and treatment of asymptomatic bacteriuria in adults," *Clinical Infectious Diseases*, vol. 40, no. 5, pp. 643–654, 2005.

[3] D. A. Wing, M. J. Fassett, and D. Getahun, "Acute pyelonephritis in pregnancy: An 18-year retrospective analysis," *American Journal of Obstetrics & Gynecology*, vol. 210, no. 3, pp. 219.e1–219.e6, 2014.

[4] F. M. Smaill and J. C. Vazquez, "Antibiotics for asymptomatic bacteriuria in pregnancy," *Cochrane Database of Systematic Reviews*, vol. 2015, no. 8, 2015.

[5] J. Schnarr and F. Smaill, "Asymptomatic bacteriuria and symptomatic urinary tract infections in pregnancy," *European Journal of Clinical Investigation*, vol. 38, no. 2, pp. 50–57, 2008.

[6] A. R. Thurman, L. L. Steed, T. Hulsey, and D. E. Soper, "Bacteriuria in pregnant women with sickle cell trait," *American Journal of Obstetrics & Gynecology*, vol. 194, no. 5, pp. 1366–1370, 2006.

[7] E. Farkash, A. Y. Weintraub, R. Sergienko, A. Wiznitzer, A. Zlotnik, and E. Sheiner, "Acute antepartum pyelonephritis in pregnancy: A critical analysis of risk factors and outcomes," *European Journal of Obstetrics & Gynecology and Reproductive Biology*, vol. 162, no. 1, pp. 24–27, 2012.

[8] American College of Obstetrics and Gynecology Committee on Obstetrical Practice, "ACOG Committee Opinion No. 91: Treatment of urinary tract infections in nonpregnant women," *Obstetrics & Gynecology*, vol. 111, no. 3, pp. 785–794, 2008.

[9] R. L. Sweet, "Bacteriuria and pyelonephritis during pregnancy," *Semin Perinatol*, pp. 1–25, 1977.

[10] C. Petersson, S. Hedges, K. Stenqvist et al., "Suppressed antibody and interleukin-6 responses to acture pyelonephritis in pregnancy," *Kidney International*, vol. 45, no. 2, pp. 571–577, 1994.

[11] American College of Obstetricians and Gynecologists Committee on Obstetric Practice, "ACOG Committee Opinion no. 485: prevention of early-onset group B streptococcal disease in newborns," *Obstetrics & Gynecology*, vol. 117, no. 4, pp. 1019–1027, 2011.

[12] B. E. Lee, H. Y. Seol, T. K. Kim et al., "Recent clinical overview of renal and perirenal abscesses in 56 consecutive cases," *Korean Journal of Internal Medicine*, vol. 23, no. 3, pp. 140–148, 2008.

[13] S. H. Lee, H. J. Jung, S. Y. Mah, and B. H. Chung, "Renal abscesses measuring 5 cm or less: Outcome of medical treatment without therapeutic drainage," *Yonsei Medical Journal*, vol. 51, no. 4, pp. 569–573, 2010.

[14] L. Dalla Palma, F. Pozzi-Mucelli, and V. Ene, "Medical treatment of renal and perirenal abscesses: CT evaluation," *Clinical Radiology*, vol. 54, no. 12, pp. 792–797, 1999.

[15] M. V. Meng, L. A. Mario, and J. W. McAninch, "Current treatment and outcomes of perinephric abscesses," *The Journal of Urology*, vol. 168, p. 1337, 2002.

[16] J. F. Siegel, A. Smith, and R. Moldwin, "Minimally invasive treatment of renal abscess," *The Journal of Urology*, vol. 155, no. 1, pp. 52–55, 1996.

[17] J. Demertzis and C. O. Menias, "State of the art: Imaging of renal infections," *Emergency Radiology*, vol. 14, no. 1, pp. 13–22, 2007.

42

Management of Bilateral Ectopic Pregnancies after Ovulation Induction Using Unilateral Salpingectomy and Methotrexate for the Remaining Ectopic with Subsequent Intrauterine Pregnancy

Quinton Katler ⓘ, Lindsey Pflugner, and Anjali Martinez

Department of Obstetrics and Gynecology, The George Washington University Hospital, Washington, DC, USA

Correspondence should be addressed to Quinton Katler; qkatler@gwu.edu

Academic Editor: Akihisa Fujimoto

Bilateral ectopic pregnancy is a rare phenomenon which is found with increased frequency when using assisted reproductive technology (ART). This diagnosis is most often made incidentally and intraoperatively, as ultrasound and serial β-hCG trends have shown poor efficacy for accurate diagnosis. Management of bilateral ectopic pregnancies is most commonly reported using bilateral surgical removal of the ectopic pregnancy (salpingostomy and/or salpingectomy). We present a case of an ART patient with incidentally found bilateral tubal ectopic pregnancies, where multiple management strategies including medical and surgical techniques were used concurrently which resulted in a subsequent spontaneous intrauterine pregnancy. While the standard of care is difficult to establish, we recommend individualizing management decisions based on the patient's reproductive goals and overall risk profile.

1. Introduction

Unilateral ectopic pregnancy is a well-known and common diagnosis in the general population [1]. Conversely, bilateral ectopic pregnancy is a much rarer phenomenon, occurring in approximately 1 per 200,000 live births [2]. While bilateral ectopic pregnancies have been documented in the literature since the 1900s, the invention of assisted reproductive technologies (ART) has led to an increase in reported cases of bilateral ectopic pregnancies [3, 4].

Given the relative frequency of bilateral ectopic pregnancies in the ART population, the importance of choosing an appropriate management strategy is further underscored given the known morbidity and potential mortality of ruptured ectopics within the context of the patient's reproductive goals. There are established criteria for management of unilateral ectopic pregnancies, which include pharmacologic, surgical, and expectant management under specific circumstances. However, there are no well-defined studies or data to suggest standard of care in the case of bilateral tubal ectopic pregnancies, particularly in the setting of one ruptured and one nonruptured ectopic pregnancy. Upon review of the existing literature, there are no reports of medical and surgical management being used simultaneously for the management of bilateral ectopic pregnancies, nor are there reports of a subsequent spontaneous intrauterine pregnancy following this treatment approach. Here we present a case of an ART patient with incidentally found bilateral tubal ectopic pregnancies, where two different management strategies were used concurrently with a successful outcome.

2. Case Report

A 32-year-old G2P0020 healthy Caucasian female initially presented to our institution for outpatient evaluation and management of secondary infertility. Her obstetric history was notable for two first-trimester miscarriages that were both managed expectantly. The couple's infertility evaluation revealed normal ovarian reserve testing and semen-analysis parameters with an unremarkable hysterosalpingogram (HSG) study, and they were diagnosed with unexplained infertility. The patient underwent ovulation induction with clomiphene citrate and HCG trigger with timed intrauterine insemination (IUI) using her partner's sperm. In

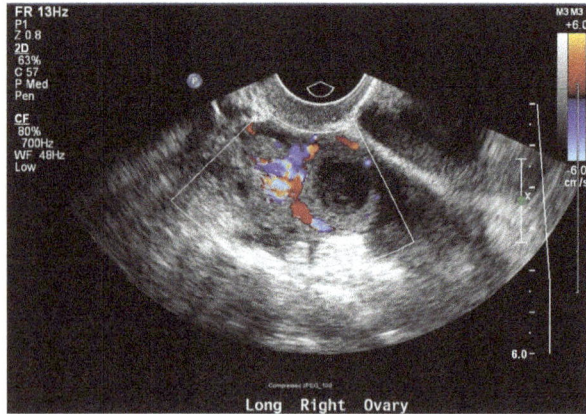

FIGURE 1: TVUS image of right adnexa with corpus luteal cyst versus ectopic gestation.

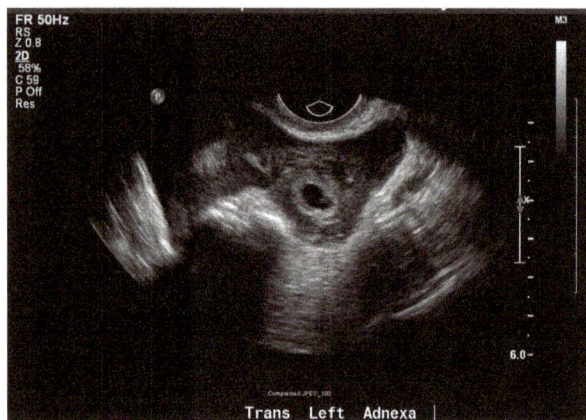

FIGURE 2: TVUS image of left adnexa with embryonic structures consistent with an ectopic pregnancy.

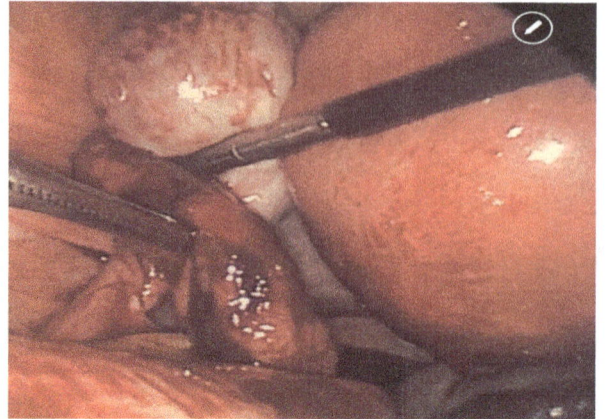

FIGURE 3: Left tubal ectopic pregnancy (active bleeding, treated with salpingectomy).

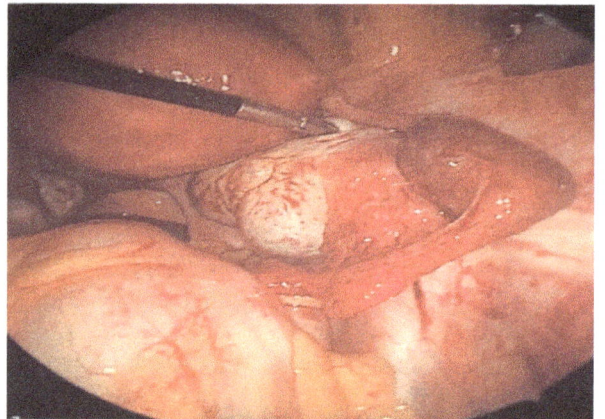

FIGURE 4: Right tubal ectopic pregnancy (treated with MTX).

the weeks following IUI, the β-hCG level rose appropriately from 641 to 971 in 48 hours. One week later, the β-hCG level rose to 3,448 and TVUS revealed a small, irregularly shaped gestational sac in the uterus without a clear yolk sac or evidence of a fetal pole. The right adnexa appeared to have two corpus luteal cysts. Of note, no free fluid was identified in the cul-de-sac and the patient was asymptomatic at that clinic visit. The plan was for a repeat β-hCG level and TVUS in 48 hours.

The patient subsequently presented to the emergency room the following morning with diffuse lower abdominal pain and vaginal bleeding. TVUS identified what appeared to be a corpus luteal cyst in the right ovary (Figure 1) and a likely ectopic pregnancy in the left adnexa (Figure 2) with a small amount of complex free fluid within the cul-de-sac. Her abdominal exam was significant for involuntary guarding of the lower quadrants bilaterally with diffuse tenderness. After discussion with the patient regarding our concern for ruptured ectopic pregnancy, the patient was amenable with the plan of proceeding with a laparoscopic unilateral salpingectomy.

A diagnostic laparoscopy was performed which revealed moderate hemoperitoneum upon abdominal entry. On pelvic survey, the left fallopian tube was noted to have a dilated distal portion, approximately 2cm in diameter with active bleeding, consistent with a ruptured left ectopic versus tubal abortion (Figure 3). Notably, the mid-portion of the right fallopian tube appeared dilated at the junction between the isthmus and the ampulla, about 3cm in diameter, without evidence of rupture or bleeding, which was concerning a concurrent second ectopic pregnancy (Figure 4).

The surgeons were then faced with a difficult decision regarding management of the unruptured contralateral tube. The patient's husband (and power of attorney) subsequently became involved with all decisions regarding the patient's plan of care. A left salpingectomy was essential given the abnormal left fallopian tube with active bleeding. Options for management of the contralateral tube were presented: right salpingectomy, right salpingostomy with Methotrexate (MTX) administration, or MTX administration alone without surgical intervention on the right fallopian tube. After thorough risk-benefit consideration, as well as intraoperative consultation with the patient's Reproductive Endocrinologist, the decision was made to retain the right fallopian tube and proceed conservatively with MTX administration (single-dose regimen of $50\,\mathrm{mg/m^2}$) due to the patient's likely desire to preserve her fallopian tube.

The patient had an uneventful recovery and her day 4 and day 7 β-hCG values confirmed an appropriate decline in β-hCG levels after MTX injection. The β-hCG level had dropped to a nonpregnant level by approximately three weeks following MTX administration. Histology of the left fallopian tube included the presence of chorionic villi, which confirmed the diagnosis of a left ectopic pregnancy. Repeat TVUS one-month following the surgery was normal without evidence of right tubal dilatation. Approximately 14 weeks after surgery, the patient had a repeat TVUS which revealed a single viable intrauterine pregnancy, which was conceived spontaneously.

3. Discussion

The general incidence of single ectopic pregnancies varies by study but according to the Center for Disease Control and Prevention accounts for about 2% of pregnancies [5]. Despite improvements in early detection and management modalities, ruptured ectopic pregnancies still account for a significant percentage of pregnancy-related mortality. Evolving data suggests that conception from ART is an independent risk factor for the development of an ectopic gestation. In literature review, studies describe a higher incidence of ectopic pregnancies after various methods of ART, ranging anywhere from 2.2 to 4.5% of ART cycles compared to spontaneous conception [6, 7]. In selected groups of patients with tubal infertility, the incidence of ectopic pregnancies after IVF may be as high as 11% [8]. A recent retrospective cohort study published by the Zhengzhou Reproductive Medical Center analyzed the incidence of ectopic pregnancies in their IVF and IUI cycles over the preceding six years [9]. The overall ectopic rate was 3% in both subgroups, suggesting an increased ectopic risk when comparing ART with spontaneous conception. Bilateral, or heterochronic, ectopics are the rarest form of ectopic pregnancy. We have witnessed a 3-fold increase in diagnosed bilateral ectopic pregnancies over the past several decades, in part due to the increasing use of ART technology [10].

When managing bilateral ectopic pregnancies, important issues arise with regard to detection and treatment. Primarily, trending the β-hCG values in bilateral ectopic pregnancies has not been shown to be an effective diagnostic practice [11]. Additionally, in most published case reports on this topic, early ultrasound use typically fails to make a diagnosis of bilateral tubal involvement. In a review of 16 case reports on bilateral ectopic pregnancies after ovulation induction, both ectopic pregnancies were identified by ultrasound imaging in only 6 of the cases prior to surgical intervention [12]. Accordingly, in a review by de los Rios et al. only 2 of 42 bilateral ectopic pregnancies were accurately diagnosed by ultrasound [13]. Commonly, ultrasound imaging identifies one ectopic pregnancy, which precipitates further investigation and subsequent management. Our case highlights this discrepancy between ultrasound results and intraoperative findings. Ultrasound may not be necessary to make the

diagnosis, and patients with significant risk factors should be counseled on the possibility of bilateral ectopic pregnancies, and decisions regarding the management algorithm should ideally be decided before surgery ensues. As a majority of bilateral ectopic pregnancies are diagnosed intraoperatively, inspection of both fallopian tubes should be standard of care in any ectopic case where the patient has risk factors for multiple gestations.

Previous studies have suggested that the same options for unilateral ectopic pregnancies be applied for bilateral ectopic pregnancies, including MTX administration or laparoscopy (with either salpingostomy or salpingectomy). However, due to the rare nature of bilateral ectopic pregnancies, there are no published guidelines to help advise management decisions. Also, data is sparse with regard to fertility outcomes and recurrent ectopic pregnancy rate after management of the concurrent ectopic pregnancy. With regard to MTX administration for bilateral ectopic pregnancies, a previously published report described treatment failure using single-dose MTX therapy, as the patient subsequently required surgery [14]. To date, there are no published reports that describe effective MTX dosage or regimen for bilateral ectopic pregnancies.

Bilateral ectopic pregnancies pose a unique dilemma in that both tubes are likely damaged, increasing the risk of future ectopic recurrence. As such, most cases of bilateral ectopic pregnancies are treated with bilateral salpingectomy. For instance, 12 of the 16 cases described by Zhu et al. involved bilateral salpingectomy [12]. In our case, the power of attorney was counseled about potential reproductive options. It was discussed that both fallopian tubes would likely have underlying damage regardless of the chosen treatment option. Discussion continued where bilateral salpingectomies would guarantee the need for IVF while a retained damaged tube would increase the rate of recurrent ectopic pregnancy. The only option that would maintain the possibility of spontaneous intrauterine pregnancy would be to retain the non-ruptured tube and to treat medically or with salpingostomy. However, with this approach, if ART was used the Reproductive Endocrinologist would likely recommend IVF in order to decrease the risk of a repeat ectopic pregnancy. This complex and rare situation emphasizes the importance of thorough evaluation of treatment options while utilizing a patient-centric approach.

When deciding between salpingostomy and salpingectomy, it is important to consider the potential impact on future fertility and subsequent ectopic pregnancy risk. RCTs comparing the two techniques in unilateral ectopics have not found significantly different rates for subsequent intrauterine pregnancies or repeat ectopic pregnancies. However, cohort studies have shown higher pregnancy rates for salpingostomy, including both intrauterine and ectopic rates [15]. Surgical management by bilateral salpingectomy should be recommended for usual indication: the patient is exhibiting hemodynamic instability or tubal bleeding. Salpingostomy or MTX administration may be considered for the remaining tube if IVF is not an option; however the patient should be counseled on the recurrence risk and the possible need for future surgery.

In the absence of established guidelines for the management of bilateral ectopic pregnancies, successful outcomes are required in order to help establish protocols for clinical care. Our case presents a unique approach to the management of the contralateral ectopic using medical therapy alone without salpingostomy while already undergoing a surgical procedure, which helped to preserve the remaining tube and allow for spontaneous pregnancy. Complete treatment was confirmed by a downtrend in the patient's β-hCG level to a nonpregnant level. Additionally, patients having a unilateral salpingectomy with Methotrexate for the remaining ectopic may consider performing a HSG remote from surgery in order to determine residual tubal patency. One limitation of our study is that tissue was not extracted from the second fallopian tube; thus histologic confirmation of the second ectopic pregnancy is not available.

In conclusion, we present a case of bilateral ectopic pregnancy which was successfully managed with unilateral salpingectomy and medical management with Methotrexate for the contralateral ectopic. As the use of ART technique may become increasingly more common, we may continue to witness a rising incidence of bilateral ectopic pregnancies. As scarce data is published on this topic, it is essential to investigate innovative diagnostic and treatment modalities in order to promote improved clinical care within this context.

Ethical Approval

According to guidelines set forth by The George Washington University Office of Human Research, IRB approval was not required for this study.

References

[1] F. Cunningham, K. Leveno, S. Bloom et al., *Ectopic Pregnancy. Williams Obstetrics*, McGraw-Hill, New York, NY, USA, 24th edition, 2013.

[2] S. Hoffmann, H. Abele, and C. Bachmann, "Spontaneous Bilateral Tubal Ectopic Pregnancy: Incidental Finding during Laparoscopy - Brief Report and Review of Literature," *Geburtshilfe und Frauenheilkunde*, vol. 76, no. 4, pp. 413–416, 2016.

[3] M. C. Edelstein and M. A. Morgan, "Bilateral simultaneous tubal pregnancy," *Obstetrical & Gynecological Survey*, vol. 44, no. 4, pp. 250–252, 1989.

[4] N. Sugawara, R. Sato, M. Kato et al., "Bilateral tubal pregnancies after a single-embryo transfer," *Reproductive Medicine and Biology*, vol. 16, no. 4, pp. 396–400, 2017.

[5] Centers for Disease Control and Prevention (CDC), "Current Trends in Ectopic pregnancy—United States, 1990-1992," *Morbidity and Mortality Weekly Report*, vol. 44, pp. 46–48, 1995.

[6] S. F. Marcus and P. R. Brinsden, "Analysis of the incidence and risk factors associated with ectopic pregnancy following in-vitro fertilization and embryo transfer," *Human Reproduction*, vol. 10, no. 1, pp. 199–203, 1995.

[7] A. Strandell, J. Thorburn, and L. Hamberger, "Risk factors for ectopic pregnancy in assisted reproduction," *Fertility and Sterility*, vol. 71, no. 2, pp. 282–286, 1999.

[8] J. B. Dubuisson, F. X. Aubriot, L. Mathieu, H. Foulot, L. Mandelbrot, and J. B. De Joliniere, "Risk factors for ectopic pregnancy in 556 pregnancies after in vitro fertilization: Implications for preventive management," *Fertility and Sterility*, vol. 56, no. 4, pp. 686–690, 1991.

[9] Z. Bu, Y. Xiong, K. Wang, and Y. Sun, "Risk factors for ectopic pregnancy in assisted reproductive technology: a 6-year, single-center study," *Fertility and Sterility*, vol. 106, no. 1, pp. 90–94, 2016.

[10] I. Stabile and J. G. Grudzinskas, "Ectopic Pregnancy," *Obstetrical & Gynecological Survey*, vol. 45, no. 6, pp. 335–347, 1990.

[11] S. K. Jena, S. Singh, M. Nayak, L. Das, and S. Senapati, "Bilateral simultaneous tubal ectopic pregnancy: a case report, review of literature and a proposed management algorithm," *Journal of Clinical and Diagnostic Research*, vol. 10, no. 3, pp. QD01–QD03, 2016.

[12] B. Zhu, G.-F. Xu, Y.-F. Liu et al., "Heterochronic bilateral ectopic pregnancy after ovulation induction," *Journal of Zhejiang University Science B*, vol. 15, no. 8, pp. 750–755, 2014.

[13] J. F. de los Ríos, J. D. Castañeda, and A. Miryam, "Bilateral ectopic pregnancy," *Journal of Minimally Invasive Gynecology*, vol. 14, no. 4, pp. 419–427, 2007.

[14] I. Marcovici and B. Scoccia, "Spontaneous bilateral tubal ectopic pregnancy and failed methotrexate therapy: A case report," *American Journal of Obstetrics & Gynecology*, vol. 177, no. 6, pp. 1545-1546, 1997.

[15] X. Cheng, X. Tian, Z. Yan et al., "Comparison of the fertility outcome of salpingotomy and salpingectomy in women with tubal pregnancy: a systematic review and meta-analysis," *PLoS ONE*, vol. 11, no. 3, p. e0152343, 2016.

43

Tumor-Like Reaction to Polypropylene Mesh from a Mid-Urethral Sling Material Resembling Giant Cell Tumor of Vagina

Ali Azadi,[1] James A. Bradley,[2] Dennis M. O'Connor,[3] Amir Azadi,[2] and Donald R. Ostergard[4]

[1] Norton Urogynecology Center, Norton Healthcare, 4001 Dutchmans Lane, Louisville, KY 40207, USA
[2] University of Louisville School of Medicine, Louisville, KY 40202, USA
[3] Clinical Pathology Associates, Norton Healthcare, 4001 Dutchmans Lane, Louisville, KY 40207, USA
[4] UCLA School of Medicine, Los Angeles, CA, USA

Correspondence should be addressed to Ali Azadi; azadoox@yahoo.com

Academic Editor: Loïc Sentilhes

Background. Polypropylene material is widely used in gynecological surgery. There are few reports regarding its carcinogenic potential. There is lack of evidence supporting tumor formation directly attributed to the use of polypropylene material. *Case.* This patient is a 49-year-old woman with a history of stress urinary incontinence which required a MiniArc® Sling who presented with a hard, tender, immobile mass on the anterior vaginal wall. Pathological analysis of the mass revealed a tumor-like reaction to the polypropylene material that resembled a giant cell tumor of soft tissue. *Conclusion.* The use of polypropylene in surgery is ubiquitous across disciplines; thus consideration for a tumor-like reaction to the material should exist for patients who present with a mass near the surgical site.

1. Introduction

Giant cell tumor of soft tissue (GCTST) is a rare lesion that has sporadically been reported in the literature as far back as the early 19th century [1, 2]. Extraossseous giant cell tumors have been reported in numerous anatomical sites, such as the breast, head, neck, vulva, and superficial and deep fascia of skeletal muscle [1]. Histologically, GCTST is comparable to its bony counterpart, giant cell tumor of the bone (GCTB), demonstrating a mixture of mononuclear cells with round to oval nuclei and osteoclast-like multinucleated giant cells. Similar to GCTB, the majority of primary GCTST is thought to be benign; however, the metastatic potential of some GCTST lesions has been highlighted in the literature, with the most common site of metastasis being the lungs [3].

Recently, it was reported that a giant cell granuloma grew around polypropylene suture that had been used in a tendon transfer procedure, and the histopathology was consistent with a foreign-body reaction to the polypropylene material. Similarly, there was a case of a suture granuloma that occurred 12 years after an open appendectomy, and several reports in the literature describe foreign-body reactions caused by suture material that mimic cancer [4]. The possible carcinogenicity of polypropylene mesh was noted by the World Health Organization in 1999 following several animal studies; however, its carcinogenicity in humans has not been established. Despite widespread use of polypropylene, there are only a limited number of reported cases to suggest carcinogenicity [5–9].

The presence of foreign bodies is known to induce inflammation, and foreign-body induced inflammation is a recognized factor known to modulate tumor progression [10]. Giant cell tumors of the vagina are extremely rare. To our knowledge, the case that we are reporting is the first case of a tumor-like reaction resembling primary giant cell tumor of the vagina in the English-language literature. A systematic

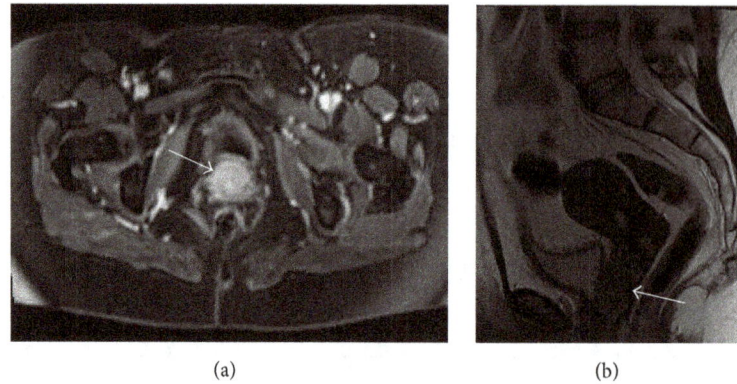

(a)   (b)

FIGURE 1: CT scan of the pelvis with (a) and without contrast (b) shows lesion on the anterior wall of the vagina, adjacent to the bladder (denoted by white arrow).

search was conducted on the Pubmed database using the search terms "giant cell tumor soft tissue," "giant cell tumor vagina," and "giant cell tumor pelvis." We report a case of a tumor-like reaction with features of benign GCTST in the vagina associated with polypropylene mesh and discuss the clinicopathological features of this lesion [1].

2. Case

A 49-year-old woman presented to clinic due to pelvic pressure and dyspareunia. Her medical history was significant for Graves' disease and tricuspid regurgitation. Her surgical history was significant for a MiniArc sling for stress urinary incontinence four years prior to presentation, endometrial ablation for abnormal uterine bleeding two years ago, remote C-section, and a laparoscopic bilateral tubal ligation. During examination, a hard, tender, and immobile mass was palpated on the anterior wall of the vagina. The epithelium covering the mass was intact and there was no discharge or bleeding noted during the examination. Due to her complaints of urinary urgency and frequency, cystourethroscopy was initially performed. No abnormality was found in the urethra by evaluation using a 0-degree cystoscope. The intravesical cavity was without any abnormal findings using a 70-degree cystoscope and with complete evaluation of the entire bladder including all edges. An MRI revealed a lesion measuring $3.1 \times 2.4 \times 2.2$ cm shown along the anterior wall of the vagina, adjacent to the base of the bladder (Figure 1).

The patient opted for removal of the vaginal mesh as dyspareunia had occurred after its placement. Vaginal excision of the mesh and surrounding mass was performed by making a vertical incision in the anterior vaginal wall, and cystourethroscopy confirmed the integrity of the bladder and urethra following the procedure. Specimens of the mesh and surrounding mass were sent to pathology for evaluation (Figure 2). It consisted of red-pink soft tissue measuring 3×2.5 cm admixed with blood clot.

Histologically, specimens demonstrated a marked fibroblast reaction with large numbers of giant cells (Figure 3(a)). Many of these giant cells exhibited osteoclastic features. Osteoid-like substance and dystrophic calcifications

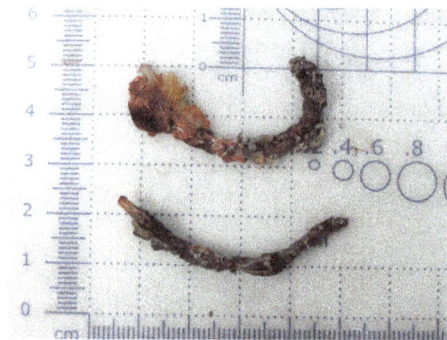

FIGURE 2: Gross specimen of sling.

resembling bone formation were noted in one specimen (Figures 3(b) and 3(c)), and several giant cells were found to surround nonpolarizable foreign material (Figure 3(d)). The proliferative nature of the fibroblasts and giant cells suggested a neoplastic characteristic with benign proliferative reactions, possibly representing a giant cell tumor of soft tissue.

3. Discussion

The use of polypropylene mesh for treatment of pelvic organ prolapse and urinary incontinence has increased over the past decade. Some controversy exists within the field regarding appropriate concerns that should be discussed with patients when considering the use of mesh in gynecological surgery. In 2011, the FDA issued a public health notification of adverse events that stated "serious complications with surgical mesh for transvaginal repair of POP are not rare." Shortly thereafter, on behalf of and endorsed by over 600 members of the Pelvic Surgeons Network, a separate review of the literature highlighted their belief that the FDA presented a biased view regarding vaginal mesh use in all repair procedures for pelvic organ prolapse [11]. Limited data exist regarding the complications of polypropylene mesh in the vagina after the body has been exposed to this material for several decades. A follow-up study of 90 women on the long-term efficacy of the tension-free vaginal tape procedure for stress urinary

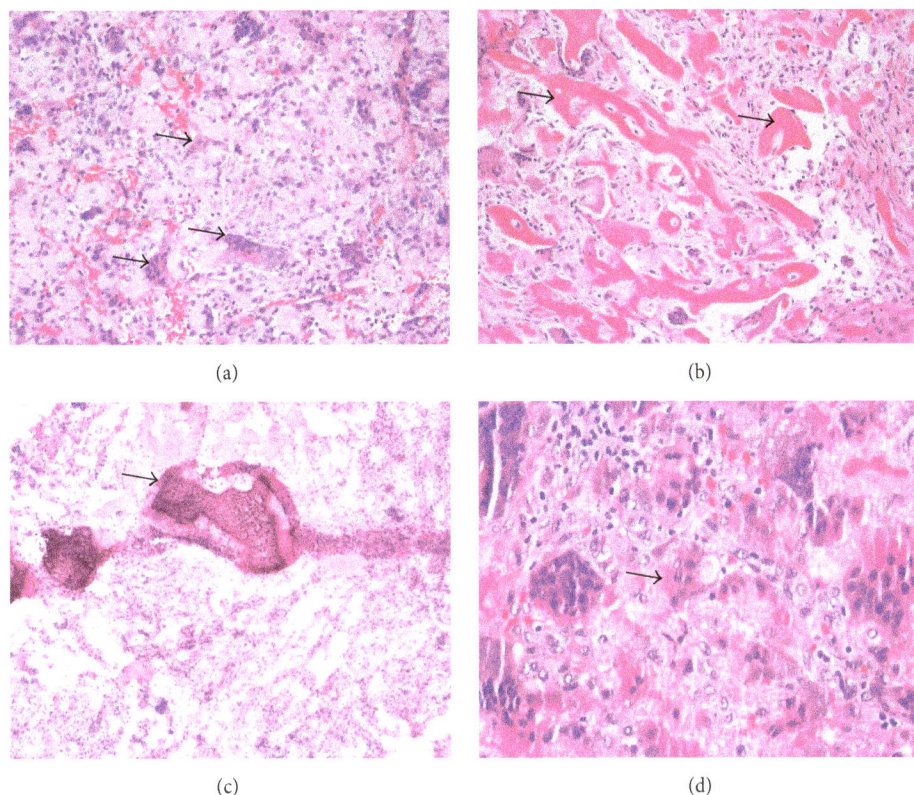

(a)

(b)

(c)

(d)

FIGURE 3: (a) Large numbers of giant cells present in a fibroblastic background (H&E stain-intermediate power; denoted by black arrows). (b) Osteoid-like material in a fibrous background (H&E stain-intermediate power; denoted by black arrows). (c) Dystrophic calcifications (H&E stain-intermediate power; denoted by a black arrow). (d) Ingestion of foreign material by a giant cell (H&E stain-high power; denoted by a black arrow).

incontinence showed an objective 90% cure rate after 11.5 years with no adverse effects from the polypropylene tape material or erosion into adjacent tissues [12]. Despite the wide use of polypropylene mesh, there has not been an established relationship between cases of human cancer attributed to the material.

Histologically, GCTST is characterized by a mixture of mononuclear cells and osteoclast-like multinucleated giant cells. Metaplastic bone formation at the periphery of the lesion is observed in 40–50% of cases [1]. Cystic changes and the formation of blood-filled lakes, changes that are similar to aneurysmal bone cystic changes, are present in approximately 30% of tumors. Foci of necrosis are very rare and cytological atypia is absent even if there is a high mitotic activity and vascular invasion. Immunohistochemically, CD68 immunoreactivity is frequently strong and diffuse in the multinucleated giant cells, whereas it is focal in the mononuclear cells. Histopathologically, GCTST should be separated from other tumors which can also exhibit giant cell components such as giant cell tumor of tendon sheath, extraskeletal osteosarcoma, or other benign reactive processes containing abundant osteoclast-like giant cells [1]. Local recurrence has been described after incomplete surgical excision, though metastases, which are characterized by nuclear atypia, pleomorphism, and atypical abundant mitoses, are extremely rare [1].

In a recent case report, recurrence of colon cancer was suspected after a suspicious lesion appeared on CT and PET scans, requiring exploratory laparotomy; a giant cell granuloma had developed around mesh used for prior abdominal hernia repair, demonstrating the ability of these lesions to mimic cancer and unavoidable surgical intervention [4].

In summary, we describe the first case of a tumor-like reaction resembling a primary GCTST in the vagina. Giant cell tumors are rare and likely underrecognized. The foreign-body reaction can make the clinical picture confusing. Consistent with the histology, the lesion in our patient could have developed as a result of the foreign-body reaction to the polypropylene mesh that had been used in the sling. Despite the benign nature of GCTST, formation of any mass can be very stressful for patients, specifically if they have had a prior diagnosis of cancer and are concerned for recurrence. Further research is warranted to better understand the inflammatory reaction to polypropylene due to its widespread use in gynecological procedures and the increased risk that patients may develop a mass late in life as a result of material used during surgery.

Consent

The authors have obtained a signed consent form from the patient discussed in this case report.

References

[1] C. D. M. Fletcher, "World Health Organization., and International Agency for Research on Cancer., WHO classification of tumours of soft tissue and bone., , World Health Organization classification of tumours," in *Proceedings of the IARC Press. 468 p*, vol. 468, p. p, Lyon, 2013.

[2] J. X. O'Connell, B. M. Wehrli, G. P. Nielsen, and A. E. Rosenberg, "Giant cell tumors of soft tissue: A clinicopathologic study of 18 benign and malignant tumors," *The American Journal of Surgical Pathology*, vol. 24, no. 3, pp. 386–395, 2000.

[3] J. G. Guccion and F. M. Enzinger, "Malignant giant cell tumor of soft parts. An analysis of 32 cases," *Cancer*, vol. 29, no. 6, pp. 1518–1529, 1972.

[4] M. A. Kassem, V. Alagiozian-Angelova, and J. Samuel, "All that glitters is not gold: Cancer-mimicking lesion in a cancer survivor," *Community Oncology*, vol. 7, no. 4, pp. 175–177, 2010.

[5] K. Moller, G. L. Mathes Jr., and W. Fowler Jr., "Primary leiomyosarcoma of the vagina: A case report involving a TVT allograft," *Gynecologic Oncology*, vol. 94, no. 3, pp. 840–842, 2004.

[6] S. Ahuja, O. Chappatte, M. Thomas, and A. Cook, "Bowel cancer and previous mesh surgery," *Journal of Gynecologic Surgery*, vol. 8, no. 2, pp. 217–221, 2011.

[7] H. Z. Lin, F. M. Wu, J. J. H. Low, K. Venkateswaran, and R. K. W. Ng, "A first reported case of clear cell carcinoma associated with delayed extrusion of midurethral tape," *International Urogynecology Journal and Pelvic Floor Dysfunction*, vol. 27, no. 3, pp. 377–380, 2016.

[8] H. B. Goldman and P. L. Dwyer, "Polypropylene mesh slings and cancer: An incidental finding or association?" *International Urogynecology Journal and Pelvic Floor Dysfunction*, vol. 27, no. 3, pp. 345-346, 2016.

[9] C. Birolini, J. G. Minossi, C. F. Lima, E. M. Utiyama, and S. Rasslan, "Mesh cancer: long-term mesh infection leading to squamous-cell carcinoma of the abdominal wall," *Hernia*, vol. 18, no. 6, pp. 897–901, 2014.

[10] R. Klopfleisch and F. Jung, "The pathology of the foreign body reaction against biomaterials," *Journal of Biomedical Materials Research Part A*, vol. 105, no. 3, pp. 927–940, 2017.

[11] M. Murphy, A. Holzberg, H. Van Raalte, N. Kohli, H. B. Goldman, and V. Lucente, "Time to rethink: An evidence-based response from pelvic surgeons to the FDA safety communication: "UPDATE on serious complications associated with transvaginal placement of surgical mesh for pelvic organ prolapse"," *International Urogynecology Journal*, vol. 23, no. 1, pp. 5–9, 2012.

[12] C. G. Nilsson, K. Palva, M. Rezapour, and C. Falconer, "Eleven years prospective follow-up of the tension-free vaginal tape procedure for treatment of stress urinary incontinence," *International Urogynecology Journal and Pelvic Floor Dysfunction*, vol. 19, no. 8, pp. 1043–1047, 2008.

44

Spontaneous Ovarian Hyperstimulation Syndrome with FSH Receptor Gene Mutation: Two Rare Case Reports

Emsal Pinar Topdagi Yilmaz,[1] Omer Erkan Yapca,[1] Yunus Emre Topdagi ⓘ,[2] Seray Kaya Topdagi,[1] and Yakup Kumtepe[1]

[1]Department of Gynecology and Obstetrics, Atatürk University School of Medicine, Erzurum, Turkey
[2]Clinic of Gynecology and Obstetrics, Nenehatun Gynecology and Obstetrics Hospital, Erzurum, Turkey

Correspondence should be addressed to Yunus Emre Topdagi; emr-topdagi@hotmail.com

Academic Editor: Kyousuke Takeuchi

Development of ovarian hyperstimulation syndrome (OHSS) is very rare in a spontaneous ovulatory cycle and it is usually seen during pregnancy. In the etiology of OHSS, higher hCG (molar pregnancies or multiple pregnancies) and thyroid-stimulating hormone (TSH) levels have been accused. In recent years, some follicle-stimulating hormone (FSH) receptor (FSHR) gene mutations have been described in patients with OHSS in the first trimester with normal hCG levels. Herein, we report two cases of FSHR gene mutation during the investigation of the etiology of spontaneous OHSS. Although OHSS is typically associated with ovulation induction, it should be kept in mind that this condition may also develop in spontaneous pregnancies.

1. Introduction

Ovarian hyperstimulation syndrome (OHSS) is a serious complication developing after the gonadotropin use for assisted reproduction methods and is observed in 10% of patients [1]. It is more common after the implantation procedure, particularly, and is accompanied by increased miscarriage rates [1–4]. The incidence of iatrogenic OHSS is 0.2 to 1%, and the risk of mortality is 1:45000-1:50000 [5].

When gonadotropin therapy is not used, the development of spontaneous OHSS is quite rare and it is usually associated with pregnancy. In the etiology of OHSS, higher hCG (molar pregnancies or multiple pregnancies) and thyroid-stimulating hormone (TSH) levels have been accused. In recent years, some follicle-stimulating hormone (FSH) receptor (FSHR) gene mutations have been described in patients with OHSS in the first trimester with normal hCG levels [6]. Clinical findings include massive ovarian growth, abdominal distension, nausea and vomiting, abdominal and inguinal pain, loss of protein rich fluid to the third space due to increased capillary permeability, extensive abdominal ascites, dyspnea, electrolyte imbalances, and the risk of thromboembolism and oliguria [3, 4]. In the differential diagnosis of

OHSS, conditions such as luteoma of pregnancy, recurrent theca lutein cysts, ovarian cancer, and hyperreactio luteinalis should be considered.

Herein, we report two cases of severe OHSS during spontaneous first trimester pregnancy in whom a FSHR gene mutation has been discovered by the genetic testing. We discuss this rare spontaneous OHSS clinical picture in the light of current data.

The test method used is as follows: the 5, 6, 7 and 10 exons in the FSHR gene and the exon/intron combination are applied. The results were analyzed using the Mutation Surveyor Program.

2. Case Report 1

A 20-year-old woman (Gravida 2/Para 1) who was unaware of the date of the last menstrual period and was evaluated during routine pregnancy follow-up presented with nonspecific complaints, such as abdominal pain, bloating, dyspepsia, and occasional respiratory distress. The medical and gynecological history of the patient was unremarkable. She had regular menstrual cycles and did not use oral contraceptives

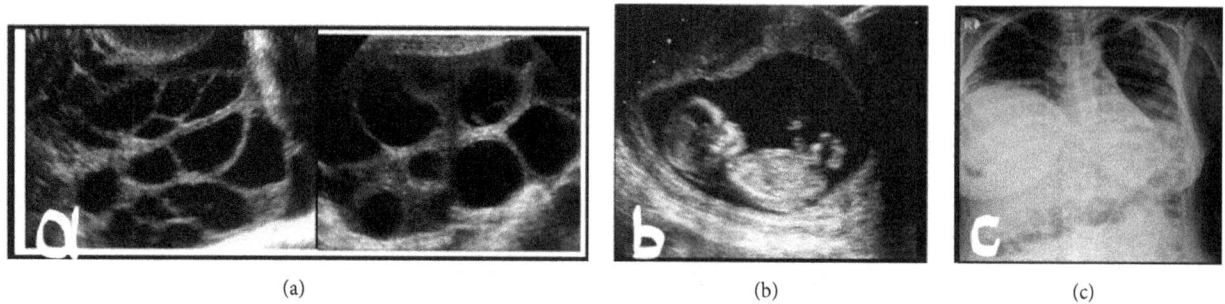

FIGURE 1: (a) Multicystic appearance in both ovaries (left ovary, 14*13 cm; right ovary, 13*12 cm). (b) A single intrauterine pregnancy with gestational age of 12 weeks according to the crown-rump length. (c) On chest X-ray, the costophrenic angles were closed with appearance of hydrothorax.

TABLE 1: The result of FSHR gene mutation in the presented two cases with spontaneous OHSS.

	c.383 C>A p.S128Y	Homozygous
	c.733 G>C p.Ala307Thr	Heterozygous
Case report 1	c.1961 G>C ve c.-29 G>A p.Ser680Asp	Polymorphism
Case report 2	c.383 C>A p.S128Y p.Ser128Tyr	Heterozygous

or any medication for the ovulation induction. An increase in the bilateral ovarian size (left side 14x13 cm and right side 13x12 cm) and a multicystic appearance were observed (Figure 1(a)). Ultrasonographic evaluation revealed a single live intrauterine fetus of 12 weeks gestation (Figure 1(b)). Extensive fluid was seen in the abdominal cavity. On chest X-ray, the costophrenic angles were closed and an appearance of hydrothorax was observed (Figure 1(c)). On physical examination, there was abdominal distension and tenderness. The laboratory tests of the patient were as follows: quantitative hCG 117740 IU/ml, TSH 3,229 μIU/ml, and free T3 and T4 were within normal ranges; hemoglobin 16,7 g/dl, hematocrit 47,6%, E2 >5000 pg/ml, PT, PTT, and fibrinogen were within normal limits; routine biochemical tests were normal (for example, total protein, albumin, creatinine, BUN, Na, K, AST, ALT, and LDH); interestingly CA-125 (564 IU/mL) was found higher, Inhibin A 861, Ristocetin cofactor (von Willebrand factor (VWF) activity) 100% (50-100%), and VWF antigen 150% (60-150%).

Serological tests (anti-HAV IgM, HBsAg, and anti-HCV) were found to be negative. Antithrombin 3, lupus anticoagulant, protein C and S activity, antiphospholipid antibodies (IgM and IgG), and anticardiolipin antibodies (IgM and IgG) were found to be within normal ranges in thrombophilia screening. Factor V Leiden mutation was not observed. Other causes of spontaneous OHSS were ruled out. In the examination of FSHR gene mutation due to investigation of spontaneous OHSS, a mutation was identified which has been previously described and reported as a disease-related mutation. The result is shown in Table 1. Doppler ultrasonography revealed normal arterial blood flow in bilateral ovaries. The patient was hospitalized with the diagnosis of Grade 2 spontaneous OHSS, according to the Golan classification [7], and conservative treatment was initiated.

Daily 75 mg of rectal indomethacin, 1500 cc/day intravenous saline infusion adjusted by considering the electrolyte balance, follow-up of fluid input and output, daily measurement of weight and waist circumference, and 3500 IU/day of low molecular weight heparin (tinzaparin sodium) for thromboembolism prophylaxis were administered. During the hospital stay, the clinical symptoms of the patient, such as abdominal pain and distention, increased. Repeated abdominal ultrasonography revealed advanced ascites in the abdomen. Approximately 2.5 to 3 L of ascites fluid was drained with a spinal needle by paracentesis. The treatment was supplemented with 20% 50cc albumin solution. Within the next three days, the laboratory parameters and clinical symptoms of the patient improved and she was discharged with suggestions of follow-up antenatal outpatient clinic visits. At 38 weeks of pregnancy, the patient gave birth of a 2,950 g healthy alive male baby, and in the first postpartum month, both ovaries were in normal appearance in transvaginal ultrasonography and in Doppler examination. The extensive abdominal ascites fluid also completely resolved. She had no complications during pregnancy and postpartum period.

3. Case Report 2

A 28-year-old woman (Gravida 3/Para 1) with unremarkable medical and gynecological history had regular menstrual cycles and did not use oral contraceptives or any medication for the ovulation induction. Ultrasonographic evaluation revealed a single live intrauterine fetus of 10-week gestation (Figure 2(a)). An increase in the bilateral ovarian size (left side 12x12,5 cm and right side 11x13 cm) and a multicystic appearance were observed (Figure 2(b)). The patient's laboratory tests were similar to those of the patient in the first

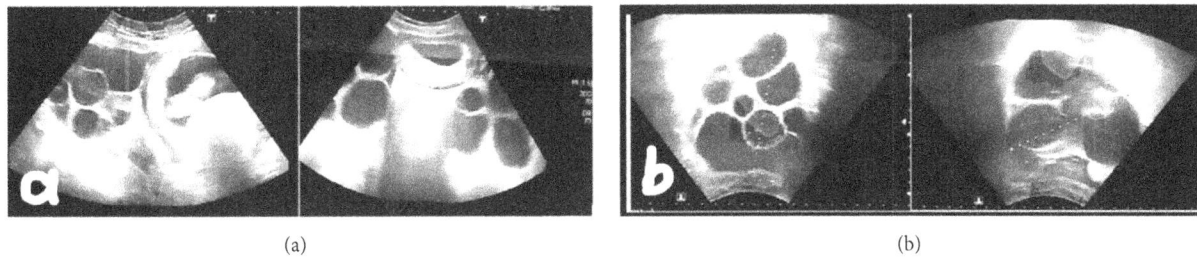

FIGURE 2: (a) Intrauterine pregnancy with gestational age of 10w and multicystic appearance in left ovary. (b) Bilateral ovaries (left ovary, 12∗12, 5cm; right ovary, 11∗13cm).

case. Other causes of spontaneous OHSS were ruled out. In the examination of FSHR gene mutation due to investigation of spontaneous OHSS, a mutation was identified which has been previously described and reported as a disease-related mutation. The result is shown in Table 1.

The patient was hospitalized with the diagnosis of Grade 2 spontaneous OHSS, according to the Golan classification, and conservative treatment was initiated. At 40 weeks of pregnancy, the patient gave birth of a 3840 g healthy alive female baby. She had no complications during pregnancy and postpartum period.

4. Discussion

Spontaneous OHSS can occur both in pregnant and non-pregnant women. De Leener classified spontaneous OHSS syndrome into three types based on clinical presentation and FSH receptor mutation. Type I is associated with the mutated FSH receptor and this type may cause recurrent spontaneous OHSS. Type II is secondary to high levels of human chorionic gonadotropin (hCG) as in hydatiform mole and multiple gestation and is the most frequent one. Type III is related to hypothyroidism[6].

Mutations in the FSH receptor (FSHR) could be activating, leading to a predisposition to OHSS, or inactivating, resulting in sterility due to poor ovarian response to gonadotropins. Polymorphisms of FSHR have been investigated and about 744 single nucleotide polymorphisms have been identified in the FSHR gene, of which only eight are located in the coding region, exons, with the rest being intronic. Ovarian response is dependent on the FSHR genotype. Clinical studies on the p.N680S polymorphism of the FSHR gene have demonstrated the homozygous Ser/Ser variant to be less sensitive to endogenous or exogenous FSH in terms of estradiol production. Polymorphism of the FSHR, Ser680Asn, in the FSHR gene is a predictor of the severity of symptoms in patients who develop OHSS [8, 9].

FSHR p.Ala307Thr and p.Ser680Asp polymorphisms have been associated with low over-reserve response and have been reported to cause prolongation of the ovulation induction period[10]. When the change in position 680 of the FSHR gene (p.Asn680Ser) is detected homozygously, however, the desired E2 level can be reached by administering a higher dose of exogenous FSH[11]. Recently, the inactivation of FSHB and FSH-R genes in animal models has been shown

to have an effect on FSH hormone levels. Mutations in FSHB and FSHR genes have also been observed in a group of patients with similar phenotypic effects[12].

FSHR-activating mutations: c.383C>A(exon 5), c.1345A>G, c.1346C>T, c.1634T>C, c1699G>A, c.1700A>G (exon 10).

FSHR-inactivating mutations: c.479T>C (exon 6), c.566C>T (exon 7), c.1255G>A, c.1555C>A, c.1717C>T, c.1760C>A, c.1801C>G (exon 10).

The knowledge about the pathophysiology of OHSS has been steadily increasing, and many agents have been suggested to play a role in the etiology of OHSS, such as estrogen, histamine, prostaglandins, aldosterone, renin, angiotensin II, and vascular endothelial growth factor (VEGF) [4]. The development of spontaneous OHSS in pregnancy is a rare clinical presentation. In recent publications, three distinct gene mutations in the FSHR have been discovered in patients with recurrent severe spontaneous OHSS. These mutated receptors are highly sensitive to hCG in vitro [13–15]. In normal pregnancy, FSHR cannot be stimulated or becomes very weak due to the very low amount of pituitary gonadotropins in the serum. In spontaneous OHSS patients, hyperstimulation develops with pregnancy-induced hCG due to increased and mutated FSHR in the growing follicle [15]. In another study of FSHR mutations, it was reported that the presence of 680FSHR mutation was predictive in determining the clinical severity of OHSS [16]. In our two cases, FSHR gene mutation was examined during the investigation of spontaneous OHSS, and it was positive. Other causes of spontaneous OHSS were ruled out.

The hCG in the blood reaches maximum level at 8th to 10th gestational weeks and starts to fall. In addition, in clinical follow-up, spontaneous OHSS develops after the 8th gestational week. However, iatrogenic OHSS cases are seen at earlier gestational weeks due to exogenous hCG stimulation [16]. In our two cases, similarly, spontaneous OHSS developed approximately at the 10th to 12th gestational week.

In the literature, there are also cases showing the coexistence of spontaneous OHSS and hypothyroidism, and polycystic ovary syndrome [16]. Possible risk factors such as molar pregnancy, multiple gestation, polycystic ovary syndrome, and hypothyroidism to explain the development of spontaneous OHSS were not found in our two cases.

In the literature, there are many studies on pregnancy and management of OHSS. Accordingly, the treatment of

OHSS should be conservative and include the regulation of intravascular volume and electrolyte balance and the prevention of complications such as hemoconcentration, hypovolemia, and coagulation disorders [17]. It has been reported that the miscarriage rates increase in pregnancies with the development of these complications. Since OHSS is usually self-limiting, the continuation of pregnancy is recommended. In almost all cases, pregnancy has reached term. Very rarely, deaths due to hypovolemia, hemorrhage, and thromboembolic events have been reported [18].

Terminating the pregnancy may be considered in cases resistant to conservative treatment, and emergency laparotomy may be necessary in conditions such as ovarian rupture, torsion, and intraperitoneal hemorrhage. Briefly, the identification of risky patients, preference for prevention strategies, bed rest, albumin levels with low salt, aspiration of ascites fluid by transvaginal ultrasonography, furosemide, low sodium intake, dopamine, close monitorization, and, recently, dopamine agonists are used in the treatment. In addition, studies are ongoing on the VEGF, which plays a major role in the pathophysiology of OHSS.

Contrary to previous studies on spontaneous OHSS management, in our two cases, the severity of OHSS was moderate and did not cause any pregnancy complication; thus, this finding supports recent publications [18]. In spontaneous OHSS cases, a rare form of OHSS, the diagnosis should be made urgently with clinical findings, unnecessary surgical procedures should be avoided, and conservative treatment for severe and life-threatening complications should be immediately initiated. Spontaneous OHSS cases are relatively more benign than iatrogenic cases. It has been reported that the probability of recurrence in later pregnancies is high. However, it has been reported that spontaneous OHSS may develop even in the patient who had a previous normal pregnancy, as in the presented case [17].

5. Conclusion

In conclusion, although OHSS is typically associated with ovulation induction, it should be kept in mind that this condition may also develop in spontaneous pregnancies. As it is usually self-limiting, continuation of the pregnancy is recommended. In general, the treatment recommendation is supportive care and anticoagulant treatment to prevent serious complications, such as pulmonary embolism due to deep venous thrombosis.

Rarity of this condition may also be due to misdiagnosis that can result in mismanagement or severe complications of this condition.

References

[1] J. G. Schenker and Y. Ezra, "Complications of assisted reproductive techniques," *Fertility and Sterility*, vol. 61, no. 3, pp. 411–422, 1994.

[2] O. A. Olatunbosun, B. Gilliland, and L. A. Brydon, "Spontaneous OHSS in four consecutive pregnancies," *Clinical and Experimental Obstetrics and Gynecology*, vol. 23, pp. 127–132, 1996.

[3] J. G. Whelan III and N. F. Vlahos, "The ovarian hyperstimulation syndrome," *Fertility and Sterility*, vol. 73, no. 5, pp. 883–896, 2000.

[4] U. Elchalal and J. G. Schenker, "The pathophysiology of ovarian hyperstimulation syndrome - Views and ideas," *Human Reproduction*, vol. 12, no. 6, pp. 1129–1137, 1997.

[5] J. Smitz, M. Camus, P. Devroey, P. Erard, A. Wisanto, and A. Van Steirteghem, "Incidence of severe ovarian hyperstimulation syndrome after GnRH agonist/HMG superovulation for in-vitro fertilization," *Human Reproduction*, vol. 5, no. 8, pp. 933–937, 1990.

[6] A. De Leener, L. Montanelli, J. Van Durme et al., "Presence and absence of follicle-stimulating hormone receptor mutations provide some insights into spontaneous ovarian hyperstimulation syndrome physiopathology," *The Journal of Clinical Endocrinology & Metabolism*, vol. 91, no. 2, pp. 555–562, 2006.

[7] A. Golan, R. Ron-El, A. Herman, Y. Soffer, Z. Weinraub, and E. Caspi, "Ovarian hyperstimulation syndrome: An update review," *Obstetrical & Gynecological Survey*, vol. 44, no. 6, pp. 430–440, 1989.

[8] B. Rizk, "Symposium: Update on prediction and management of OHSS - Genetics of ovarian hyperstimulation syndrome," *Reproductive BioMedicine Online*, vol. 19, no. 1, pp. 14–27, 2009.

[9] G. Vassart, L. Pardo, and S. Costagliola, "A molecular dissection of the glycoprotein hormone receptors," *Trends in Biochemical Sciences*, vol. 29, no. 3, pp. 119–126, 2004.

[10] T. Borgbo, J. Jeppesen, I. Lindgren, Y. Lundberg Giwercman, L. Hansen, and C. Yding Andersen, "Effect of the FSH receptor single nucleotide polymorphisms (FSHR 307/680) on the follicular fluid hormone profile and the granulosa cell gene expression in human small antral follicles," *MHR: Basic science of reproductive medicine*, vol. 21, no. 3, pp. 255–261, 2015.

[11] S. S. Desai, S. K. Achrekar, S. R. Paranjape, S. K. Desai, V. S. Mangoli, and S. D. Mahale, "Association of allelic combinations of FSHR gene polymorphisms with ovarian response," *Reproductive BioMedicine Online*, vol. 27, no. 4, pp. 400–406, 2013.

[12] E. T. Siegel, H.-G. Kim, H. K. Nishimoto, and L. C. Layman, "The molecular basis of impaired follicle-stimulating hormone action: Evidence from human mutations and mouse models," *Reproductive Sciences*, vol. 20, no. 3, pp. 211–233, 2013.

[13] G. Smits, O. Olatunbosun, A. Delbaere, R. Pierson, G. Vassart, and S. Costagliola, "Ovarian hyperstimulation syndrome due to a mutation in the follicle-stimulating hormone receptor," *The New England Journal of Medicine*, vol. 349, no. 8, pp. 760–766, 2003.

[14] C. Vasseur, P. Rodien, I. Beau et al., "A chorionic gonadotropin-sensitive mutation in the follicle-stimulating hormone receptor as a cause of familial gestational spontaneous ovarian hyperstimulation syndrome," *The New England Journal of Medicine*, vol. 349, no. 8, pp. 753–759, 2003.

[15] L. Montanelli, A. Delbaere, C. Di Carlo et al., "A Mutation in the Follicle-Stimulating Hormone Receptor as a Cause of Familial Spontaneous Ovarian Hyperstimulation Syndrome,"

The Journal of Clinical Endocrinology & Metabolism, vol. 89, no. 3, pp. 1255–1258, 2004.

[16] C. Daelemans, G. Smits, V. De Maertelaer et al., "Prediction of severity of symptoms in iatrogenic ovarian hyperstimulation syndrome by follicle-stimulating hormone receptor Ser680Asn polymorphism," *The Journal of Clinical Endocrinology & Metabolism*, vol. 89, no. 12, pp. 6310–6315, 2004.

[17] H. D. Chae, E. J. Park, S. H. Kim, C. H. Kim, B. M. Kang, and Y. S. Chang, "Ovarian hyperstimulation syndrome complicating a spontaneous singleton pregnanc: a case report," *Journal of Assisted Reproduction and Genetics*, vol. 18, no. 2, p. 120, 2001.

[18] A. Delbaere, G. Smits, A. De Leener, S. Costagliola, and G. Vassart, "Understanding ovarian hyperstimulation syndrome," *Endocrine Journal*, vol. 26, no. 3, pp. 285–289, 2005.

45

Two Cases of Dedifferentiated Endometrioid Carcinoma: Case Presentation and Brief Review of the Literature

Sachiko Morioka ⓘ,[1] **Yasuhito Tanase,**[1] **Ryuji Kawaguchi,**[1]
Tomoko Uchiyama,[2] **and Hiroshi Kobayash**[1]

[1]*Department of Obstetrics and Gynecology, Nara Medical University, Nara, Japan*
[2]*Department of Diagnostic Pathology, Nara Medical University, Nara, Japan*

Correspondence should be addressed to Sachiko Morioka; morioka.sac@gmail.com

Academic Editor: Maria Grazia Porpora

Endometrioid carcinoma is the most common histological type of uterine endometrial cancer and particularly dedifferentiated endometrioid carcinomas (DEC) are less commonly observed. Silva et al. reported the biological features of UC based on the undifferentiated component of DEC, although the component represented only 20% of undifferentiated carcinoma. In this study, we report two cases of DEC with different presentation. Case 2 presented with the invasion to the bladder, rectum, and LN metastases. In contrast, the tumor in case 1 advanced into the endometrial cavity, similar to an endometrial polyp, without myometrial invasion. Hence, the diagnosis was established early. While we strive to improve the diagnosis of DEC, it is also crucial to better assess the prognosis and the appropriate treatment for the patients with established diagnosis of DEC.

1. Introduction

Endometrioid carcinoma is the most common histological type of uterine endometrial cancer, whereas serous, clear cell, undifferentiated, and particularly dedifferentiated endometrioid carcinomas (DEC) are less commonly observed. Silva et al. first reported the patients with undifferentiated uterine carcinoma (UC) coexisting with low-grade endometrioid carcinoma (grades 1 or 2) as having DEC in 2006 [1]. They reported the biological features of UC based on the undifferentiated component of DEC, although the component represented only 20% of UC. In this study, we report two cases diagnosed as DEC with different presentations. In the first case, the tumor developed on the surface of an endometrial polyp; in the second case, the tumor presented as an advanced cancer with metastasis in multiple lymph nodes.

2. Case Presentation

Case 1. A 68-year-old postmenopausal woman (gravida 2; body mass index [BMI], 32.4 kg/m^2) presented at a local gynecology clinic 20 months ago with a chief complaint of vaginal spotting. Transvaginal ultrasonography showed no thickness of the endometrium, and endometrial cytology was negative. At the three-month follow-up visit, a repeat endometrial cytology was also negative. However, vaginal bleeding persisted, and the patient visited the clinic again a month ago. At this time, pelvic magnetic resonance imaging (MRI) was performed, which revealed irregularity and endometrial thickening, and the patient was referred to our institution—Nara Medical University, Kashihara, Nara, Japan—for further evaluation. Endometrial curettage was performed that revealed atypical cells with large nuclei and conspicuous nucleoli without gland formation, which appeared to be consistent with high-grade endometrioid carcinoma or UC. The level of tumor markers was not elevated: CA125, 17 U/ml; CA19-9, 9 U/ml; CA72-4, 2.9 U/ml; CEA, 1.1 ng/ml; and SCC, 0.9 ng/ml. Chest and abdominal contrast-enhanced computed tomography (CECT) revealed no metastatic lesions. Pelvic contrast-enhanced MRI showed multiple myomas and a 30 mm polyp-like mass projecting into the endometrial cavity without myometrial invasion. The patient underwent abdominal total hysterectomy, bilateral salpingo-oophorectomy, pelvic lymphadenectomy,

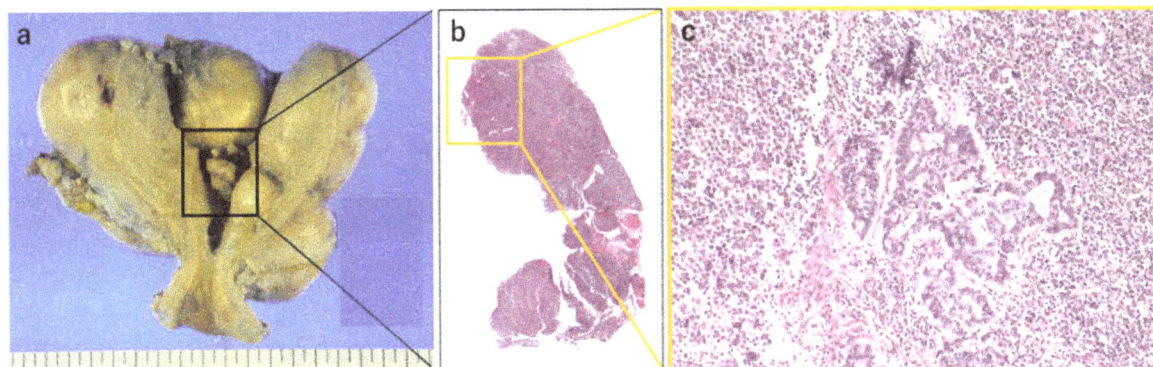

FIGURE 1: Case 1. (a) On gross examination a polypoid mass filled the endometrial cavity. (b, c) The tumor comprised well-differentiated endometrioid carcinoma and UC whose component represented about 80% of the whole neoplasm (hematoxylin and eosin [HE]).

para-aortic lymphadenectomy, and omentectomy. The surgical specimen of the uterus showed a 35 mm polypoid tumor developing from the uterine posterior wall. Microscopically, the polypoid tumor comprised well-differentiated endometrioid carcinoma, grades 1-2, and UC. The well-differentiated endometrioid carcinoma was confirmed on the surface of the endometrial polyp, and the coexisting UC showed a diffuse proliferation of atypical cells (Figure 1). Pancytokeratin (AE1/AE3) was diffusely expressed in the differentiated carcinoma component and was focally expressed in the UC component. Estrogen receptor (ER) and progesterone receptor (PR) were well expressed only in the differentiated carcinoma component (Figure 2). The UC component represented about 80% of the whole neoplasm. Endometrium invasion or lymph node (LN) metastasis was not observed. Based on these findings, the patient was diagnosed with DEC located on the endometrial polyp. The final Federation of Obstetrics and Gynecology (FIGO) stage was IA. The patient was treated with adjuvant chemotherapy (TC protocol: paclitaxel, 175 mg/m^2 + carboplatin AUC 6, every three weeks, and six cycles). She has been disease-free for 15 months after the initial surgery.

Case 2. A 58-year-old woman (BMI, 22.9 kg/m^2), who had been hospitalized for several months with a diagnosis of bipolar disorder, reported that she has been experiencing atypical vaginal bleeding for >1 year, which had worsened over time. An abdominal CECT showed a large pelvic mass, and she was transferred to our institution for further evaluation. Pelvic MRI revealed a bulky mass in the whole uterine corpus, which spread to the bladder and rectum. Chest and abdominal CECT revealed multiple LN metastases, which extended from the para-aortic to pelvic LNs. Endometrial curettage revealed the foci of atypical cells arranged in sheets with numerous mitotic figures. There was no sarcoma component, and the histological pattern represented that of only a carcinoma. ER and PR tumor cell were focally expressed. As tumor markers, CA19-9, CEA, and SCC levels had risen (CA19-9, 43 U/ml; CEA, 13.9 ng/ml; SCC, 80.4 ng/ml); CA125 and CA72-4 levels were within normal range (CA125, 12 U/ml; CA72-4, 2.5 U/ml). Although the pathological diagnosis

remained uncertain, based on the overall findings, the patient was diagnosed with stage IVA uterine endometrial cancer. Because of the presence of mental disorder and poor general condition (performance status 4), best supportive care was selected as the optimal treatment. However, the patient died in three months. Autopsy revealed uterine tumor invasion to the bladder, rectum, and pelvic wall with the involvement of the greater omentum and small intestine. The metastases to the pelvic and para-aortic LNs were observed. Microscopically, endometrioid carcinoma (grade 2) and UC components were present. Pancytokeratin (AE1/AE3) was diffusely expressed in the differentiated carcinoma component and focally expressed in the UC component (Figure 3). ER and PR tumor cells were expressed only in the differentiated carcinoma component. There were bone marrow hyperplasia and neutrophil infiltration in the lung and myocardium. The patient died of sepsis due to urinary tract infection secondary to the tumor invasion. The final diagnosis was DEC with FIGO stage IVB.

3. Discussion

DEC is defined as a tumor wherein the components of well-differentiated and UC are present. The transition between the two tumor components is abrupt with a sharp border. This histological pattern has also been reported in bone and soft tissue tumors such as chondrosarcoma [2], osteosarcoma [3], and liposarcoma [4]. In 2005, Silva et al. proposed classification criteria for endometrial uterine cancer [5]. In the following year, the authors presented the clinicopathological features of 25 cases of low-grade endometrioid carcinoma-associated UC and designated them as DEC [1]. They further examined the prognosis of these patients and concluded that DEC was associated with unfavorable prognosis, although the UC component was <20% of the whole neoplasm.

In 2014, the WHO classification of tumors of female reproductive organs (4th edition) added DEC as one of the pathological subtype of endometrial carcinoma [6]. Because the pathological diagnosis of DEC has only been established recently, the clinical features of the disease, including incidence, treatment, and prognosis, are unknown.

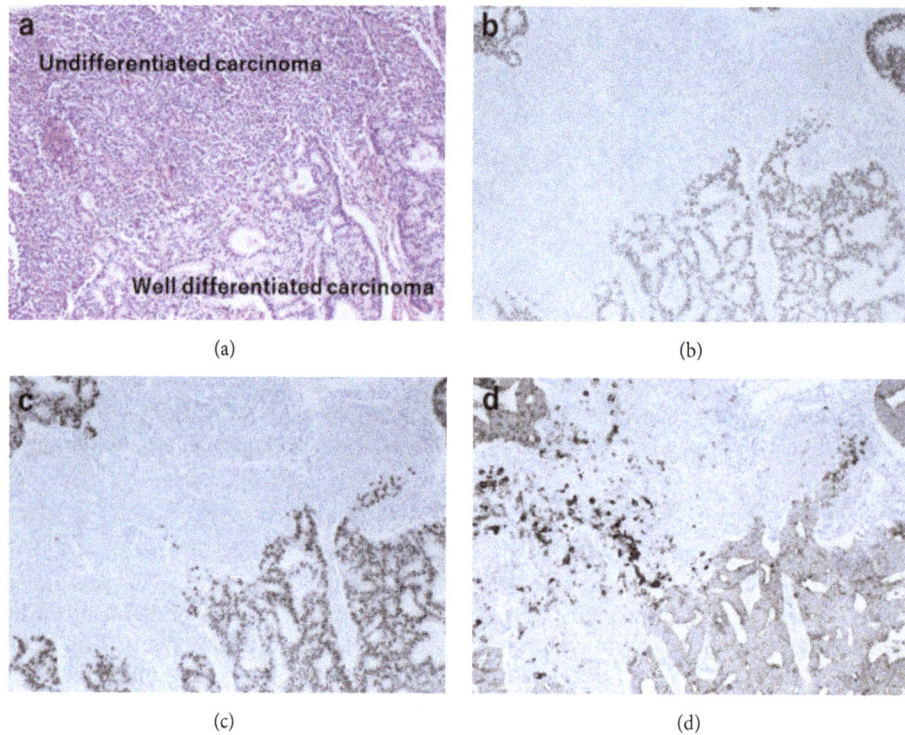

FIGURE 2: Case 1. (a) The tumor was composed of well-differentiated endometrioid carcinoma and UC with a sharp border (HE). ((b) ER, (c) PR) Differentiated components were strongly positive for ER and PR, whereas undifferentiated areas were not stained. (d) Pancytokeratin (AE1/AE3) was diffusely expressed in the well-differentiated carcinoma component and focally expressed in the UC component.

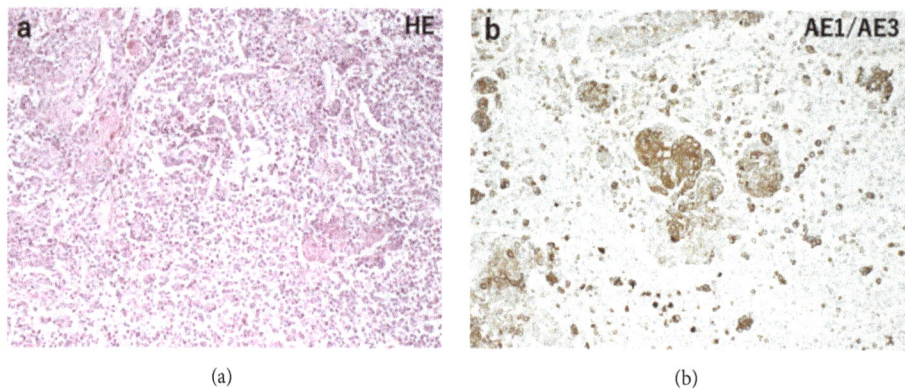

FIGURE 3: Case 2. (a) The tumor comprised moderately DEC and UC. (b) Pancytokeratin (AE1/AE3) was diffusely expressed in the well-differentiated carcinoma component and focally expressed in the UC component.

In the present study, we reviewed 68 cases associated with diagnosed DEC (Table 1) [1, 7–15]. Advanced cancer stages were higher among these patients than those observed in usual endometrial uterine cancers; 30 patients had stages I and II, and 38 patients had stages III and IV. Excluding the 30 cases that were not referred for the treatment, of the 38 remaining patients, hysterectomy was performed in 36 patients, leading to the definitive diagnosis of DEC. In two cases, the diagnosis of DEC was established by endometrial biopsy. Of the 68 cases, only one case was diagnosed with DEC after a bone metastasis was detected.

Lymphadenectomy was performed in only eight patients during the surgery; of these, four were of pelvic and four were of pelvic and para-aortic LNs. Adjuvant treatment was instituted in 25 cases; of these, 17 received only chemotherapy, four received only radiotherapy, and four received chemotherapy and radiation therapy. There was no consensus associated with the regimen of adjuvant chemotherapy for DEC, and the patients received one of the following regimens: cisplatin + anthracycline + taxane, taxane + carboplatin, cisplatin + anthracycline, or cisplatin + anthracycline + cyclophosphamide. For the two cases presented in our study, case 1 received systemic adjuvant chemotherapy with taxane + carboplatin and case 2 received best supportive care due to direct tumor invasion to the bladder and rectum and distant metastases.

TABLE 1: Cases of dedifferentiated endometrial carcinoma (DEC).

Author	Year	No. cases	Age	Stage (cases)	Treatment (cases)	Adjuvant therapy (cases)	UC component, %	Outcome (cases)
J. Han [7]	2017	4	54	I	ATH+BSO+PLA+PALA	Not treated	30	NED (19 monhts)
			77	II	ATH+BSO+PLA	Not treated	20	DOD (7 weeks)
			52	II	ATH+BSO+PLA+PALA	Radiation (EBRT+ICR)	60	NED (39 months)
			60	III	SRH+BSO	Chemotherapy (CDDP+ADM+CPA) and Radiation (EBRT+ICR)	90	DOD (10 months)
R. Yokomizo [8]	2017	3	66	I	ATH+BSO+PLA+PALA	Chemotherapy (CDDP+ADM)	45	NED (24 months)
			48	III	ATH+BSO+OMX+ Right hemicolectomy+ Hartmann operation	Chemotherapy (PTX+CBDCA)	90	DOD (5 months)
			48	IV	ATH+BSO+OMX+PLA+PALA	Radiation (EBRT)	60	DOD (7 months)
Z. Li [9]	2016	13	61 (median)	I/II (1) III/IV (12)	NA NA	Chemotherapy	NA	NA DFI(>3 months) 10%
C. J. Stewart [10]	2015	17	68.5 (mean) (range: 49-86)	I (7) II (1) III/IV (9)	NA	NA	NA	NA
E. S. Wu [11]	2013	1	62	IV	T10-T12 laminectomy	Radiation and hormonal therapy (TAM)	NA	NA
R. Berretta [12]	2013	1	67	IV	ATH+BSO+Adrenalectomy	Chemotherapy (PTX+CBDCA)	NA	NA
Y. Shen [13]	2012	1	51	II	ATH+BSO+PLA	Vaginal radiation and chemotherapy (CDDP+DTX+Taxane)	20	NED (11 months)
G. Giordano [14]	2012	2	83	I	ATH+BSO+PLA	NA	almost all	AWD (12 months)
			61	III	ATH+BSO+PLA	NA	85	DOD (3 months)
G. Vita [15]	2011	1	45	III	ATH+BSO	Chemotherapy (CDDP+anthracycline+taxane)	40	NA
E. G. Silva [1]	2006	25	51 (median) (range: 30-82)	I (14) II (1) III (6) IV (4)	ATH+BSO (24)	Chemothrapy (18) Radiation (4) Not treated (3)	20-90	DOD (median 7 months)(15) AWD (6) NA (3) NED (104 months)(1)

Of the 34 cases with outcome data (including the two cases described in this study), 21 patients (62%) died as the result of the tumor, 7 (20%) were alive with the tumors, and 6 (18%) were disease-free. Case 1 was disease-free for 15 months after the initial surgery, and case 2, who had advanced disease, died a month after being admitted to the hospital. Zaibo et al. also reported the outcome data for 10 of 13 patients with DEC [9]. Of these, nine cases had recurrent or metastatic diseases within 3 years since their diagnosis. From this report, it is possible that DEC is associated with worse prognosis compared with the findings in our study.

Preoperative diagnosis of DEC is difficult by only endometrial curettage [8]. Our literature review showed that almost all cases were diagnosed by surgical specimens and only two cases were diagnosed by endometrial biopsy. In our study, endometrial curettage failed to establish the diagnosis of DEC; the pretreatment diagnosis for case 1 was adenocarcinoma and for case 2 was carcinoma. Considering the diagnosis criteria of DEC, it is difficult to establish the diagnosis by endometrial curettage sometimes. While the differentiated components of the tumor can be seen on the surface, the UC components are seen deeper in the myometrium; hence, the definitive diagnosis of DEC needs to be established from a specimen sample large enough.

For the diagnosis of DEC, it is important to differentiate UC component from high-grade endometrial cancer. The point is whether to have a foci of gland formation, and immunohistochemical studies are beneficial in conducting differential diagnosis. Differentiated components are strongly positive for keratins, epithelial membrane antigen (EMA), ER, and PR, whereas undifferentiated areas show almost complete loss of expression of these markers or only focal staining for keratins and EMA [6, 9].

The following entities should be considered in the differential diagnosis of the undifferentiated component of DEC: high-grade endometrial carcinoma, neuroendocrine carcinoma, unclassified sarcoma, and carcinosarcoma [13, 16]. The lack of focal expression for keratin or EMA in a tumor composed of oval cell of medium or large size arranged in sheets can be misinterpreted as an evidence of sarcoma. Most sarcomas, however, are composed of epithelioid and spindle cells. In addition, the expression of desmin, caldesmon, and smooth muscle actin is the key for differentiating sarcomas from the UC component of DEC because these markers are positive in sarcomas but negative in the UC component of DEC. Carcinosarcoma is composed of high-grade endometrioid carcinoma, with serous carcinoma being the most frequently observed histological type, which mainly comprises spindle-cell proliferation. In contrast, gland forming components are confirmed in DEC; these components indicate low-grade endometrioid carcinoma. The UC components of DEC can show neuroendocrine feature by expressing highly focal neuroendocrine-related markers. In contrast, neuroendocrine carcinoma shows strong and diffuse staining for neuroendocrine markers.

An association between DEC and Lynch syndrome has been previously reported [6]. Yokomizo et al. examined the immunohistochemistry for DNA mismatch-repair (MMR) proteins in three cases diagnosed as DEC and demonstrated the loss of MMR protein expression in the UC components of these patients [8]. Thus, the authors emphasized the importance of assessing the genetic background of patients with DEC. The two cases in our study had no family history of cancer.

DEC expresses aggressive clinical features, and the prognosis of these patients is poor [1, 17]. In our study, case 2 presented with the invasion to the bladder, rectum, and LN metastases. In contrast, the tumor in case 1 advanced into the endometrial cavity, similar to an endometrial polyp, without myometrial invasion. Hence, the diagnosis was established early. However, because DEC is typically associated with poor prognosis, we will continue to closely monitor this patient.

Because the criteria of DEC have been established recently, the incidence of DEC is unknown yet. Most studies have reported an incidence of UC to be approximately 1%–2% [18]. However, Altrabulsi et al. reported an incidence of 9%. They found that most cases of endometrium UC were mixed with endometrioid carcinoma; of the 56 cases of UC in the study, 40 (71%) were mixed with endometrioid carcinoma [5]. This evidence reinforces the need of a specimen sample to accurately establish the diagnosis of DEC. When surgery is not indicated due to advanced disease, the correct diagnosis of DEC may only be established through autopsy, as it occurred in case 2; it also can be diagnosis from the specimen of hysterectomy. Laura J et al. examined 32 carcinomas with UC components (26 endometrial and 6 of ovarian origin). Of the 26 endometrial cases, 10 (38.5%) showed the presence of an adjacent well-differentiated carcinoma [19]. DEC might be under recognized, and it is possible that the incidence of DEC is much higher than that previously reported.

4. Conclusion

Based on these studies, it is possible that there are cases of uterine endometrial cancer with DEC that are still undiagnosed due to advanced disease or aggressive tumor behavior, suggesting that the incidence of DEC is higher than that reported in previous studies. While we strive to improve the diagnosis of DEC, it is also crucial to better assess the prognosis and the appropriate treatment for the patients with established diagnosis of DEC.

Authors' Contributions

Sachiko Morioka handled data collection and writing. Yasuhito Tanase and Ryuji Kawaguchi were responsible for data analysis. Tomoko Uchiyama conducted pathological analysis. Hiroshi Kobayash proofread the manuscript.

References

[1] E. G. Silva, M. T. Deavers, D. C. Bodurka, and A. Malpica, "Association of low-grade endometrioid carcinoma of the

uterus and ovary with undifferentiated carcinoma: A new type of dedifferentiated carcinoma?" *International Journal of Gynecological Pathology*, vol. 25, no. 1, pp. 52–58, 2006.

[2] D. C. Dahlin and J. W. Beabout, "Dedifferentiation of low-grade chondrosarcomas," *Cancer*, vol. 28, no. 2, pp. 461–466, 1971.

[3] K. K. Unni, D. C. Dahlin, R. A. McLeod, and D. J. Pritchard, "Intraosseous well-differentiated osteosarcoma," *Cancer*, vol. 40, no. 3, pp. 1337–1347, 1977.

[4] H. L. Evans, "Liposarcoma. A study of 55 cases with a reassessment of its classification," *The American Journal of Surgical Pathology*, vol. 3, no. 6, pp. 507–523, 1979.

[5] B. Altrabulsi, A. Malpica, M. T. Deavers, D. C. Bodurka, R. Broaddus, and E. G. Silva, "Undifferentiated carcinoma of the endometrium," *The American Journal of Surgical Pathology*, vol. 29, no. 10, pp. 1316–1321, 2005.

[6] R. J. Kurman, M. L. Carcangiu, C. S. Herrington, and R. H. Young, *WHO Classification of Tumours of Female Reproductive Organs*, World Health Organization, 4th edition, 2014.

[7] J. Han, E. Y. Ki, S. E. Rha, S. Hur, and A. Lee, "Dedifferentiated endometrioid carcinoma of the uterus: Report of four cases and review of literature," *World Journal of Surgical Oncology*, vol. 15, no. 1, article no. 17, 2017.

[8] R. Yokomizo, K. Yamada, Y. Iida et al., "Dedifferentiated endometrial carcinoma: A report of three cases and review of the literature," *Molecular and Clinical Oncology*, vol. 7, no. 6, pp. 1008–1012, 2017.

[9] Z. Li and C. Zhao, "Clinicopathologic and immunohistochemical characterization of dedifferentiated endometrioid adenocarcinoma," *Applied Immunohistochemistry & Molecular Morphology*, vol. 24, no. 8, pp. 562–568, 2016.

[10] C. J. R. Stewart and M. L. Crook, "Fascin expression in undifferentiated and dedifferentiated endometrial carcinoma," *Human Pathology*, vol. 46, no. 10, pp. 1514–1520, 2015.

[11] E. S. Wu, I. Shih, and T. P. Díaz-Montes, "Dedifferentiated endometrioid adenocarcinoma: An under-recognized but aggressive tumor?" *Gynecologic Oncology Reports*, vol. 5, pp. 25–27, 2013.

[12] R. Berretta, T. S. Patrelli, R. Faioli et al., "Dedifferentiated endometrial cancer: an atypical case diagnosed from cerebellar and adrenal metastasis: case presentation and review of literature," *International Journal of Clinical and Experimental Pathology*, vol. 6, no. 8, pp. 1652–1657, 2013.

[13] Y. Shen, Y. Wang, Y. Shi, J. Liu, and Y. Liu, "Clinicopathologic study of endometrial dedifferentiated endometrioid adenocarcinoma: A case report," *International Journal of Clinical and Experimental Pathology*, vol. 5, no. 1, pp. 77–82, 2012.

[14] G. Giordano, T. D'Adda, L. Bottarelli et al., "Two cases of low-grade endometriod carcinoma associated with undifferentiated carcinoma of the uterus (dedifferentiated carcinoma): A molecular study," *Pathology & Oncology Research*, vol. 18, no. 2, pp. 523–528, 2012.

[15] G. Vita, L. Borgia, L. Di Giovannantonio, and M. Bisceglia, "Dedifferentiated endometrioid adenocarcinoma of the uterus: A Clinicopathologic study of a case," *International Journal of Surgical Pathology*, vol. 19, no. 5, pp. 649–652, 2011.

[16] E. G. Silva, M. T. Deavers, and A. Malpica, "Undifferentiated carcinoma of the endometrium: A review," *Pathology*, vol. 39, no. 1, pp. 134–138, 2007.

[17] K. Ueda, K. Yamada, M. Urashima et al., "Association of extracellular matrix metalloproteinase inducer in endometrial carcinoma with patient outcomes and clinicopathogenesis using monoclonal antibody 12C3," *Oncology Reports*, vol. 17, no. 4, pp. 731–735, 2007.

[18] R. J. Kurman, L. H. Ellenson, and B. M. Ronnet, *Blaustein's Pathology of the Female Genital Tract*, New York, NY, USA, 5th edition, 2002.

[19] L. J. Tafe, K. Garg, I. Chew, C. Tornos, and R. A. Soslow, "Endometrial and ovarian carcinomas with undifferentiated components: clinically aggressive and frequently underrecognized neoplasms," *Modern Pathology*, vol. 23, no. 6, pp. 781–789, 2010.

46

Laparoendoscopic Single-Site Surgery for Management of Heterotopic Pregnancy: A Case Report and Review of Literature

Shadi Rezai [ID],[1,2] Richard A. Giovane,[3] Heather Minton,[4] Elise Bardawil,[2] Yiming Zhang,[5] Ninad M. Patil [ID],[6] Cassandra E. Henderson [ID],[7] and Xiaoming Guan [ID][2]

[1]Department of Obstetrics and Gynecology, Southern California Kaiser Permanente, Kern County, 1200 Discovery Drive, Bakersfield, CA 93309, USA

[2]Division of Minimally Invasive Gynecologic Surgery, Department of Obstetrics and Gynecology, Baylor College of Medicine, 6651 Main Street, 10th Floor, Houston, TX 77030, USA

[3]University of Alabama, Department of Family Medicine, 801 Campus Drive, Tuscaloosa, AL 35487, USA

[4]University of Birmingham, School of Medicine, 1720 2nd Avenue, Birmingham, AL 35294, USA

[5]Division of Reproductive Medicine, Jinan Central Hospital Group, 105 Jiefang Road, Jinan City, Shandong Province 250013, China

[6]Department of Pathology & Immunology, Baylor College of Medicine, 6651 Main Street, 4th Floor, Houston, TX 77030, USA

[7]Maternal and Fetal Medicine, Department of Obstetrics and Gynecology, Lincoln Medical and Mental Health Center, 234 East 149th Street, Bronx, NY 10451, USA

Correspondence should be addressed to Xiaoming Guan; xiaoming@bcm.edu

Academic Editor: Erich Cosmi

Background. Heterotopic pregnancy occurs when two pregnancies occur simultaneously in the uterus and an ectopic location. Treatment includes removal of the ectopic pregnancy with preservation of the intrauterine pregnancy. Treatment is done laparoscopically with either a Laparoendoscopic Single-Site Surgery (LESS) or a multiport laparoscopic surgery. *Case.* We present a case of a first trimester heterotopic pregnancy in a 42-year-old gravida 5, para 0-1-3-1 female with previous history of left salpingectomy, who underwent laparoscopic right salpingectomy and lysis of adhesions (LOA) via Single-Incision Laparoscopic Surgery (SILS). *Conclusion.* Although LESS for benign OB/GYN cases is feasible, safe, and equally effective compared to the conventional laparoscopic techniques, studies have suggested no clinically relevant advantages in the frequency of perioperative complications between LESS and conventional methods. No data on the cost effectiveness of LESS versus conventional methods are available. LESS utilizes only one surgical incision which may lead to decreased pain and better cosmetic outcome when compared to multiport procedure. One significant undesirable aspect of LESS is the crowding of the surgical area as only one incision is made. Therefore, all instruments go through one port, which can lead to obstruction of the surgeon's vision and in some cases higher rate of procedure failure resulting in conversion to multiport procedure.

1. Background

Heterotopic pregnancy is defined as two simultaneous pregnancies that occur at different sites of implantation, most commonly uterine cavity and fallopian tube [1, 2]. The incidence of heterotopic pregnancy is 1 in 30,000. However, patients with fallopian tube disease have a greater risk of having heterotopic pregnancy [3]. Presentation is similar to an ectopic pregnancy, including flank pain, vaginal bleeding, and, in severe cases, hemodynamic instability [4]. Diagnosis is often made via transvaginal ultrasound [4]. Treatment includes removal of the ectopic pregnancy with preservation of the intrauterine pregnancy [3, 4]. Frequent management is to remove the ectopic pregnancy via a laparoscopic approach using a single incision or multiple port approach [5, 6]. Employing the single-site laparoscopic procedure can be a more favorable approach due to its simplicity [7].

Laparoendoscopic Single-Site Surgery (LESS) is a form of surgery in which a single incision is made, usually at the umbilicus [8–10]. Although this technique has been referred to by different names, LESS is now the accepted name of this procedure by consensus [11]. LESS has been used for different procedures such as cholecystectomy, appendectomy, and ectopic pregnancy [12]. LESS is generally a more favored approach than laparotomy due to the patient having less post-operative pain, better cosmetic results, and shorter hospital stay [13]. Furthermore, as LESS uses a single port for surgery, there is less of a risk for infection and blood loss [14]. There are, however, disadvantages to this technique such as only having one port for placement of the camera and instruments, which hinders depth perception and decreases the field of view [15].

2. Presentation of the Case

Our patient is a 42-year-old, obese, gravida 5, para 0-1-3-1 woman, who was referred to our clinic for laparoscopic management of heterotopic pregnancy. The patient had a history of adverse perinatal outcome and poor obstetric history with one preterm classical cesarean delivery at 25 6/7 weeks in 2014. The patient was diagnosed with female infertility of unspecified origin in 2012 that was being managed by the Reproductive Endocrinology and Infertility (REI) service with the use of stored eggs and in vitro fertilization (IVF). Of note, the patient was also being managed by the Maternal-Fetal Medicine (MFM) service for a history of first trimester recurrent pregnancy losses (RPL) at 4 weeks, 6 weeks, and 11 weeks of gestational age (GA) that included a twin gestation. The RPL work-up revealed a clotting disorder (MTHFR C677T single copy) and hypothyroidism. Relevant surgical history for the patient was a left salpingectomy in 2000.

The patient was planning to attempt embryo transfer in July 2017 using stored eggs from previous in vitro fertilization (IVF) cycle.

Obstetrics ultrasound [**Figures 1(a), 1(b), and 1(c)**] revealed one intrauterine pregnancy (IUP) (Twin A) at 10 4/7 weeks with fetal heart rate (FHR) of 175 BPM with Crown-Rump Length (CRL) of 36 mm corresponding to the 56th percentile [**Figure 1(a)**], as well as one right ectopic tubal pregnancy (Twin B) at 9 3/7 weeks with CRL of 26.5 mm corresponding to less than 5th percentile with FHR of 188 BPM [**Figure 1(b)**].

The patient underwent laparoscopic right salpingectomy and lysis of adhesions (LOA) via Single-Incision Laparoscopic Surgery (SILS) with estimated blood loss of 10 ml [**Figure 2**]. SILS was done via inserting a single-site laparoscopy device at a 15 mm umbilical port [16]. The right fallopian tube with ectopic pregnancy was identified and LOA performed using the ENSEAL® articulating tissue sealer and the Endo Shears. Slight bleeding from the tube was controlled using the bipolar device. The fallopian tube was transected near the cornua.

Following surgery, the specimen was opened with identification of the presence of fetus and placental tissue. Transvaginal ultrasound (TVUS) following surgery confirmed the presence of a detectable fetal heart beat in the intrauterine pregnancy at 165 BPM and the presence of positive fetal movement. The patient did not require anti-D immune globulin as the patient had an O Rh positive blood type. The patient had an uncomplicated recovery course and was discharged on postoperative day 1.

The pathology specimen was examined with disrupted right fallopian tube with tubally implanted placenta and embryo that were consistent with a diagnosis of ectopic pregnancy [**Table 1**].

Regarding the intrauterine pregnancy (Twin A), the patient underwent repeat cesarean delivery at 36 5/7 weeks of gestation due to previous classical cesarean delivery and microscopic placenta accreta. Estimated blood loss (EBL) was 1000 ml. The patient gave birth to a healthy baby with weight of 2820 grams and APGAR scores of 8 and 9 at 1 and 5 minutes, respectively. The postoperative course was uncomplicated after her cesarean delivery, with hospital discharge occurring on postoperative day 3.

3. Discussions

Heterotopic pregnancy is two simultaneous pregnancies in which one occurs in the uterus and the other occurs in an ectopic location [2]. Patients who have tubal disease and increased levels of estrogen and progesterone have an increased risk of developing heterotopic pregnancy [17]. Patient presentation may be variable. They generally present with abdominal or flank pain, vaginal bleeding, or, in advanced cases, shock. Differentiating heterotopic pregnancy from ectopic pregnancy is of critical importance as management will differ. Ultrasound is used to differentiate ectopic from heterotopic pregnancy, due to the presence of an additional gestational sac in the uterine cavity [18, 19]. The use of measured beta-human chorionic gonadotrophin has little utility in diagnosing a heterotopic pregnancy as levels will reflect that of the intrauterine pregnancy [11]. Management is surgical with the goal of removing the ectopic pregnancy [6, 20, 21]. The choice of laparotomy versus a laparoscopic procedure is dependent on the patient's hemodynamic stability. Furthermore, a LESS approach versus multiport approach is dependent on certain factors as outlined below.

LESS was first introduced for ectopic pregnancy treatment by Ghezzi et al. [17]. Although the management can include medical management through the use of methotrexate, situations arise when surgical management is the only option such as when the patient is hemodynamically unstable or fetal heart beats are detected. The decision to use LESS versus multiple ports depends on different factors pertaining to the patient. One absolute contraindication for LESS is if the patient has an abdominal mesh from a prior umbilical hernia repair [22]. Theoretically, LESS is a simpler procedure as only one incision is made; however, a major drawback to this surgery as that only one port is placed so there is difficulty maneuvering instruments in the abdomen as well as gauging depth perception [23, 24]. Comparing LESS to multiport surgeries is important when determining which method to use. Regarding length of time to completion of surgery, LESS has been shown to require less time to complete than multiport surgery in ectopic pregnancy [15, 17]. Regarding adverse events, LESS had comparable events to multiport surgeries [25, 26]. However, it is suggested that LESS has an increased rate of umbilical hernia when compared to multiport surgery

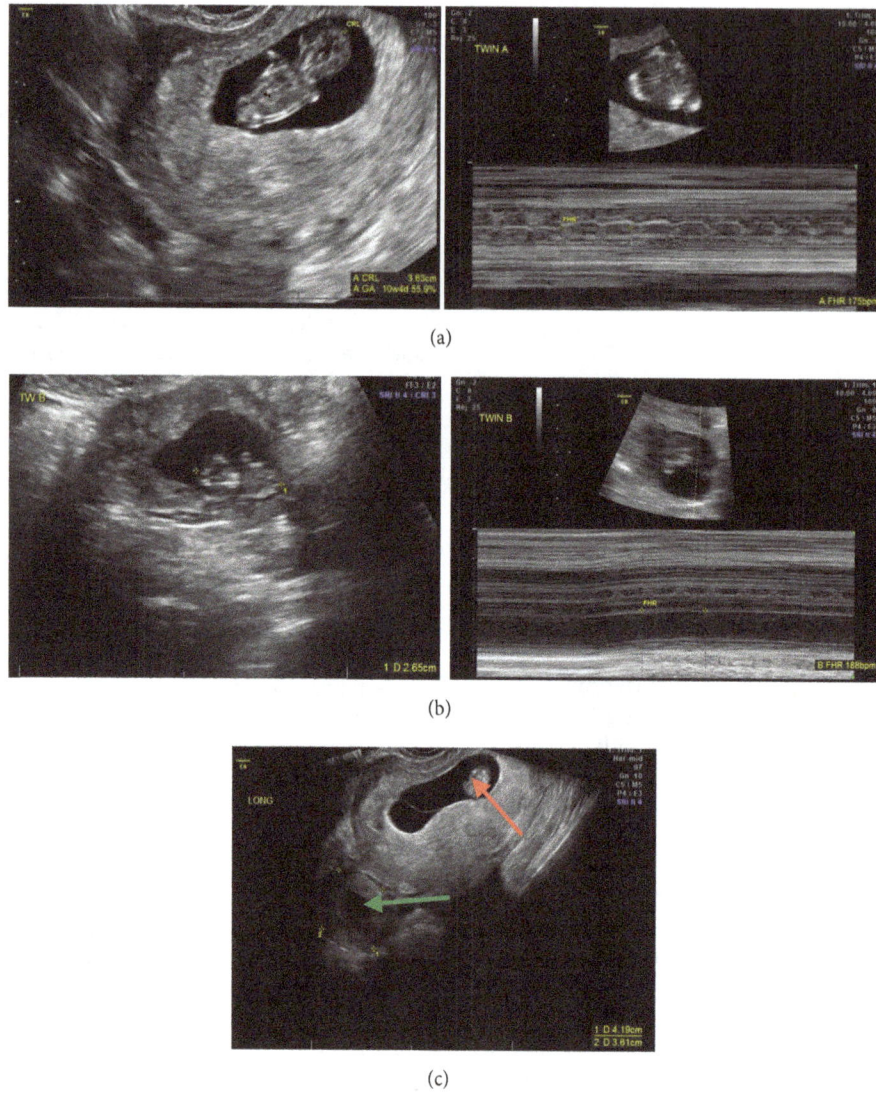

(a)

(b)

(c)

Figure 1: Official ultrasound showing positive FHR for Twin A, intrauterine pregnancy (IUP) (**a**); for Twin B, right tubal ectopic pregnancy (EP) (**b**); and presence of both **Twin A [intrauterine pregnancy (IUP)] (red arrow)** and **Twin B [ectopic pregnancy (EP)] (green arrow)** (**c**).

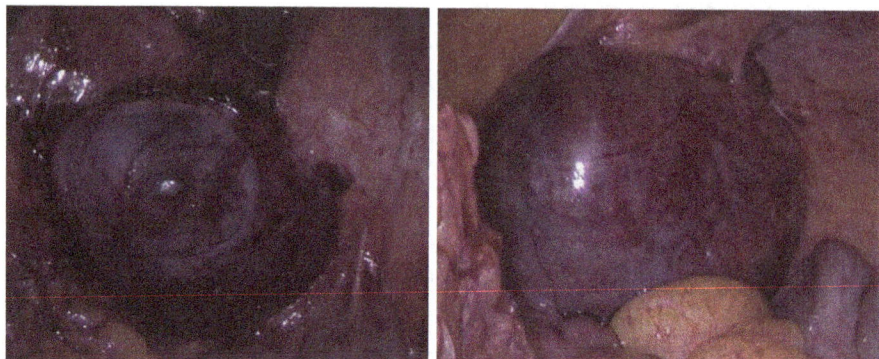

Figure 2: Intraoperative laparoscopic images of heterotopic pregnancy showing right tubal heterotopic pregnancy.

TABLE 1: Pathology macroscopic and microscopic images of right fallopian tube with implanted placenta and fetus, consistent with ectopic pregnancy.

Slide Number	Slide	Explanations
3A.		Right fallopian tube with implanted placenta, (bottom left) attached by umbilical cord to fetus.
3B		Fetal skeletal elements (Microscopy: hematoxylin and eosine stain).
3C.		Placental chorionic villi (top left) with ectopic implantation (center) in tubal mucosa (bottom). (Microscopy: hematoxylin and eosine stain)

[18, 26]. Regarding hospital stay and postoperative pain, patients undergoing LESS have shorter hospital stay and have less pain [15]. Furthermore, patients who underwent LESS had more favorable cosmetic results [15].

4. Conclusion

Heterotopic pregnancy is a rare form of pregnancy in which two simultaneously pregnancies occur, one intrauterine and one in an ectopic location. Treatment is directed at removing the ectopic pregnancy while trying to preserve the intrauterine pregnancy. Removal of the ectopic pregnancy is done laparoscopically if the patient is hemodynamically stable. LESS has become a viable option, as only it requires only one incision which leads to fewer surgical complications such as bleeding, infection, postoperative pain [27, 28], and hospital stay.

Although LESS for benign OB/GYN cases is feasible, safe, and equally effective compared to the conventional laparoscopic techniques [16, 29], studies have suggested no clinically relevant advantages in the frequency of perioperative complications between LESS and conventional methods [29, 30]. No data on the cost effectiveness of LESS versus conventional methods are available [29].

LESS utilizes only one surgical incision which may lead to decreased pain and better cosmetic outcome when compared to multiport procedure.

Disadvantages associated with LESS include possible difficulty in maneuvering instruments in one port due to loss of triangulation as well as obstruction of view and in some cases higher rate of procedure failure resulting in conversion to multiport procedure [29]. A case by case approach must be adopted when deciding to do LESS in a patient with heterotopic pregnancy. As far as future pregnancy for patient with history of heterotopic pregnancy, preconceptional counseling and planned pregnancy with early ultrasound imaging are recommended to ensure proper uterine implantation.

References

[1] N. Rojansky and J. G. Schenker, "Heterotopic pregnancy and assisted reproduction—an update," *Journal of Assisted Reproduction and Genetics*, vol. 13, no. 7, pp. 594–601, 1996.

[2] A. Chadee, S. Rezai, C. Kirby et al., "Spontaneous Heterotopic Pregnancy: Dual Case Report and Review of Literature," *Case Reports in Obstetrics and Gynecology*, vol. 2016, pp. 1–5, 2016.

[3] H. B. Clayton, L. A. Schieve, H. B. Peterson, D. J. Jamieson, M. A. Reynolds, and V. C. Wright, "A comparison of heterotopic and intrauterine-only pregnancy outcomes after assisted reproductive technologies in the United States from 1999 to 2002," *Fertility and Sterility*, vol. 87, no. 2, pp. 303–309, 2007.

[4] E. Reece, R. H. Petrie, M. F. Sirmans, M. Finster, and W. Todd, "Combined intrauterine and extrauterine gestations: A review," *American Journal of Obstetrics & Gynecology*, vol. 146, no. 3, pp. 323–330, 1983.

[5] M. A. Bedaiwy, J. Volsky, N. Lazebnik, and J. Liu, "Laparoscopic single-site linear salpingostomy for the management of heterotopic pregnancy: a case report," *J Reprod Med*, vol. 59, no. (9-10), pp. 522–524, 2014.

[6] A. Z. Loh, M. P. Torrizo, and Y. W. Ng, "Single Incision Laparoscopic Surgery for Surgical Treatment of Tubal Ectopic Pregnancy: A Feasible Alternative to Conventional Laparoscopy," *Journal of Gynecologic Surgery*, vol. 33, no. 2, pp. 61–67, 2017.

[7] B. Ramesh, M. Vidyashankar, and P. Sharma Dimri, *Single Port Laparoscopic Surgery in Gynecology, Section 2: LESS in Gynecology*, vol. 82 of *Laparoendoscopic Single-Site Surgery for Ectopic Pregnancy*, Chapter 12, Jaypee Brothers Medical Pub, 1st edition, 2013.

[8] P. F. Escobar, A. N. Fader, M. F. Paraiso, J. H. Kaouk, and T. Falcone, "Robotic-Assisted Laparoendoscopic Single-Site Surgery in Gynecology: Initial Report and Technique," *Journal of Minimally Invasive Gynecology*, vol. 16, no. 5, pp. 589–591, 2009.

[9] S. A. Scheib and A. N. Fader, "Gynecologic robotic laparoendoscopic single-site surgery: prospective analysis of feasibility, safety, and technique," *American Journal of Obstetrics & Gynecology*, vol. 212, no. 2, pp. 179.e1–179.e8, 2015.

[10] L. S. Bradford and D. M. Boruta, "Laparoendoscopic Single-Site Surgery in Gynecology," *Obstetrical & Gynecological Survey*, vol. 68, no. 4, pp. 295–304, 2013.

[11] I. S. Gill, A. P. Advincula, M. Aron et al., "Consensus statement of the consortium for laparoendoscopic single-site surgery," *Surgical Endoscopy*, vol. 24, no. 4, pp. 762–768, 2010.

[12] M. A. Bedaiwy, T. Farghaly, W. Hurd et al., "Laparoendoscopic Single-Site Surgery for Management of Ovarian Endometriomas," *JSLS: Journal of the Society of Laparoendoscopic Surgeons*, vol. 18, no. 2, pp. 191–196, 2014.

[13] J. M. Marks, M. S. Phillips, R. Tacchino et al., "Single-incision laparoscopic cholecystectomy is associated with improved cosmesis scoring at the cost of significantly higher hernia rates: 1-year results of a prospective randomized, multicenter, single-blinded trial of traditional multiport laparoscopic cholecystectomy vs single-incision laparoscopic cholecystectomy," *Journal of the American College of Surgeons*, vol. 216, no. 6, pp. 1037–1047, 2013.

[14] A. Habana, A. Dokras, J. L. Giraldo, and E. E. Jones, "Cornual heterotopic pregnancy: Contemporary management options," *American Journal of Obstetrics & Gynecology*, vol. 182, no. 5, pp. 1264–1270, 2000.

[15] S. Seong, H. Park, C. Park, B. Yoon, and I. Kim, "Single Port Versus Conventional Laparoscopic Salpingectomy for Surgical Treatment of Tubal Pregnancy," *Journal of Minimally Invasive Gynecology*, vol. 16, no. 6, p. S129, 2009.

[16] X. Guan, J. Liu, Y. Wang, J. Gisseman, Z. Guan, and C. Kleithermes, "Laparoscopic Single-Incision Supracervical Hysterectomy for an Extremely Large Uterus with Bag Tissue Extraction," *Journal of Minimally Invasive Gynecology*, 2017.

[17] F. Ghezzi, A. Cromi, M. Fasola, and P. Bolis, "One-trocar salpingectomy for the treatment of tubal pregnancy: a 'marionette-like' technique," *BJOG: An International Journal of Obstetrics & Gynaecology*, vol. 112, no. 10, pp. 1417–1419, 2005.

[18] M. A. Bedaiwy, P. F. Escobar, J. Pinkerton, and W. Hurd, "Laparoendoscopic Single-Site Salpingectomy in Isthmic and Ampullary Ectopic Pregnancy: Preliminary Report and Technique," *Journal of Minimally Invasive Gynecology*, vol. 18, no. 2, pp. 230–233, 2011.

[19] K. K. Yamoah and Z. Girn, "Heterotopic pregnancy: should we instrument the uterus at laparoscopy for ectopic pregnancy," *BMJ Case Reports*, vol. 2012, 2012.

[20] A. Takeda, S. Hayashi, S. Imoto, C. Sugiyama, and H. Nakamura, "Pregnancy outcomes after emergent laparoscopic surgery for acute adnexal disorders at less than 10 weeks of gestation," *Journal of Obstetrics and Gynaecology Research*, vol. 40, no. 5, pp. 1281–1287, 2014.

[21] J. Eze, "Successful Intrauterine Pregnancy following salpingostomy; Case Report," *Nigerian Journal of Medicine*, vol. 17, no. 3, 2008.

[22] C. C. Gunderson, J. Knight, J. Ybanez-Morano et al., "The risk of umbilical hernia and other complications with laparoendoscopic single-site surgery," *Journal of Minimally Invasive Gynecology*, vol. 19, no. 1, pp. 40–45, 2012.

[23] A. Fader, K. Levinson, C. Gunderson, A. Winder, and P. Escobar, "Laparoendoscopic single-site surgery in gynaecology: A new frontier in minimally invasive surgery," *Journal of Minimal Access Surgery*, vol. 7, no. 1, pp. 71–77, 2010.

[24] P. F. Escobar, D. Starks, A. N. Fader, M. Catenacci, and T. Falcone, "Laparoendoscopic single-site and natural orifice surgery

in gynecology," *Fertility and Sterility*, vol. 94, no. 7, pp. 2497–2502, 2010.

[25] A. N. Fader, L. Rojas-Espaillat, O. Ibeanu, F. C. Grumbine, and P. F. Escobar, "Laparoendoscopic single-site surgery (LESS) in gynecology: A multi-institutional evaluation," *American Journal of Obstetrics & Gynecology*, vol. 203, no. 5, pp. 501–e6, 2010.

[26] A. N. Fader, S. Cohen, P. F. Escobar, and C. Gunderson, "Laparoendoscopic single-site surgery in gynecology," *Current Opinion in Obstetrics and Gynecology*, vol. 22, no. 4, pp. 331–338, 2010.

[27] C. Kliethermes, K. Blazek, B. Nijjar, K. Ali, S. Kliethermes, and X. Guan, "Abdominal Binder Use Following Single-Incision Laparoscopic Surgery," *Journal of Minimally Invasive Gynecology*, vol. 24, no. 7, p. S156, 2017.

[28] C. Kliethermes, K. Blazek, K. Ali, J. B. Nijjar, S. Kliethermes, and X. Guan, "Postoperative Pain After Single-Site Versus Multiport Hysterectomy," *JSLS : Journal of the Society of Laparoendoscopic Surgeons*, vol. 21, no. 4, p. e2017.00065, 2017.

[29] E. M. Sandberg, C. F. la Chapelle, M. M. van den Tweel, J. W. Schoones, and F. W. Jansen, "Laparoendoscopic single-site surgery versus conventional laparoscopy for hysterectomy: a systematic review and meta-analysis," *Archives of Gynecology and Obstetrics*, vol. 295, no. 5, pp. 1089–1103, 2017.

[30] L. Yang, J. Gao, L. Zeng, Z. Weng, and S. Luo, "Systematic review and meta-analysis of single-port versus conventional laparoscopic hysterectomy," *International Journal of Gynecology & Obstetrics*, vol. 133, no. 1, pp. 9–16, 2016.

47

Atypical Amniotic Fluid Embolism Managed with a Novel Therapeutic Regimen

Shadi Rezai,[1] **Alexander C. Hughes,**[2] **Tracy B. Larsen,**[3]
Paul N. Fuller,[1] **and Cassandra E. Henderson**[4]

[1]*Department of Obstetrics and Gynecology, Kaiser Permanente Southern California, 1200 Discovery Drive, Bakersfield, Kern County, CA 93309, USA*
[2]*School of Medicine, St. George's University, St. George's, Grenada*
[3]*Department of Anesthesiology, Adventist Health Bakersfield, 2615 Chester Avenue, Bakersfield, CA 93301, USA*
[4]*Department of Obstetrics and Gynecology, Lincoln Medical and Mental Health Center, 234 East 149th Street, Bronx, NY 10451, USA*

Correspondence should be addressed to Shadi Rezai; rezsha@sgu.edu
and Cassandra E. Henderson; cassandra.henderson@nychhc.org

Academic Editor: Edi Vaisbuch

Amniotic fluid embolism (AFE) is the second leading cause of maternal mortality in the USA with an incidence of 1 : 15,200 births. The case fatality rate and perinatal mortality associated with AFE are 13–30% and 9–44%, respectively. This rare but devastating complication can be difficult to diagnose as many of the early signs and symptoms are nonspecific. Compounding this diagnostic challenge is a lack of effective treatment regimens which to date are mostly supportive. We present the case of a 26-year-old woman who suffered from suspected AFE and was successfully treated with the novel regimen of Atropine, Ondansetron, and Ketorolac (A-OK). The authors acknowledge that this case does not meet the new criteria proposed, by Clark in 2016, but feel that it is important to share this case report, due to dramatic patient response to the provided supportive therapy presented in this case report. We hope this case report will prompt further research into this novel approach to treating AFE with Atropine, Ondansetron, and Ketorolac.

1. Introduction

Amniotic fluid embolism (AFE) is a rare, unpredictable, and potentially devastating complication of childbirth, in which amniotic fluid, fetal cells, hair, or other types of debris enter into the maternal pulmonary circulation, causing cardiovascular collapse [1, 2]. The incidence of AFE ranges from 1 : 15,200 to 1 : 53,800 [3–5]. AFE is the second leading direct cause of maternal death in the USA and Europe [3–6]. Conde-Agudelo and Romero found the percent total maternal deaths due to AFE to be 13.7%, slightly higher than the previous widely held 10% [5].

Early recognition and initiation of treatment of AFE are essential to increase the likelihood of patient survival [1, 7]. This can be a challenge, as AFE is a diagnosis of exclusion with no universal pathological or serological markers [1, 8, 9]. Transesophageal echocardiography (TEE) can be used to determine cardiac dysfunction due to pulmonary hypertension but may not be widely available on obstetric units [7, 10]. AFE is traditionally diagnosed clinically, in a woman early during labor with ruptured membranes, by a trio of symptoms: acute respiratory distress, cardiovascular collapse, and coagulopathy [3–5, 8, 9, 11]. Other symptoms include hypotension, frothing from the mouth, fetal heart rate abnormalities, loss of consciousness, bleeding, uterine atony, and seizure like activity [8, 12]. However, as a diagnosis of exclusion, the AFE triad is neither sensitive nor specific and should be considered once other diagnoses have been ruled out. Clark has recently proposed diagnostic criteria for AFE case report in order to prevent over reporting, but the Society for Maternal Fetal Medicine (SMFM) continues to support the current clinical diagnosis [11, 13].

With a greater understanding of the pathophysiology of AFE, new therapies have shown potential [4, 5]. Copper et al.

have reported "that antiserotonin, antithromboxane, and vagolytic therapy" were the mechanisms for the restoration of a patients' circulation and led to successful resuscitation [14]. We present a similar case of a 26-year-old woman with suspected AFE who was successfully managed with traditional therapy and a novel regimen of Atropine, Ondansetron, and Ketorolac (A-OK) [4, 14].

2. Case History

A 26-year-old Hispanic female, G2P1001, at 38 1/7 weeks of gestation complicated by obesity (BMI of 41) and gestational diabetes (GDM2) presented to the emergency room complaining of shortness of breath for approximately 8 hours. On exam she was noted to have a fever (102.2 degrees Fahrenheit or 39.0 degrees Celsius), blood pressure of 119/73 mm Hg, maternal tachycardia (144 beats per minute (BPM)), tachypnea (24 breaths/minute), oxygen saturation of 97%, and fetal tachycardia (211 BPM). The cervical exam was 1 cm cervical dilatation, zero percent effacement, long and posterior position fetus in vertex presentation, and intact amniotic fluid membrane (i.e., 1 cm/long/posterior, vertex, and intact). Urine toxicology screen was negative. Intravenous hydration was initiated and the patient was started on broad spectrum antibiotics for the empirical treatment of sepsis (Piperacillin/Tazobactam, Vancomycin). The patient underwent stat primary low transverse cesarean delivery due to nonreactive tracing and fetal tachycardia with minimal variability (category 2 tracing) under general endotracheal intubation anesthesia with rapid sequence intubation. A total of 200 mg of Propofol with 100 mg of succinylcholine were rapidly infused, and blood pressure at that time was 80/40 mg Hg. A size 7.0 endotracheal tube (ETT) was placed under direct laryngoscopy with clear view of tube passing the vocal cords. Intubation was atraumatic with a grade 1 view. Endotracheal tube was taped and secured at 21 cm. Bilateral breath sounds were obtained by auscultation and positive CO_2 per anesthesia monitor were used to confirm placement.

Patient delivered an infant with Apgar of 9 and 9 in one and five minutes, respectively, with meconium amniotic fluid. Immediately after delivery of the infant and before the extraction of placenta, the patient's heart rate remained in 140 beats per minute (BPM), but the patient's oxygen saturation decreased to 72%, blood pressure lowered to 72/48 mm Hg, and end-tidal CO2 (ETCO2) as per the anesthesia monitor fell from 32 to 0 mm Hg. Normal reference range for ETCO2 is between 35 and 45 mm Hg. The anesthesia equipment was rapidly checked to confirm that there was no equipment leak or disconnection as the phenylephrine IVP was administered with an initial dose of 200 mcg and repeated several times for a total of 1800 mcg (see Table 1 for summary). The patient was evaluated by the obstetrics team for hysterotomy extensions, lacerations, or uncontrolled bleeding (suggestive of DIC) which was found to be negative.

The anesthesia team initiated A-OK AFE protocol within one minute of onset of the listed symptoms. A-OK consisting of 0.2 mg Atropine, 8 mg Ondansetron, and 15 mg Ketorolac were all given as intravenous push. Within 2-3 minutes the patient's oxygen saturation recovered to 97% and blood

TABLE 1

Time/dose phenylephrine given
(1) 19:48: 200 mcg/ml
(2) 20:00: 200 mcg/ml
(3) 20:15: 400 mcg/ml
(4) 20:30: 400 mcg/ml
(5) 20:45: 400 mcg/ml
Total: 1800 mcg/ml

pressure increased to 138/68 mm Hg, CO2 returned per monitor to 32 mm Hg, but tachycardia remained with a heart rate of approximately 140 BPM (see Figure 2 and Table 2). Patient's oxygen saturation and blood pressure responded to medical management by the anesthesia team with intravenous fluids, Atropine, Ondansetron, and Ketorolac. As the patient responded to medical management, her blood pressures and oxygen saturation quickly improved. To treat uterine atony and intraoperative hemorrhage, the patient received 50 units of Oxytocin and 2 doses of Carboprost, 3 units of packed red blood cells (PRBCs), 1 unit of fresh frozen plasma (FFP), and 3,500 ml intravenous fluid. She had 2,000 ml estimated blood loss (EBL).

Once stabilized, she remained intubated and was transported to the intensive care unit (ICU) for further monitoring. Postoperative chest computed tomography (CT) scan with and without contrast did not show any evidence of pulmonary embolism (PE) but showed bibasilar atelectasis with no evidence of definite consolidation and/or pneumonia. Lower extremity Doppler ultrasound showed negative results for deep venous thrombosis (DVT). Intraoperative and postoperative laboratory blood works were also negative for DIC with PT, PTT, and INR within normal limits. Blood culture, urine culture, and sputum cultures were taken and later found to be negative. Chest X-ray was done that showed no acute pathology. Placental pathology was negative for chorioamnionitis, placental abruption, and retroplacental hematoma.

The patient was extubated on postoperative day one. Antibiotics were switched to Cefazolin. The patient remained afebrile and asymptomatic with stable vital signs. The patient and newborn had an uneventful postoperative recovery course and were both discharged on postoperative day 3 with a follow-up appointment at our clinic.

3. Discussion

The case described is a woman, with no known risk factors for AFE (summarized in Table 3), presenting to the emergency room in distress with subsequent rapid decomposition after delivery [17, 18]. The clinical diagnosis of AFE was made and differential diagnoses were ruled out. The patient was managed with traditional cardiovascular support and administration of PRBCs and FFP while the anesthesia team initiated the A-OK therapy. Shortly after A-OK therapy and phenylephrine, the patient experienced a rapid reversal of symptoms and stabilization [7, 19].

TABLE 2: Patient vital signs as demonstrated in Figure 2.

Event	Time	Minutes	EtCO$_2$	RR	BP	Pulse	O$_2$ saturation
Initial patient presentation to ED	11/29/16 16:59:00	0	NA	24	119/73	144	97% (room air)
	11/29/2016 19:15	16		21	128/50	133	99% (room air)
C-section procedure start	11/29/16 19:55:00	56	32	ETT	128/75	120	96% (on ETT)
Delivery of baby	11/29/16 19:56:00	57	0	ETT	72/48	140	72% (on ETT)
A-OK therapy initiated	11/29/16 19:57:00	58		ETT	80/50	130	94% (on ETT)
(Effect of) A-OK therapy	11/29/16 20:00:00	61	35	ETT	138/68	140	97% (on ETT)
Operating room timeout	11/29/16 21:20:00	81	37	21	140/94	140	94% (on ventilator)

TABLE 3: Risk factors and odd ratios for AFE. Abenhaim et al.

Risk factors	Odds ratio
Placenta previa	30.4
Preeclampsia	7.3
Cesarean section	5.7
Forceps delivery	4.3
Maternal age > 35 yrs	2.2
Vacuum delivery	1.9
All other methods of induction	1.5

AFE has traditionally been a diagnosis of exclusion made in an emergency situation [11]. Recently, Clark et al. have proposed diagnostic criteria for scientific research but this has not yet been widely adopted [13, 20]. The Society for Maternal Fetal Medicine (SFMFM) which continues to endorse AFE is a clinical diagnosis with an emphasis on maintaining cardiovascular function and hemodynamic stability [11]. In this case the criteria outlined in Clark et al. 2016 (see Table 4) were not met. The main exclusion criteria, from Clark et al.'s proposed guidelines, were the presence of fever on admission and during the C section [13]. Clark et al. suggested that cases with fever should be excluded in order to eliminate infectious causes of cardiovascular collapse seen in sepsis/systemic inflammatory response syndrome (SIRS) [13], but this patient was found to have negative blood cultures and no source of infection. We acknowledge Clark's much needed proposal of universal criteria for reporting research cases but see the limitations of these criteria in clinical practice and case presentations. The authors therefore would like to acknowledge this as an atypical presentation of AFE. This clinical diagnosis is supported by ruling out other likely diagnoses (see Table 5). The rapid return of functional status of pulmonary and cardiovascular systems are congruent with Leighton's findings in 2013 which similarly described the dramatic return of cardiovascular function

with the use of A-OK in AFE [4, 14]. However, adding to the diagnostic uncertainty is the large dose of phenylephrine used in this case. Although not part of the AOK regime phenylephrine the dose used in this case may have contributed to resuscitation and hemodynamic stabilization rather than Atropine, Ondansetron, and Ketorolac.

The current recommendations from the Society for Maternal Fetal Medicine suggest the use of Sildenafil, Dobutamine, Milrinone, inhaled nitrous oxide, Prostacyclin, and Norepinephrine when managing AFE [21]. Sympathomimetic medications help maintain blood pressure, but the mechanism of action of these agents does not address the potential underlying mechanisms of ventricular dysfunction. Historically, studies have suggested mechanical obstruction as the main mechanism for pulmonary hypertension [7]. However, more recent animal models have suggested serotonin and thromboxane act synergistically to cause platelet dysfunction, platelet degranulation, and pulmonary hypertension [14, 21, 22]. According to these models, pulmonary hypertension begins with serotonin stimulation of 5-HT receptors causing pulmonary vasoconstriction [21, 23]. Platelets are entrapped due to the pulmonary vasoconstriction and activated by thromboxane (TXA$_2$) [14]. The thromboxane causes the recruitment and activation of additional platelets, compounding pulmonary hypertension with the release of more serotonin mediators causing a self-perpetuating cycle (Figure 1) [4, 14, 21]. Leaños et al. suggested these same mediators, while causing local vasoconstriction, cause systemic vagal stimulation leading to a fall in systemic vasomotor tone [21]. Finally, some animal models have suggested that consumptive coagulopathy occurs due to the activation of platelets, factor III, factor X, and amniotic fluid tissue factor leading to disseminated intravascular coagulation (DIC). However contradictory results have been reported [5, 7, 9].

Some authors have suggested the ventricular dysfunction is secondary to either pulmonary hypertension caused by serotonin and thromboxane or systemic hypotension caused

TABLE 4

Proposed criteria for research reporting of amniotic fluid embolism [12]

(1) Sudden onset of cardiorespiratory arrest or both hypotension (systolic blood pressure < 90 mm Hg) and respiratory compromise (dyspnea, cyanosis, or peripheral capillary oxygen saturation [SpO2] < 90%)

(2) Documentation of overt DIC following appearance of these initial signs or symptoms, using scoring system of Scientific and Standardization Committee on DIC of the ISTH, modified for pregnancy Coagulopathy must be detected prior to loss of sufficient blood to itself account for dilutional or shock-related consumptive coagulopathy

(3) Clinical onset during labor or within 30 min of delivery of placenta

(4) No fever (38.0°C) during labor

TABLE 5

Differential diagnosis for AFE [5]

Pulmonary thromboembolism; more common later postpartum, chest CT was clear and lower limb Doppler was clear

Anesthetic complications; hypoxia was not associated with administration of any medication

Drug-induced allergic anaphylaxis; no rash or wheeze was observed

Myocardial infarction; no ECG changes and negative troponins

Cardiac arrhythmia; the intraoperative anesthesia record reports sinus tachycardia throughout monitoring

Aspiration of gastric contents; patient was had ETT tube inserted with cuff inflated preventing aspiration

Reaction to local anesthetic drugs; patients' condition deterioration does not correlate with any medications given

Sepsis: sepsis is ruled out since there was no source of infection, and patient had clear chest CT scan with SOB; there were no evidence of pneumonia, blood, and urine cultures which were negative

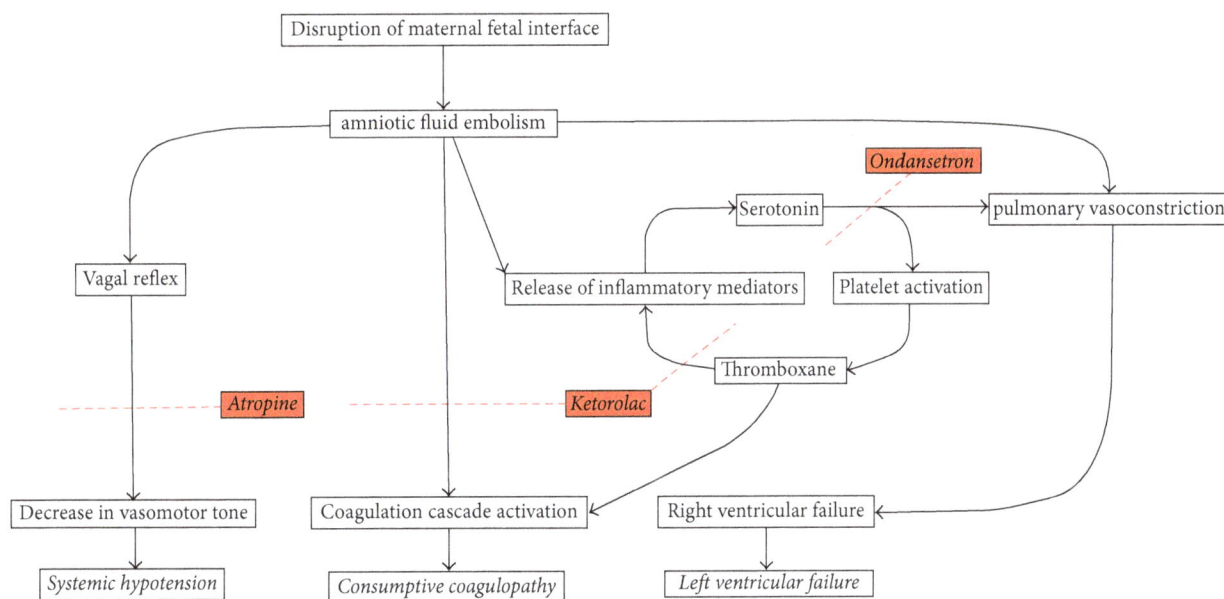

FIGURE 1: Proposed mechanism for Atropine, Ondansetron, and Ketorolac (A-OK) protocol.

by vagal stimulation [1, 11]. It has been proposed that Atropine and Ondansetron may act to block serotonin and vagal stimulation improving cardiovascular function rather than simply providing cardiovascular support [11]. Additionally, the A-OK regimen rather than replacing the consumed factors blocks the proposed cause of coagulopathy by inhibiting thromboxane with Ketorolac [1, 11] (see Table 6).

4. Summary

Traditionally the prognosis for AFE is poor, with a mortality rate ranging from 13 to 44% [1, 3]. Current recommended treatment for AFE includes pulmonary vasodilators, prostaglandins, sympathomimetics, and a host of other interventions [5, 10, 15, 21]. Along with these systemic mediators,

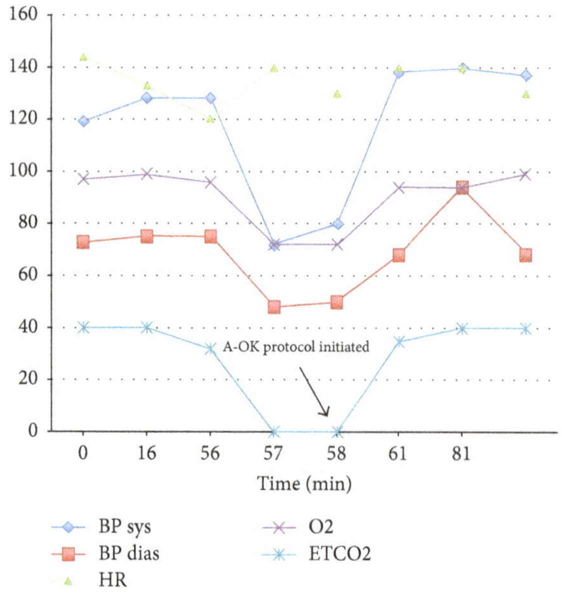

FIGURE 2: Graph of patient's vital signs prior and after initiation of A-OK therapy.

TABLE 6: Shamshirsaz and Clark in SOAP 2013 also describe this A-OK therapy with the addition of metoclopramide, which was not used in our patient [15]. The atropine is used to treat vagal overstimulation and improve vasomotor tone while Ondansetron blocks serotonin receptors inhibiting the release of further mediators [4, 16]. The Ketorolac blocks thromboxane production thereby preventing coagulopathy [4].

A-OK medication regimen [3]
Atropine 1 mg (vagolytic)
Ondansetron 8 mg (5-HT3 antagonist)
Ketorolac 30 mg (cyclooxygenase inhibitor)

large amounts of blood products such as FFP and PRBC are rapidly infused to combat DIC [1]. Other management methods such as bypass and exchange transfusion, by cardiovascular surgery, have also been reported in several cases [10, 16, 24–27].

The authors acknowledge that this case does not meet Clark's proposed criteria for AFE [12]. With AFE affecting many women across the globe and being a significant contributor to maternal mortality, efforts should be made to find effective treatments. We hope this case will prompt future investigation into novel treatments such as A-OK, which can be used in conjunction with traditional supportive measures.

Acknowledgments

The authors would like to thank Ms. Judith Wilkinson, Medical Librarian at Lincoln Medical and Mental Health Center Science Library, for providing the reference articles.

References

[1] C. S. Sundin and L. B. Mazac, "Amniotic fluid embolism," *MCN, The American Journal of Maternal/Child Nursing*, vol. 42, no. 1, pp. 29–35, 2017.

[2] K. Kaur, M. Bhardwaj, P. Kumar, S. Singhal, T. Singh, and S. Hooda, "Amniotic fluid embolism," *Journal of Anaesthesiology Clinical Pharmacology*, vol. 32, no. 2, p. 153, 2016.

[3] C. Thongrong, P. Kasemsiri, J. Hofmann et al., "Amniotic fluid embolism," *International Journal of Critical Illness & Injury Science*, vol. 3, no. 1, p. 51, 2013.

[4] B. L. Leighton, "Amniotic Fluid Embolism, March of Dimes," 2013, http://www.marchofdimes.org/pdf/missouri/AFE_11-21-13.pdf.

[5] A. Conde-Agudelo and R. Romero, "Amniotic fluid embolism: an evidence-based review," *American Journal of Obstetrics & Gynecology*, vol. 201, no. 5, pp. 445.e1–445.e13, 2009.

[6] N. McDonnell, M. Knight, M. J. Peek et al., "Amniotic fluid embolism: an Australian-New Zealand population-based study," *BMC Pregnancy and Childbirth*, vol. 15, no. 1, 2015.

[7] L. S. Dean, R. P. Rogers, R. A. Harley, and D. D. Hood, "Case Scenario," *Anesthesiology*, vol. 116, no. 1, pp. 186–192, 2012.

[8] S. L. Clark, "Amniotic fluid embolism," *Obstetrics & Gynecology*, vol. 123, no. 2, Part 1, pp. 337–348, 2014.

[9] S. L. Clark, F. J. Montz, and J. P. Phelan, "Hemodynamic alterations associated with amniotic fluid embolism: a reappraisal," *American Journal of Obstetrics & Gynecology*, vol. 151, no. 5, pp. 617–621, 1985.

[10] B. K. Ray, M. C. Vallejo, M. D. Creinin et al., "Amniotic fluid embolism with second trimester pregnancy termination: a case report," *Canadian Journal of Anesthesia*, vol. 51, no. 2, Article ID 1482654637, pp. 139–144, Feb 2004, http://download.springer.com/static/pdf/879/art%253A10.1007%252FBF03018773.pdf.

[11] L. D. Pacheco, G. Saade, G. D. Hankins, and S. L. Clark, "Amniotic fluid embolism: diagnosis and management," *American Journal of Obstetrics & Gynecology*, vol. 215, no. 2, pp. B16–B24, 2016.

[12] S. L. Clark, "Amniotic fluid embolism," *Clinical Obstetrics and Gynecology*, vol. 53, no. 2, pp. 322–328, 2010.

[13] S. L. Clark, R. Romero, G. A. Dildy et al., "Proposed diagnostic criteria for the case definition of amniotic fluid embolism in research studies," *American Journal of Obstetrics & Gynecology*, vol. 215, no. 4, pp. 408–412, 2016.

[14] P. L. Copper, M. P. Otto, and B. L. Leighton, "Successful management of cardiac arrest from amniotic fluid embolism with ondansetron, metoclopramide, atropine, and ketorolac: a case report," *SOAP 2013*, 2013.

[15] A. A. Shamshirsaz and S. L. Clark, "Amniotic fluid embolism," *Obstetrics and Gynecology Clinics of North America*, vol. 43, no. 4, pp. 779–790, 2016.

[16] P. Sultan, K. Seligman, and B. Carvalho, "Amniotic fluid embolism," *Current Opinion in Anaesthesiology*, vol. 29, no. 3, pp. 288–296, 2016.

[17] H. A. Abenhaim, L. Azoulay, M. S. Kramer, and L. Leduc, "Incidence and risk factors of amniotic fluid embolisms: a population-based study on 3 million births in the United States," *American Journal of Obstetrics & Gynecology*, vol. 199, no. 1, pp. 49–e8, 2008.

[18] M. Knight, C. Berg, P. Brocklehurst et al., "Amniotic fluid embolism incidence, risk factors and outcomes: a review and recommendations," *BMC Pregnancy and Childbirth*, vol. 12, no. 1, 2012.

[19] A. Rafael and M. Benson, "Amniotic fluid embolism: then and now," *Obstetric Medicine: The Medicine of Pregnancy*, vol. 7, no. 1, pp. 34–36, 2014.

[20] O. Erez, "Proposed diagnostic criteria for the case definition of amniotic fluid embolism in research studies," *American Journal of Obstetrics & Gynecology*, vol. 217, no. 2, pp. 228-229, 2017.

[21] O. Leaños, E. Hong, and J. Amezcua, "Reflex circulatory collapse following intrapulmonary entrapment of activated platelets: mediation via 5-HT3 receptor stimulation," *British Journal of Pharmacology*, vol. 116, no. 3, pp. 2048–2052, 1995.

[22] D. Armstrong and S. Miller, "The role of platelets in the reflex tachypnoeic response to miliary pulmonary embolism in anaesthetized rabbits," *Experimental Physiology*, vol. 75, no. 6, pp. 791–800, 1990.

[23] X. Jiang, L. Yuan, P. Li et al., "Effect of Simvastatin on 5-HT and 5-HTT in a rat model of pulmonary artery hypertension," *Cellular Physiology and Biochemistry*, vol. 37, no. 5, pp. 1712–1724, 2015.

[24] Y. Todo, N. Tamura, H. Itoh, T. Ikeda, and N. Kanayama, "Therapeutic application of C1 esterase inhibitor concentrate for clinical amniotic fluid embolism: a case report," *Clinical Case Reports*, vol. 3, no. 7, pp. 673–675, 2015.

[25] E. M. Wise, R. Harika, and F. Zahir, "Successful recovery after amniotic fluid embolism in a patient undergoing vacuum-assisted vaginal delivery," *Journal of Clinical Anesthesia*, vol. 34, pp. 557–561, 2016.

[26] S. L. Clark, G. D. Hankins, D. A. Dudley, G. A. Dildy, and T. Porter, "Amniotic fluid embolism: analysis of the national registry," *American Journal of Obstetrics & Gynecology*, vol. 172, no. 4, pp. 1158–1169, 1995.

[27] S. Yufune, M. Tanaka, R. Akai et al., "Successful resuscitation of amniotic fluid embolism applying a new classification and management strategy," *Journal of Anesthesia, Clinical Reports*, vol. 1, no. 1, 2015.

Permissions

The contributors of this book come from diverse backgrounds, making this book a truly international effort. This book will bring forth new frontiers with its revolutionizing research information and detailed analysis of the nascent developments around the world.

We would like to thank all the contributing authors for lending their expertise to make the book truly unique. They have played a crucial role in the development of this book. Without their invaluable contributions this book wouldn't have been possible. They have made vital efforts to compile up to date information on the varied aspects of this subject to make this book a valuable addition to the collection of many professionals and students.

This book was conceptualized with the vision of imparting up-to-date information and advanced data in this field. To ensure the same, a matchless editorial board was set up. Every individual on the board went through rigorous rounds of assessment to prove their worth. After which they invested a large part of their time researching and compiling the most relevant data for our readers.

The editorial board has been involved in producing this book since its inception. They have spent rigorous hours researching and exploring the diverse topics which have resulted in the successful publishing of this book. They have passed on their knowledge of decades through this book. To expedite this challenging task, the publisher supported the team at every step. A small team of assistant editors was also appointed to further simplify the editing procedure and attain best results for the readers.

Apart from the editorial board, the designing team has also invested a significant amount of their time in understanding the subject and creating the most relevant covers. They scrutinized every image to scout for the most suitable representation of the subject and create an appropriate cover for the book.

The publishing team has been an ardent support to the editorial, designing and production team. Their endless efforts to recruit the best for this project, has resulted in the accomplishment of this book. They are a veteran in the field of academics and their pool of knowledge is as vast as their experience in printing. Their expertise and guidance has proved useful at every step. Their uncompromising quality standards have made this book an exceptional effort. Their encouragement from time to time has been an inspiration for everyone.

The publisher and the editorial board hope that this book will prove to be a valuable piece of knowledge for researchers, students, practitioners and scholars across the globe.

List of Contributors

S. Read
UConn Health, Department of OB/GYN, Farmington, CT, USA

J. Mullins
Hartford Hospital, Department of OB/GYN, Hartford, CT, USA

Daisuke Katsura, Yuichiro Takahashi, Shigenori Iwagaki, Rika Chiaki, Kazuhiko Asai, Masako Koike, Shunsuke Yasumi and Madoka Furuhashi
Department of Fetal-Maternal Medicine, Nagara Medical Centre, 1300-7, Nagara, Gifu 502-8558, Japan

Svetha Rao
Liverpool Hospital, Australia

Supuni Kapurubandara and Anbu Anpalagan
Westmead Hospital, Australia

Filipa de Castro Coelho
Gynecology Department, Hospital Dr. NélioMendonça, Serviço de Saúde da Região Autónoma daMadeira, EPE, Funchal, Portugal

Maria Amaral and Augusta Borges
Internal Medicine Department, Maternidade Dr. Alfredo da Costa, Centro Hospitalar Lisboa Central, Lisboa, Portugal

Lúcia Correia
Gynecology Department, Instituto Português de Oncologia de Lisboa Francisco Gentil, EPE, Lisboa, Portugal

Maria João Nunes Campos, Tereza Paula and Jorge Borrego
Gynecology Department, Maternidade Dr. Alfredo da Costa, Centro Hospitalar Lisboa Central, Lisboa, Portugal

Jean V. Storey and Deirdre M. McCullough
Department of Obstetrics and Gynecology, Brooke Army Medical Center, 3551 Roger Brooke Drive, Fort Sam Houston, San Antonio, TX 78234, USA

Steven H. Craig, and Christian L. Carlson and Timothy B. Dinh
Department of Radiology, Brooke Army Medical Center, 3551 Roger Brooke Drive, Fort Sam Houston, San Antonio, TX 78234, USA

Chunyan Zeng, Chunhua Wu and Juan Liu
Key Laboratory for Major Obstetric Diseases of Guangdong Province, Key Laboratory of Reproduction and Genetics of Guangdong Higher Education Institutes, Department of Obstetrics and Gynecology, The Third Affiliated Hospital of Guangzhou Medical University, No. 63 Duobao Road, Liwan District, Guangzhou, Guangdong 510150, China

Feng Yang and Junlin Zhu
Department of Ultrasound Medicine, Laboratory of Ultrasound Molecular Imaging, The Third Affiliated Hospital of Guangzhou Medical University, No. 63 Duobao Road, Liwan District, Guangzhou, Guangdong 510150, China

Xiaoming Guan
Division of Minimally Invasive Gynecologic Surgery, Department of Obstetrics and Gynecology, Baylor College of Medicine, 6651Main Street, 10th Floor, Houston, Texas 77030, USA

Yasuyuki Kawagoe, Tetsuo Nakayama, Satoshi Matuzawa, Kazuko Fukushima, Junji Onishi and Hiroshi Sameshima
Department of Obstetrics and Gynecology, Faculty of Medicine, University of Miyazaki, 5200 Kihara, Kiyotake, Miyazaki 889-1692, Japan

Yuichiro Sato
Department of Diagnostic Pathology, University of Miyazaki Hospital, Faculty of Medicine, University of Miyazaki, 5200 Kihara, Kiyotake, Miyazaki 889-1692, Japan

Kimihiro Nagai
Department of Palliative Care, Miyazaki Medical Association Hospital, 738-1 Funado, Shinbeppu, Miyazaki City, Miyazaki 889-0834, Japan

Yoko Matsuda, Yoshitsugu Chigusa, Eiji Kondoh, Yusuke Ueda and Masaki Mandai
Department of Gynecology and Obstetrics, Kyoto University, 54 Shogoin Kawahara-cho, Sakyo-ku, Kyoto 606-8507, Japan

Isao Ito
Department of Respiratory Medicine, Kyoto University, 54 Shogoin Kawahara-cho, Sakyo-ku, Kyoto 606-8507, Japan

Edgar Gulavi and Steve Kyende Mutiso
Obstetrics and Gynecology, Aga Khan University Hospital, Nairobi, Kenya

Charles Mariara Muriuki
Kijabe Mission Hospital, Kiambu, Kenya

Abraham Mukaindo Mwaniki
Aga Khan University Hospital, Nairobi, Kenya

Rotem Sadeh, Yakir Segev, Meirav Schmidt and Ofer Lavie
Division of Gynecology Oncology, Department of Obstetrics and Gynecology, Carmel Medical Center, Haifa, Israel

Jacob Schendler and Tamar Baruch
Department of Pathology, Carmel Medical Center, Haifa, Israel

Antonella Vimercati, Vittoria Del Vecchio, Annarosa Chincoli and Ettore Cicinelli
Department of Biomedical and Human Oncological Science (DIMO), 2nd Unit of Obstetrics and Gynaecology, University of Bari, Bari, Italy

Antonio Malvasi
Santa Maria Hospital, GVM Care and Research, Bari, Italy

Anna Walch
Doctor of Medicine (MD), Griffith University, Australia
Lecturer, School of Medicine, Griffith University, Australia
Obstetrics and Gynaecology Principal House Officer, Gold Coast University Hospital, Australia

Madeline Duke
Bachelor of Medicine and Bachelor of Surgery (MBBS), Bond University, Australia
Obstetric Medicine Fellow, Royal Brisbane and Women's Hospital, Australia
Endocrine Advanced Trainee, Royal Brisbane and Women's Hospital, Australia

Travis Auty
Lecturer, School of Medicine, Griffith University, Australia
Bachelor of Medicine and Bachelor of Surgery (MBBS), Griffith University, Australia
Intensive Care Unit Registrar, Gold Coast University Hospital, Australia

Audris Wong
Obstetrics and Gynaecology Staff Specialist, Gold Coast University Hospital, Australia

FRANZCOG (Fellowship of the Royal Australian and New Zealand College of Obstetricians and Gynaecologists), Australia
MRCOG (Membership of the Royal college of Obstetricians and Gynaecologist), UK
MRCPI (Membership of the Royal College of Physicians in Ireland (Obstetrics and Gynaecology and General Medicine)), Ireland

L. Di Tizio
Department of Obstetrics and Gynecology, SS Annunziata Hospital, Chieti, Italy

M. R. Spina
Department of Obstetrics and Gynecology, SS Annunziata Hospital, Chieti, Italy
Department of Medicine and Aging Sciences University "G. d'Annunzio" of Chieti-Pescara, Italy

S. Gustapane
Department of Obstetrics and Gynecology, Casa di Cura Salus srl, Brindisi, Italy

F. D'Antonio
Women's Health and Perinatology Research Group, Department of Clinical Medicine, Faculty of Health Sciences, UiT-The Arctic University of Norway, Tromsø, Norway
Department of Obstetrics and Gynaecology, University Hospital of Northern Norway, Tromsø, Norway

M. Liberati
Department of Obstetrics and Gynecology, SS Annunziata Hospital, Chieti, Italy
Department of Medicine and Aging Sciences University "G. d'Annunzio" of Chieti-Pescara, Italy
"G. d'Annunzio" University, Chieti, Italy

Nanami Tsukasaki, Takuro Yamamoto, Akihisa Katayama, Nozomi Ogiso and Tomoharu Okubo
Department of Obstetrics and Gynecology, Japanese Red Cross Society Kyoto Daiichi Hospital, 15-749 Honmachi, Higashiyama-ku, Kyoto 605-0981, Japan

Pınar Yalcin Bahat, Gokce Turan and Berna Aslan Cetin
Department of Obstetrics and Gynecology, Kanuni Sultan Suleyman Training and Research Hospital, Istanbul Health Sciences University, Istanbul, Turkey

Athanase Lilungulu
Department of Obstetrics and Gynecology, Dodoma University, College of Health Sciences, Dodoma, Tanzania

Willy Mwibea
Department of Obstetrics and Gynaecology, Kibaha Clinical Officer Training College, Coast Regional, Tanzania

Mzee Nassoro
Department of Obstetrics and Gynaecology, Dodoma Regional Referral Hospital, Dodoma, Tanzania

Balthazar Gumodoka
Department of Obstetrics and Gynaecology, Catholic University of Health and Allied Sciences, Bugando Medical Centre, Mwanza, Tanzania

Amanda Lino de Faria, CinthiaMoreno Garcia and Gabriela de Andrade Rodrigues
Federal University of São Paulo (UNIFESP), São Paulo, Brazil

Lais Helena Dumbra Toloni dos Santos, Gabriela B. K. Uyeda, Simone Elias, Marair G. F. Sartori, Afonso Celso Pinto Nazário and Gil Facina
Department of Gynecology, Federal University of São Paulo (UNIFESP), São Paulo, Brazil

Hiroaki Takagi, Emi Takata, Jinichi Sakamoto, Satoko Fujita, Masahiro Takakura and Toshiyuki Sasagawa
Department of Obstetrics and Gynecology, Kanazawa Medical University, School of Medicine, Japan

Hisako Yagi, Yoshino Kinjyo, Yukiko Chinen, Hayase Nitta, Tadatsugu Kinjo, Keiko Mekaru, Hitoshi Masamoto and Yoichi Aoki
Department of Obstetrics and Gynecology, Graduate School of Medicine, University of the Ryukyus, 207 Uehara, Nishihara, Okinawa 903-0215, Japan

Hideki Goya and Tomohide Yoshida
Department of Pediatrics, Graduate School of Medicine, University of the Ryukyus, 207 Uehara, Nishihara, Okinawa 903-0215, Japan

Naoya Sanabe
Department of Digestive and General Surgery, Graduate School of Medicine, University of the Ryukyus, 207 Uehara, Nishihara, Okinawa 903-0215, Japan

Michelle Nguyen and Maria Raquel Kronen
Department of Obstetrics and Gynecology, White Memorial Medical Center, Los Angeles, CA 90033, USA

Alex Nhan
University of Central Florida College of Medicine, Orlando, FL 32827, USA

Antonio Liu
Department of Neurology, White Memorial Medical Center, Los Angeles, CA 90033, USA

Jaimin Shah and Cristina Wallace-Huff
Department of Obstetrics, Gynecology and Reproductive Sciences, McGovern Medical School, The University of Texas Health Science Center at Houston, Houston, TX, USA

Eduardo Matta
Department of Diagnostic and Interventional Imaging, McGovern Medical School, The University of Texas Health Science Center at Houston, Houston, TX, USA

Fernando Acosta and Natalia Golardi
Department of Pathology and Laboratory Medicine, McGovern Medical School, The University of Texas Health Science Center at Houston, Houston, TX, USA

Jessica Parrott and Marium Holland
Division of Maternal Fetal Medicine, Department of Obstetrics and Gynecology, University of Kansas School of Medicine, 3901 Rainbow Boulevard, Kansas City, KS 66160, USA

Victoria Sampson, Oluremi Mogekwu, Ammar Ahmed and Farida Bano
Department of Obstetrics and Gynaecology, Queen's Hospital, Romford, UK

Anis Haddad, Olfa Zoukar, Awatef Hajjeji and Raja Faleh
Department of Obstetrics and Gynecology, Fattouma Bourguiba Teaching Hospital of Monastir. Rue 1er Juin 1955, 5000Monastir, Tunisia

Houda Mhabrich
Department of Radiology, Fattouma Bourguiba Teaching Hospital of Monastir. Rue 1er Juin 1955, 5000Monastir, Tunisia

Anastasia Mikuscheva, Elliot McKenzie and Adel Mekhail
Department of Gynecology and Obstetrics, Dunedin University Hospital, Dunedin, New Zealand

Nicholas A. Leyland
Department of Obstetrics and Gynecology, McMaster University, 1280 Main St.West, Hamilton, Ontario L8S4L8, Canada

Katerina Pizzuto, Kathleen Tafler, Sarah Scattolon and Michelle Morais
School of Medicine, McMaster University, 1280 Main St. West, Hamilton, Ontario L8S4K1, Canada

Department of Obstetrics and Gynecology, McMaster University, 1280 Main St. West, Hamilton, Ontario L8S4L8, Canada

Cory Ozimok
School of Medicine, McMaster University, 1280 Main St.West, Hamilton, Ontario L8S4K1, Canada
Department of Radiology, McMaster University, 1200 Main St.West, Hamilton, Ontario L8N3Z5, Canada

Radenka Bozanovic
School of Medicine, McMaster University, 1280 Main St. West, Hamilton, Ontario L8S4K1, Canada
Department of Pathology, McMaster University, 1200 Main St. West, Hamilton, Ontario L8N 3Z5, Canada

Cristina Ramalho, Mónica Pires and Almerinda Petiz
Department of Gynecology, Francisco Gentil Portuguese Oncology Institute, Porto, Portugal

Maria Inês Raposo
Department of Gynecology, Francisco Gentil Portuguese Oncology Institute, Porto, Portugal
Department of Gynecology, Hospital of Divino Espírito Santo of Ponta Delgada, EPER, São Miguel, Azores, Portugal

Mariana Cardoso and Mariana Ormonde
Department of Gynecology, Hospital of Divino Espírito Santo of Ponta Delgada, EPER, São Miguel, Azores, Portugal

Catarina Meireles and Mariana Afonso
Department of Pathology, Francisco Gentil Portuguese Oncology Institute, Porto, Portugal

Joan Tymon-Rosario
Montefiore Medical Center, Department of Obstetrics and Gynecology and Women's Health, Bronx, NY, USA

Meleen Chuang
Montefiore Medical Center, Department of Obstetrics and Gynecology and Women's Health, Bronx, NY, USA
Albert Einstein College of Medicine, Bronx, NY, USA

Chiara Di Tucci, Daniele Di Mascio, Michele Carlo Schiavi, Giorgia Perniola, Ludovico Muzii and Pierluigi Benedetti Panici
Department of Gynecological and Obstetric Sciences, and Urological Sciences, University of Rome "Sapienza", Umberto I Hospital, Rome, Italy

Angelika Kaufmann, Raj Naik and Ann Fisher
Northern Gynaecological Oncology Centre, Gateshead NHS Foundation Trust, Queen Elizabeth Hospital, Sheriff Hill, Gateshead NE9 6SX, UK

Christina Founta
Northern Gynaecological Oncology Centre, Gateshead NHS Foundation Trust, Queen Elizabeth Hospital, Sheriff Hill, Gateshead NE9 6SX, UK
Musgrove Park Hospital, Taunton and Somerset NHS Foundation Trust, Taunton TA1 5DA, UK

Emmanouil Papagiannakis
DYSIS Medical Ltd, Edinburgh, UK

Clare E. Thiele
Royal Brisbane and Women's Hospital, Cnr Butterfield St. and Bowen Bridge Rd, Herston QLD 4029, Australia

Lamiaa Elsebay
Specialized Medical Center Hospital, Riyadh, Saudi Arabia
Alfaisal University, Riyadh, Saudi Arabia
SCFHS, Riyadh, Saudi Arabia

Mariam Ahmed Galal
Specialized Medical Center Hospital, Riyadh, Saudi Arabia
Alfaisal University, Riyadh, Saudi Arabia

Rati Chadha
Department of Obstetrics and Gynecology; Division of Maternal Fetal Medicine, Foothills Medical Center, University of Calgary, Calgary, AB, Canada

Rita Shats
Department of Obstetrics and Gynecology, Richmond University Medical Center, 355 Bard Avenue, Staten Island, NY 10310, USA

Brittany van Staalduinen, Andrew Stahler, Catherine Abied and Nisha A. Lakhi
Department of Obstetrics and Gynecology, Richmond University Medical Center, 355 Bard Avenue, Staten Island, NY 10310, USA
Department of Obstetrics and Gynecology, New York Medical College, Valhalla, New York, USA

A. MacGibbon and Y.M. Ius
Department of Obstetrics and Gynaecology, John Hunter Hospital. Newcastle, New South Wales, Australia

Barbara Monard and Nicolas Mottet
Obstetrics and Gynecology Department, Besancon University Medical Center, 3 boulevard Alexandre Fleming, 25000 Besancon, France

Rajeev Ramanah and Didier Riethmuller
Obstetrics and Gynecology Department, Besancon University Medical Center, 3 boulevard Alexandre Fleming, 25000 Besancon, France

University of Franche-Comte, Hauts de Chazal, 19 rue Ambroise Paré, 25000 Besancon, France

E. Thornton
ST1 Obstetrics and Gynaecology, Royal Bolton Hospital, Bolton, UK

L. Tripathi
North Manchester General Hospital, Manchester, UK

S. Shebani
Glenfield Hospital, Leicester, UK

I. Bruce
Department of Rheumatology, Manchester Royal Infirmary, Manchester, UK

L. Byrd
St Mary's Hospital, Manchester, UK

Valerie John-Cole, Mike Kamara and Alimamy Philip Koroma
Department of Obstetrics and Gynecology, Princess Christian Maternity Hospital (PCMH), University Teaching Hospitals Complex, University of Sierra Leone, Freetown, Sierra Leone

Mariatu Binta Leigh
Department of Obstetrics and Gynecology, Princess Christian Maternity Hospital (PCMH), University Teaching Hospitals Complex, University of Sierra Leone, Freetown, Sierra Leone
Center for Internal Medicine I, Department for Angiology, Medical School Brandenburg Theodor Fontane (MHB), Campus Brandenburg, Brandenburg, Germany

Peter Bramlage and Ivo Buschmann
Center for Internal Medicine I, Department for Angiology, Medical School BrandenburgTheodor Fontane (MHB), Campus Brandenburg, Brandenburg, Germany

Michael Momoh Koroma
Department of Anesthesia, Princess Christian Maternity Hospital (PCMH), University Teaching Hospitals Complex, University of Sierra Leone, Freetown, Sierra Leone

Edward Ejiro Emuveyan
Department of Obstetrics and Gynecology, Princess Christian Maternity Hospital (PCMH), University Teaching Hospitals Complex, University of Sierra Leone, Freetown, Sierra Leone
Department of Obstetrics and Gynecology, College of Medicine, University of Lagos, Akoka, Lagos, Nigeria

Kristen Stearns
Medical College of Wisconsin and Affiliated Hospitals, Department of Obstetrics and Gynecology, 9200 W. Wisconsin Ave, Milwaukee, WI 53226, USA

Antoun Al Khabbaz
University of Illinois College of Medicine-Rockford, Department of Obstetrics and Gynecology, 1601 Parkview Ave, Rockford, IL 61101, USA

B. Wormald, S. Elorbany, H. Hanson, J. W. Williams and S. Heenan
St George's Hospital, UK

D. P. J. Barton
St George's Hospital and the Royal Marsden Hospital, UK

Sharon J. Kim, Amanda N. King and Mary L.Marnach
Mayo Clinic, Department of Obstetrics and Gynecology, Rochester, MN, USA

Pavan Parikh
Mayo Clinic, Department of Obstetrics and Gynecology, Division of Maternal Fetal Medicine, Rochester, MN, USA

Quinton Katler, Lindsey Pflugner and Anjali Martinez
Department of Obstetrics and Gynecology, The George Washington University Hospital, Washington, DC, USA

Ali Azadi
Norton Urogynecology Center, Norton Healthcare, 4001 Dutchmans Lane, Louisville, KY 40207, USA

James A. Bradley and Amir Azadi
University of Louisville School of Medicine, Louisville, KY 40202, USA

Dennis M. O'Connor
Clinical Pathology Associates, Norton Healthcare, 4001 Dutchmans Lane, Louisville, KY 40207, USA

Donald R. Ostergard
UCLA School of Medicine, Los Angeles, CA, USA

Emsal Pinar Topdagi Yilmaz, Omer Erkan Yapca, Seray Kaya Topdagi and Yakup Kumtepe
Department of Gynecology and Obstetrics, Atatürk University School of Medicine, Erzurum, Turkey

Yunus Emre Topdagi
Clinic of Gynecology and Obstetrics, Nenehatun Gynecology and Obstetrics Hospital, Erzurum, Turkey

Sachiko Morioka, Yasuhito Tanase, Ryuji Kawaguchi and Hiroshi Kobayash
Department of Obstetrics and Gynecology, Nara Medical University, Nara, Japan

Tomoko Uchiyama
Department of Diagnostic Pathology, Nara Medical University, Nara, Japan

Shadi Rezai
Department of Obstetrics and Gynecology, Southern California Kaiser Permanente, Kern County, 1200 Discovery Drive, Bakersfield, CA 93309, USA
Division of Minimally Invasive Gynecologic Surgery, Department of Obstetrics and Gynecology, Baylor College of Medicine, 6651 Main Street, 10th Floor, Houston, TX 77030, USA

Elise Bardawil and Xiaoming Guan
Division of Minimally Invasive Gynecologic Surgery, Department of Obstetrics and Gynecology, Baylor College of Medicine, 6651 Main Street, 10th Floor, Houston, TX 77030, USA

Richard A. Giovane
University of Alabama, Department of Family Medicine, 801 Campus Drive, Tuscaloosa, AL 35487, USA

Heather Minton
University of Birmingham, School of Medicine, 1720 2nd Avenue, Birmingham, AL 35294, USA

Yiming Zhang
Division of Reproductive Medicine, Jinan Central Hospital Group, 105 Jiefang Road, Jinan City, Shandong Province 250013, China

Ninad M. Patil
Department of Pathology and Immunology, Baylor College of Medicine, 6651 Main Street, 4th Floor, Houston, TX 77030, USA

Cassandra E. Henderson
Maternal and Fetal Medicine, Department of Obstetrics and Gynecology, Lincoln Medical and Mental Health Center, 234 East 149th Street, Bronx, NY 10451, USA

Index

www.ingramcontent.com/pod-product-compliance
Lightning Source LLC
Chambersburg PA
CBHW080510200326
41458CB00012B/4159